clinical evidence

Cardiovascular Disorders
Second Edition

The international source of the
best available evidence for
cardiovascular health care

BMJ
Publishing
Group

Reprinted from *Clinical Evidence*, Issue 8, 2002, published by the BMJ Publishing Group

Editorial Office
BMJ Publishing Group, BMA House, Tavistock Square, London, WC1H 9JR, United Kingdom.
Tel: +44 (0)20 7387 4499 • Fax: +44 (0)20 7383 6242 • www.bmjpg.com

Clinical Evidence Cardiovascular Disorders
Please email us at CEfeedback@bmjgroup.com to register interest in future updates of *Clinical Evidence Cardiovascular Disorders* or complete the feedback card provided in this book

Subscription prices for *Clinical Evidence*
Clinical Evidence and *Clinical Evidence Concise* (with companion CD-ROM) are both published six monthly (June/December) by the BMJ Publishing Group. The annual subscription rates for both publications (December, Issue 8, and June, Issue 9) are:

Personal: £85 • €135 • US$135 • Can$200
Institutional: £175 • €280 • US$280 • Can$420
Student/nurse: £40 • €65 • US$65 • Can$95

The above rates are for either the full print or the concise formats. The combined rates, for both formats, are:

Personal £120 • €190 • US$190 • Can$285
Institutional £235 • €375 • US$375 • Can$560
Student/nurse £65 • €105 • US$105 • Can$155

For further subscription information please visit the subscription pages of our website www.clinicalevidence.com or email us at CEsubscriptions@bmjgroup.com (UK and ROW) or clinevid@pmds.com (Americas). You may also telephone us or fax us on the following numbers:

UK and ROW Tel: +44 (0)20 7383 6270 • Fax: +44 (0)20 7383 6402
Americas Tel: +1 800 373 2897/240 646 7000 • Fax: +1 240 646 7005

Bulk subscriptions for societies and organisations
The Publishers offer discounts for any society or organisation buying bulk quantities for their members/specific groups. Please contact Miranda Lonsdale, Sales Manager (UK) at mlonsdale@bmjgroup.com or Diane McCabe, Sales and Marketing Manager (USA) at dmccabe@bmjgroup.com.

Contributors
If you are interested in becoming a contributor to *Clinical Evidence* please contact us at clinicalevidence@bmjgroup.com.

Rights
For information on translation rights, please contact Daniel Raymond-Barker at draymond-barker@bmjgroup.com.

British Library Cataloguing in Publication Data
A catalogue record for this book is available from the British Library: ISBN 0 7279 1788 9

Permission to reproduce
Please contact Josephine Woodcock at jwoodcock@bmjgroup.com when requesting permission to reprint all or part of any contribution in *Clinical Evidence*.

Legal Disclaimer
Care has been taken to confirm the accuracy of the information presented and to describe generally accepted practices. However, the authors, editors, and publishers are not responsible for errors or omissions or for any consequences from application of the information in this book and make no warranty, express or implied, with respect to the contents of the publication.

Categories presented in *Clinical Evidence* indicate a judgement about the strength of the evidence available and the relative importance of benefits and harms. The categories do not indicate whether a particular treatment is generally appropriate or whether it is suitable for individuals.

Printed and bound in Great Britain by Thanet Press Limited, Margate, Kent

Team and Advisors

Contents

Clinical Evidence Cardiovascular Disorders

Welcome to this collection of cardiovascular reprints from *Clinical Evidence*, a compendium of the best available evidence to guide clinical practice in specific cardiovascular disorders. This book is aimed primarily at cardiologists, clinical pharmacologists, generalist physicians, nurses, and physicians' assistants who care for people with cardiovascular disorders or who promote the prevention of cardiovascular disease. In addition, we believe that this book will be useful for adults with cardiovascular conditions, as well as for healthcare managers involved in organising cardiovascular services.

We decided to publish a *Clinical Evidence* version devoted solely to cardiovascular disorders for several reasons. Despite multiple advances in prevention and treatment, cardiovascular disorders remain the leading cause of morbidity, disability, and mortality in most western countries. Cardiovascular experts have long been stalwart standard bearers for rigorous evaluations of treatments. Literally, thousands of randomised controlled trials have evaluated hundreds of different prevention and treatment options for various cardiovascular disorders. New treatments are constantly being developed and tested, and some old treatments are discarded if better alternatives are found. Practitioners need quick, reliable knowledge about the optimum treatments for cardiovascular disorders, but they are overwhelmed by the variety of available options and the rapid accumulation of research evidence. We hope to help practicing clinicians who care for people with cardiovascular conditions by finding, sorting, critiquing, and summarising the best available research evidence.

About Clinical Evidence

Clinical Evidence is a continuously updated international source of evidence on the effects of clinical interventions. It summarises the current state of knowledge, ignorance, and uncertainty about the prevention and treatment of clinical conditions, based on thorough searches and appraisal of the literature. It purposely emphasises rigorous evidence about treatment and prevention that has been derived from randomised controlled trials and systematic reviews of the trials. It is neither a textbook of medicine nor a book of guidelines. It describes the best available evidence, and where there is no good evidence it says so. *Clinical Evidence* is regularly expanded to include new summaries of evidence on additional diseases, syndromes, and clinical questions.

A UNIQUE RESOURCE

Clinical Evidence joins a growing number of sources of evidence-based information for clinicians. But it has several features that make it unique.

- Its contents are driven by questions rather than by the availability of research evidence. Rather than start with the evidence and summarise what is there, we have tried to identify important clinical questions, and then to search for and summarise the best available evidence to answer them.
- It identifies but does not try to fill important gaps in the evidence. In a phrase used by Jerry Osheroff, who has led much of the recent research on clinicians' information needs, *Clinical Evidence* presents the dark as well as the light side of the moon. We feel that it will be helpful for clinicians to know when their uncertainty stems from gaps in the evidence rather than gaps in their own knowledge.
- It is updated every 6 months in print and monthly online. *Clinical Evidence Concise* is also available with companion CD-ROM.
- It specifically aims not to make recommendations. We feel that simply summarising the evidence will make it more widely useful. The experience of the clinical practice guideline movement has shown that it is nearly impossible to make recommendations that are appropriate in every situation. Differences in individual patients' baseline risks and preferences, and in the local availability of interventions, will always mean that the evidence must be individually interpreted rather than applied across the board. *Clinical Evidence* provides the raw material for developing locally applicable clinical practice guidelines, and for clinicians and patients to make up their own minds on the best course of action. We supply the evidence, you make the decisions.

A WORK IN PROGRESS

Clinical Evidence is an evolving project. We knew before we started that we were undertaking an enormous task, but the more we worked the more we realised its enormity. We recognise that there is some mismatch between what we aim eventually to achieve and what we have achieved so far. Although we have made every effort to ensure that the searches are thorough and that the appraisals of studies are objective, we will inevitably have missed some important studies. In order not to make unjustified claims about the accuracy of the information, we use phrases such as "we found no systematic review" rather than "there is no systematic review". In order to be as explicit as possible about the methods used for each contribution, we have asked each set of contributors to provide a brief methods section, describing the searches that were performed and how individual studies were selected.

For more information about our methods and processes, visit our website at www.clinicalevidence.com

Cindy Mulrow
Professor of Medicine
University of Texas
Health Science Center

The book is arranged by common cardiovascular topics. We include evidence relevant to both prevention and treatment of cardiovascular disease, and address a variety of associated risk factors such as dyslipidaemia, sedentary lifestyle, tobacco use, hypertension, unhealthy diets, and obesity.

SUMMARY PAGE

The summary page for each topic presents the questions addressed, some key messages, and a list of the interventions covered, categorised according to whether they have been found to be effective or not. We have developed the categories of effectiveness from one of the Cochrane Collaboration's first and most popular products, *A guide to effective care in pregnancy and childbirth*.[1] The categories we now use are explained in the table below:

TABLE	Categorisation of treatment effects in *Clinical Evidence*
Beneficial	Interventions for which effectiveness has been demonstrated by clear evidence from RCTs, and for which expectation of harms is small compared with the benefits.
Likely to be beneficial	Interventions for which effectiveness is less well established than for those listed under "beneficial".
Trade off between benefits and harms	Interventions for which clinicians and patients should weigh up the beneficial and harmful effects according to individual circumstances and priorities.
Unknown effectiveness	Interventions for which there are currently insufficient data or data of inadequate quality.
Unlikely to be beneficial	Interventions for which lack of effectiveness is less well established than for those listed under "likely to be ineffective or harmful"
Likely to be ineffective or harmful	Interventions for which ineffectiveness or harmfulness has been demonstrated by clear evidence.

CATEGORISING THE EVIDENCE

Categorising the effectiveness of interventions is not straightforward. First, evidence is often limited. Interventions may have been tested only in narrow groups of people, such as those who are at particularly high risk for an outcome. Interventions may have been tested in tightly controlled circumstances that are not easily replicable in general practice, and direct comparisons of important alternative treatments may not be available. Second, finding no good evidence that a treatment works is not the same as saying that the treatment doesn't work. Statements of effectiveness necessarily are a reflection of currently available evidence and ideally distinguish between lack of benefit and lack of evidence of benefit. Third, several dimensions must be considered simultaneously when making decisions about effectiveness. These include the following: types, magnitudes, and frequency of expected benefits; types, magnitudes, and frequency of expected harms; level or rigor of evidence relevant to expected benefits and harms; and degree of certainty around expected benefits and harms.

INFORMATION ABOUT THE CONDITION

After each summary page, we present up-to-date, quantified, and referenced information about the condition. We define the clinical problem or condition of interest; describe its incidence, aetiology, risk factors, and prognosis; state the primary aims of treatment and/or prevention; and delineate the major outcomes of interest. Clinical outcomes, such as survival, heart attacks and strokes, symptoms, disability, and quality of life are emphasised. We then note the methods of our summaries, including the dates of the most recent searches and appraisal of evidence for each topic.

THE FILTERED EVIDENCE

The core of *Clinical Evidence* follows. We present pertinent clinical questions and list multiple different therapeutic and/or preventive options. High quality evidence regarding the potential benefits and harms associated with the different options is summarised. Comments are supplied on the quality of the evidence, applicability of the results for different subgroups of people, and on any trials that are known to be in progress. Finally, we define important terms in glossaries and list the selected references. Decisions about treatment and prevention require judgements about the trade offs between benefits and harms, and between alternative priorities. The best people to make these decisions are individuals and their personal healthcare providers; therefore, we talk about the effects of interventions, both positive and negative, rather than the effectiveness. For each question or intervention option we present evidence on benefits and harms under separate headings. We make no systematic attempt to provide information on drug dosages, formulations, indications, and contraindications. For this information, we refer readers to their national drug formularies. We also do not include information on cost or cost effectiveness of interventions as costs can vary greatly both within and between countries.

FEEDBACK

We hope that clinicians find *Clinical Evidence Cardiovascular Disorders* useful. We value your feedback on *Clinical Evidence Cardiovascular Disorders*, and in particular whether you would like to receive regular updates in print. Please email us at CEfeedback@bmjgroup.com or complete and return the feedback card provided in this book.

REFERENCES

1. Enkin M, Keirse M, Renfrew M, et al. A guide to effective care in pregnancy and childbirth. Oxford: Oxford University Press, 1998.

Glossary

Absolute risk (AR) The probability that an individual will experience the specified outcome during a specified period. It lies in the range 0 to 1, or is expressed as a percentage. In contrast to common usage, the word "risk" may refer to adverse events (such as myocardial infarction) or desirable events (such as cure).

Absolute risk increase (ARI) The absolute difference in risk between the experimental and control groups in a trial. It is used when the risk in the experimental group exceeds the risk in the control group, and is calculated by subtracting the AR in the control group from the AR in the experimental group. This figure does not give any idea of the proportional increase between the two groups: for this, relative risk (RR) is needed (see below).

Absolute risk reduction (ARR) The absolute difference in risk between the experimental and control groups in a trial. It is used when the risk in the control group exceeds the risk in the experimental group, and is calculated by subtracting the AR in the experimental group from the AR in the control group. This figure does not give any idea of the proportional reduction between the two groups: for this, relative risk (RR) is needed (see below).

Allocation concealment A method used to prevent selection bias by concealing the allocation sequence from those assigning participants to intervention groups. Allocation concealment prevents researchers from (unconsciously or otherwise) influencing which intervention group each participant is assigned to.

Applicability The application of the results from clinical trials to individual people. A randomised trial only provides direct evidence of causality within that specific trial. It takes an additional logical step to apply this result to a specific individual. Individual characteristics will affect the outcome for this person.

Baseline risk The risk of the event occurring without the active treatment. Estimated by the baseline risk in the control group.

Bias Systematic deviation of study results from the true results, because of the way(s) in which the study is conducted.

Blinding/blinded A trial is fully blinded if all the people involved are unaware of the treatment group to which trial participants are allocated until after the interpretation of results. This includes trial participants and everyone involved in administering treatment or recording trial results.

Block randomisation Randomisation by a pattern to produce the required number of people in each group.

Case control study A study design that examines a group of people who have experienced an event (usually an adverse event) and a group of people who have not experienced the same event, and looks at how exposure to suspect (usually noxious) agents differed between the two groups. This type of study design is most useful for trying to ascertain the cause of rare events, such as rare cancers.

Case series Analysis of series of people with the disease (there is no comparison group in case series).

Clinically significant A finding that is clinically important. Here, "significant" takes its everyday meaning of "important" (compared with statistically significant; see below). Where the word "significant" or "significance" is used without qualification in the text, it is being used in its statistical sense.

Cluster randomisation A cluster randomised study is one in which a group of participants are randomised to the same intervention together. Examples of cluster randomisation include allocating together people in the same village, hospital, or school. If the results are then analysed by individuals rather than the group as a whole bias can occur.

Cohort study A non-experimental study design that follows a group of people (a cohort), and then looks at how events differ among people within the group. A study that examines a cohort, which differs in respect to exposure to some suspected risk factor (e.g. smoking), is useful for trying to ascertain whether exposure is likely to cause specified events (e.g. lung cancer). Prospective cohort studies (which track participants forward in time) are more reliable than retrospective cohort studies.

Completer analysis Analysis of data from only those participants who remained at the end of the study. Compare with intention to treat analysis, which uses data from all participants who enrolled (see below).

Confidence interval (CI) The 95% confidence interval (or 95% confidence limits) would include 95% of results from studies of the same size and design in the same population. This is close but not identical to saying that the true size of the effect (never exactly known) has a 95% chance of falling within the confidence interval. If the 95% confidence interval for a relative risk (RR) or an odds ratio (OR) crosses 1, then this is taken as no evidence of an effect. The practical advantages of a confidence interval (rather than a P value) is that they present the range of likely effects.

Controls In a randomised controlled trial (RCT), controls refer to the participants in its comparison group. They are allocated either to placebo, no treatment, or a standard treatment.

Crossover randomised trial A trial in which participants receive one treatment and have outcomes measured, and then receive an alternative treatment and have outcomes measured again. The order of treatments is randomly assigned. Sometimes a period of no treatment is used before the trial starts and in between the treatments (washout periods) to minimise interference between the treatments (carry over effects). Interpretation of the results from crossover randomised controlled trials (RCTs) can be complex.

Cross sectional study A study design that involves surveying a population about an exposure, or condition, or both, at one point in time. It can be used for assessing prevalence of a condition in the population.

Effect size (standardised mean differences) In the medical literature, effect size is used to refer to a variety of measures of treatment effect. In *Clinical Evidence* it refers to a standardised mean difference: a statistic for combining continuous variables (such as pain scores or height), from different scales, by dividing the difference between two means by an estimate of the within group standard deviation.

Event The occurrence of a dichotomous outcome that is being sought in the study (such as myocardial infarction, death, or a four-point improvement in pain score).

Experimental study A study in which the investigator studies the effect of intentionally altering one or more factors under controlled conditions.

Factorial design A factorial design attempts to evaluate more than one intervention compared with control in a single trial, by means of multiple randomisations.

False negative A person with the target condition (defined by the gold standard) who has a negative test result.

False positive A person without the target condition (defined by the gold standard) who has a positive test result.

Fixed effects The "fixed effects" model of meta-analysis assumes, often unreasonably, that the variability between the studies is exclusively because of a random sampling variation around a fixed effect (see random effects below).

Hazard ratio (HR) Broadly equivalent to relative risk (RR); useful when the risk is not constant with respect to time. It uses information collected at different times. The term is typically used in the context of survival over time. If the HR is 0.5 then the relative risk of dying in one group is half the risk of dying in the other group.

Heterogeneity In the context of meta-analysis, heterogeneity means dissimilarity between studies. It can be because of the use of different statistical methods (statistical heterogeneity), or evaluation of people with different characteristics, treatments or outcomes (clinical heterogeneity). Heterogeneity may render pooling of data in meta-analysis unreliable or inappropriate.

Homogeneity Similarity (see heterogeneity above).

Incidence The number of new cases of a condition occurring in a population over a specified period of time.

Intention to treat analysis Analysis of data for all participants based on the group to which they were randomised and not based on the actual treatment they received.

Likelihood ratio The ratio of the probability that an individual with the target condition has a specified test result to the probability that an individual without the target condition has the same specified test result.

Meta-analysis A statistical technique that summarises the results of several studies in a single weighted estimate, in which more weight is given to results of studies with more events and sometimes to studies of higher quality.

Morbidity Rate of illness but not death.

Mortality Rate of death.

Negative likelihood ratio (NLR) The ratio of the probability that an individual with the target condition has a negative test result to the probability that an individual without the target condition has a negative test result. This is the same as the ratio (1-sensitivity/specificity).

Negative predictive value (NPV) The chance of not having a disease given a negative test result (not to be confused with specificity, which is the other way round; see below).

Not significant/non-significant (NS) In *Clinical Evidence*, not significant means that the observed difference, or a larger difference, could have arisen by chance with a probability of more than 1/20 (i.e. 5%), assuming that there is no underlying difference. This is not the same as saying there is no effect, just that this experiment does not provide convincing evidence of an effect. This could be because the trial was not powered to detect an effect that does exist, because there was no effect, or because of the play of chance.

Number needed to harm (NNH) One measure of treatment harm. It is the average number of people from a defined population you would need to treat with a specific intervention for a given period of time to cause one additional adverse outcome. NNH can be calculated as 1/ARI. In *Clinical Evidence*, these are usually rounded downwards.

Number needed to treat (NNT) One measure of treatment effectiveness. It is the number of people you would on average need to treat with a specific intervention for a given period of time to prevent one additional adverse outcome or achieve one additional beneficial outcome. NNT can be calculated as 1/ARR (see appendix 2). In *Clinical Evidence*, NNTs are usually rounded upwards.

NNT for a meta-analysis Absolute measures are useful at describing the effort required to obtain a benefit, but are limited because they are influenced by both the treatment and also by the baseline risk of the individual. If a meta-analysis includes individuals with a range of baseline risks, then no single NNT will be applicable to the people in that meta-analysis, but a single relative measure (odds ratio or relative risk) may be applicable if there is no heterogeneity. In *Clinical Evidence*, an NNT is provided for meta-analysis, based on a combination of the summary odds ratio (OR) and the mean baseline risk observed in average of the control groups.

Odds The odds of an event happening is defined as the probability that an event will occur, expressed as a proportion of the probability that the event will not occur.

Odds ratio (OR) One measure of treatment effectiveness. It is the odds of an event happening in the experimental group expressed as a proportion of the odds of an event happening in the control group. The closer the OR is to one, the smaller the difference in effect between the experimental intervention and the control intervention. If the OR is greater (or less) than one, then the effects of the treatment are more (or less) than those of the control treatment. Note that the effects being measured may be adverse (e.g. death or disability) or desirable (e.g. survival). When events are rare the OR is analogous to the relative risk (RR), but as event rates increase the OR and RR diverge.

Odds reduction The complement of odds ratio (1-OR), similar to the relative risk reduction (RRR) when events are rare.

Placebo A substance given in the control group of a clinical trial, which is ideally identical in appearance and taste or feel to the experimental treatment and believed to lack any disease specific effects. In the context of non-pharmacological interventions, placebo is usually referred to as sham treatments (see sham treatment below).

Positive likelihood ratio (LR+) The ratio of the probability that an individual with the target condition has a positive test result to the probability that an individual without the target condition has a positive test result. This is the same as the ratio (sensitivity/1-specificity).

Positive predictive value (PPV) The chance of having a disease given a positive test result (not to be confused with sensitivity, which is the other way round; see below).

Power A study has adequate power if it can reliably detect a clinically important difference (i.e. between two treatments) if one actually exists. The power of a study is increased when it includes more events or when its measurement of outcomes is more precise.

Pragmatic study An RCT designed to provide results that are directly applicable to normal practice (compared with explanatory trials that are intended to clarify efficacy under ideal conditions). Pragmatic RCTs recruit a population that is representative of those who are normally treated, allow normal compliance with instructions (by avoiding incentives and by using oral instructions with advice to follow manufacturers instructions), and analyse results by "intention to treat" rather than by "on treatment" methods.

Prevalence The proportion of people with a finding or disease in a given population at a given time.

Publication bias Occurs when the likelihood of a study being published varies with the results it finds. Usually, this occurs when studies that find a significant effect are more likely to be published than studies that do not find a significant effect, so making it appear from surveys of the published literature that treatments are more effective than is truly the case.

P value The probability that an observed or greater difference occurred by chance, if it is assumed that there is in fact no real difference between the effects of the interventions. If this probability is less than 1/20 (which is when the P value is less than 0.05), then the result is conventionally regarded as being "statistically significant".

Quasi randomised A trial using a method of allocating participants to different forms of care that is not truly random; for example, allocation by date of birth, day of the week, medical record number, month of the year, or the order in which participants are included in the study (e.g. alternation).

Random effects The "random effects" model assumes a different underlying effect for each study and takes this into consideration as an additional source of variation, which leads to somewhat wider confidence intervals than the fixed effects model. Effects are assumed to be randomly distributed, and the central point of this distribution is the focus of the combined effect estimate (see fixed effects above).

Randomised controlled trial (RCT) A trial in which participants are randomly assigned to two or more groups: at least one (the experimental group) receiving an intervention that is being tested and another (the comparison or control group) receiving an alternative treatment or placebo. This design allows assessment of the relative effects of interventions.

Regression analysis Given data on a dependent variable and one or more independent variables, regression analysis involves finding the "best" mathematical model to describe or predict the dependent variable as a function of the independent variable(s). There are several regression models that suit different needs. Common forms are linear, logistic, and proportional hazards.

Relative risk (RR) The number of times more likely (RR > 1) or less likely (RR < 1) an event is to happen in one group compared with another. It is the ratio of the absolute risk (AR) for each group. It is analogous to the odds ratio (OR) when events are rare.

Relative risk increase (RRI) The proportional increase in risk between experimental and control participants in a trial.

Relative risk reduction (RRR) The proportional reduction in risk between experimental and control participants in a trial. It is the complement of the relative risk (1-RR).

Sensitivity The chance of having a positive test result given that you have a disease (not to be confused with positive predictive value [PPV], which is the other way around; see above).

Sensitivity analysis Analysis to test if results from meta-analysis are sensitive to restrictions on the data included. Common examples are large trials only, higher quality trials only, and more recent trials only. If results are consistent this provides stronger evidence of an effect and of generalisability.

Sham treatment An intervention given in the control group of a clinical trial, which is ideally identical in appearance and feel to the experimental treatment and believed to lack any disease specific effects (e.g. detuned ultrasound or random biofeedback).

Significant By convention, taken to mean statistically significant at the 5% level (see statistically significant below). This is the same as a 95% confidence interval not including the value corresponding to no effect.

Specificity The chance of having a negative test result given that you do not have a disease (not to be confused with negative predictive value [NPV], which is the other way around; see above).

Standardised mean difference (SMD) A measure of effect size used when outcomes are continuous (such as height, weight, or symptom scores) rather than dichotomous (such as death or myocardial infarction). The mean differences in outcome between the groups being studied are standardised to account for differences in scoring methods (such as pain scores). The measure is a ratio; therefore, it has no units.

Statistically significant Means that the findings of a study are unlikely to have arisen because of chance. Significance at the commonly cited 5% level (P < 0.05) means that the observed difference or greater difference would occur by chance in only 1/20 similar cases. Where the word "significant" or "significance" is used without qualification in the text, it is being used in this statistical sense.

Subgroup analysis Analysis of a part of the trial/meta-analysis population in which it is thought the effect may differ from the mean effect.

Systematic review A review in which specified and appropriate methods have been used to identify, appraise, and summarise studies addressing a defined question. It can, but need not, involve meta-analysis (see meta-analysis). In *Clinical Evidence*, the term systematic review refers to a systematic review of RCTs unless specified otherwise.

True negative A person without the target condition (defined by a gold standard) who has a negative test result.

True positive A person with the target condition (defined by a gold standard) who also has a positive test result.

Validity The soundness or rigour of a study. A study is internally valid if the way it is designed and carried out means that the results are unbiased and it gives you an accurate estimate of the effect that is being measured. A study is externally valid if its results are applicable to people encountered in regular clinical practice.

Weighted mean difference (WMD) A measure of effect size used when outcomes are continuous (such as symptom scores or height) rather than dichotomous (such as death or myocardial infarction). The mean differences in outcome between the groups being studied are weighted to account for different sample sizes and differing precision between studies. The WMD is an absolute figure and so takes the units of the original outcome measure.

Search date October 2001

Gregory Y H Lip, Sridhar Kamath, and Bethan Freestone

QUESTIONS

INTERVENTIONS

Key Messages

Heart rate control

- **Digoxin** Two RCTs found that digoxin versus placebo significantly reduced ventricular rate after 30 minutes or 18 hours in people with atrial fibrillation.

- **Diltiazem** One RCT in people with atrial fibrillation or atrial flutter found that intravenous diltiazem (a calcium channel blocker) versus placebo significantly reduced heart rate over 15 minutes. Another RCT in people with acute atrial fibrillation or atrial flutter found that intravenous diltiazem versus intravenous digoxin significantly reduced heart rate within 5 minutes.

- **Timolol** One small RCT in people with atrial fibrillation found that intravenous timolol (a β blocker) versus placebo significantly reduced ventricular rate within 20 minutes.

- **Verapamil** Two RCTs found that intravenous verapamil (a calcium channel blocker) versus placebo significantly reduced heart rate at 10 or 30 minutes in people with atrial fibrillation or atrial flutter. One RCT found no significant difference in rate control or measures of systolic function with intravenous verapamil versus intravenous diltiazem in people with atrial fibrillation or atrial flutter, but verapamil caused hypotension in some people.

Conversion to sinus rhythm

- **DC cardioversion** We found no RCTs of DC cardioversion in acute atrial fibrillation. It may be unethical to conduct RCTs.

- **Digoxin** Three RCTs found no significant difference in conversion to sinus rhythm with digoxin versus placebo in people with atrial fibrillation.

- **Timolol** One small RCT found that intravenous timolol (a β blocker) versus placebo increased conversion to sinus rhythm in people with atrial fibrillation, but the difference was not significant.

Prevention of embolism

- **Antithrombotic treatment prior to cardioversion** We found no RCTs of aspirin, heparin, or warfarin as thromboprophylaxis prior to cardioversion in acute atrial fibrillation.

DEFINITION Acute atrial fibrillation is the sudden onset of rapid, irregular, and chaotic atrial activity, and the 48 hours after that onset. It includes both the first symptomatic onset of persistent atrial fibrillation (see glossary, p 9) and episodes of paroxysmal atrial fibrillation (see glossary, p 8). It is sometimes difficult to distinguish episodes of new onset atrial fibrillation from newly diagnosed atrial fibrillation. Atrial fibrillation within 72 hours of onset is sometimes called recent onset atrial fibrillation. By contrast, chronic atrial fibrillation (see glossary, p 8) is a more sustained form of atrial fibrillation, which in turn can be described as paroxysmal, persistent, or permanent atrial fibrillation (see glossary, p 8). If the atrial fibrillation recurs intermittently, with sinus rhythm between recurrences and with spontaneous recurrences/termination, then it is designated as paroxysmal atrial fibrillation. More sustained atrial fibrillation, which can be successfully reverted back to sinus rhythm (cardioversion), is designated persistent atrial fibrillation. If cardioversion is inappropriate, then atrial fibrillation is designated as permanent atrial fibrillation. In this review we have excluded episodes of atrial fibrillation that arise during or soon after cardiac surgery, and we have excluded the management of chronic atrial fibrillation.

INCIDENCE/ PREVALENCE We found limited evidence of the incidence or prevalence of acute atrial fibrillation. Extrapolation from the Framingham study[1] suggests an incidence in men of 3/1000 person years at age 55 years, rising to 38/1000 person years at 94 years. In women, the incidence was 2/1000 person years at age 55 years and 32.5/1000 person years at 94 years. The prevalence of atrial fibrillation ranged from 0.5% for people aged 50–59 years to 9% in people aged 80–89 years. Among acute emergency medical admissions in the UK, 3–6% have atrial fibrillation and about 40% were newly diagnosed.[2,3] Among acute hospital admissions in New Zealand, 10% (95% CI 9% to 12%) had documented atrial fibrillation.[4]

AETIOLOGY/ RISK FACTORS Paroxysms of atrial fibrillation are more common in athletes.[5] Age increases the risk of developing acute atrial fibrillation. Men are more likely to develop atrial fibrillation than women (38 years' follow up from the Framingham Study, RR after adjustment for age and known predisposing conditions 1.5).[6] Atrial fibrillation can occur in association with underlying disease (both cardiac and non-cardiac) or can arise in the absence of any other condition. Epidemiological surveys have found that risk factors for the development of acute atrial fibrillation include ischaemic heart disease, hypertension, heart failure, valve disease, diabetes, alcohol abuse, thyroid disorders, and disorders of the lung and pleura.[1] In a UK survey of acute hospital admissions with atrial fibrillation, a history of ischaemic heart disease was present in 33%, heart failure in 24%, hypertension in 26%, and rheumatic heart disease in 7%.[3] In some populations, the acute effects of alcohol explain a large proportion of the incidence of acute atrial fibrillation.

PROGNOSIS We found no evidence about the proportion of people with acute atrial fibrillation who develop more chronic forms of atrial fibrillation (e.g. paroxysmal, persistent, or permanent atrial fibrillation). Observational studies and placebo arms of RCTs have found that more than 50% of people with acute atrial fibrillation revert spontaneously within 24–48 hours, especially atrial fibrillation associated with an identifiable precipitant such as alcohol or myocardial infarction. We found little evidence about the effects on mortality and morbidity of acute atrial fibrillation where no underlying cause is found. Acute atrial fibrillation during myocardial infarction is an independent predictor of both short term and long term mortality.[7] Onset of atrial fibrillation reduces cardiac output by 10–20% irrespective of the underlying ventricular rate[8,9] and can contribute to heart failure. People with acute atrial fibrillation who present with heart failure have worse prognosis. Acute atrial fibrillation is associated with a risk of imminent stroke.[10 13] One case series used transoesophageal echocardiography in people who had developed acute atrial fibrillation within the preceding 48 hours; it found that 15% had atrial thrombi.[14] An ischaemic stroke associated with atrial fibrillation is more likely to be fatal, have a recurrence, and leave a serious functional deficit among survivors, than a stroke not associated with atrial fibrillation.[15]

AIMS To reduce symptoms, morbidity, and mortality, with minimum adverse effects.

OUTCOMES Major outcomes include measures of symptoms, recurrent stroke or transient ischaemic attack, thromboembolism, mortality, and major bleeding. Proxy measures include heart rhythm, ventricular rate, and timing to restoration of sinus rhythm. Frequent spontaneous reversion to sinus rhythm makes it difficult to interpret short term studies of rhythm; treatments may accelerate restoration of sinus rhythm without increasing the proportion of people who eventually convert. The clinical importance of changes in mean heart rate is also unclear.

METHODS *Clinical Evidence* search and appraisal October 2001. Current Contents, textbooks, review articles, and recent abstracts were reviewed. Many studies were not solely in people with acute atrial fibrillation. The text indicates where results have been extrapolated from studies of paroxysmal, persistent, or permanent atrial fibrillation. Atrial fibrillation that follows coronary surgery has been excluded.

QUESTION **What are the effects of treatments for acute atrial fibrillation?**

OPTION **ANTITHROMBOTIC TREATMENT PRIOR TO CARDIOVERSION**

We found no RCTs on use of aspirin, heparin, or warfarin as thromboprophylaxis prior to cardioversion in acute atrial fibrillation.

Benefits: We found no RCTs on use of aspirin, heparin, or warfarin as thromboprophylaxis prior to cardioversion in acute atrial fibrillation.

Acute atrial fibrillation

Harms: We found no RCTs.

Comment: For acute atrial fibrillation, there is consensus to give heparin to people undergoing cardioversion within 48 hours of arrhythmia onset.[16] Warfarin is not used as an anticoagulant in acute atrial fibrillation because of its slow onset of action. One transoesophageal echocardiography study in people with a recent embolic event found left atrial thrombus in 15% of people with acute atrial fibrillation of less than 3 days' duration.[14] This would suggest that people with atrial fibrillation of less than 3 days' duration may benefit from formal anticoagulation or require evaluation by transoesophageal echocardiography before safe cardioversion. One ongoing trial comparing low molecular weight and unfractionated heparin in people with atrial fibrillation of more than 2 days duration undergoing transoesophageal echocardiographically guided early electrical or chemical cardioversion, will recruit 200 people to assess the feasibility and effects of such a strategy.[17]

OPTION	DC CARDIOVERSION

We found no RCTs on use of DC cardioversion in acute atrial fibrillation. It may be unethical to conduct RCTs of DC cardioversion in people with acute atrial fibrillation and haemodynamic compromise.

Benefits: We found no RCTs on use of DC cardioversion in acute atrial fibrillation. It may be unethical to conduct RCTs on use of DC cardioversion in people with acute atrial fibrillation and haemodynamic compromise.

Harms: We found no RCTs on use of DC cardioversion in acute atrial fibrillation. Adverse events from synchronised DC cardioversion include those associated with a general anaesthetic, generation of a more serious arrhythmia, superficial burns, and thromboembolism. Cardioversion may be unsuccessful. The atrial fibrillation may recur.

Comment: It may be unethical to conduct RCTs on the use of DC cardioversion in people with acute atrial fibrillation and haemodynamic compromise. The evidence for DC cardioversion in acute atrial fibrillation can only be extrapolated from its use in chronic atrial fibrillation (see glossary, p 8). DC cardioversion has been used for the treatment of atrial fibrillation since the 1960s.[18] There is a consensus[16] that immediate DC cardioversion for acute atrial fibrillation should be attempted only if there are signs of haemodynamic compromise. Otherwise full anticoagulation is recommended (warfarin for 3 weeks prior to and 4 weeks following cardioversion) to reduce the risk of thromboembolism in people with acute atrial fibrilation of more than 48 hours' duration.[16] We found no clear evidence on whether cardioversion or rate control is superior for acute atrial fibrillation.

OPTION   DIGOXIN

Three RCTs found no significant difference in conversion to sinus rhythm with digoxin versus placebo in people with atrial fibrillation. Two RCTs found that digoxin versus placebo significantly reduced ventricular rate after 30 minutes and 18 hours in people with atrial fibrillation.

Benefits: We found no systematic review but found three RCTs.[19–21] **Versus placebo:** One RCT (239 people within 7 days of onset of atrial fibrillation, mean age 66 years, mean ventricular rate 122 beats/min) found that intravenous digoxin (mean 0.88 mg) versus placebo did not increase the restoration of sinus rhythm by 16 hours (51% with digoxin v 46% with placebo).[19] It found a rapid and clinically important reduction in ventricular rate at 2 hours (to 105 beats/min with digoxin v 117 beats/min with placebo; P = 0.0001). The second RCT (40 people within 7 days of the onset of atrial fibrillation, mean age 64 years, 23 men) compared high dose intravenous digoxin (1.25 mg) versus placebo. Restoration to sinus rhythm was not significantly different (9/19 [47%] with digoxin v 8/20 [40%] with placebo; P = 0.6). The ventricular rate after 30 minutes was significantly lower with digoxin versus placebo (P < 0.02).[20] The third RCT (36 people within 7 days of the onset of atrial fibrillation) compared oral digoxin (doses of 0.6, 0.4, 0.2, and 0.2 mg at 0, 4, 8, and 14 h, or until conversion to sinus rhythm, whichever occurred first) versus placebo. Conversion to sinus rhythm by 18 hours was not significantly different (50% with digoxin v 44% with placebo; ARR +6%, 95% CI −11% to +22%).[21]

Harms: In one RCT some people developed asymptomatic bradycardia and one person with previously undiagnosed hypertrophic cardiomyopathy suffered circulatory distress.[19] In the second RCT, two people developed bradyarrhythmias.[20] No adverse effects were stated in the third RCT.[21] Digoxin at toxic doses may result in visual, gastrointestinal, and neurological symptoms; heart block; and arrhythmias.

Comment: The peak action of digoxin is delayed: taking 6–12 hours to reduce mean ventricular rate below 100 beats/minute. We found one systematic review and RCTs of digoxin versus placebo in people with chronic atrial fibrillation (see glossary, p 8), which found that control of the ventricular rate during exercise was poor unless a β blocker or rate limiting calcium channel blocker (verapamil or diltiazem) was used in combination.[22–24] The evidence suggests that digoxin is no better than placebo at restoring sinus rhythm in people with recent onset atrial fibrillation.

OPTION   DILTIAZEM

One RCT found that intravenous diltiazem (a calcium channel blocker) versus placebo significantly reduced heart rate in people with atrial fibrillation or atrial flutter. One RCT found that intravenous diltiazem versus intravenous digoxin significantly reduced heart rate within 5 minutes in people with acute atrial fibrillation and atrial flutter.

Benefits: We found no systematic review but found three RCTs.[25–27] **Versus placebo:** One RCT (113 people; 89 with atrial fibrillation and 24 with [atrial flutter — see glossary, p 8]; ventricular rate > 120 beats/min;

systolic blood pressure ≥ 90 mm Hg without severe heart failure; 108 people with at least one underlying condition that may explain atrial arrhythmia; mean age 64 years) compared intravenous diltiazem (a calcium channel blocker) versus placebo.[25] Following randomisation, a dose of intravenous diltiazem (or equivalent placebo) 0.25 mg/kg every 2 minutes was given; if the first dose had no effect after 15 minutes, then the code was broken and diltiazem 0.35 mg/kg every 2 minutes was given regardless of randomisation. The RCT found that intravenous diltiazem versus placebo significantly decreased heart rate during a 15 minute observation period (ventricular rate below 100 beats/min 42/56 [75%] with diltiazem v 4/57 [7%] with placebo; P < 0.001; average decrease in heart rate, 22% with diltiazem v 3% with placebo; median time from start of drug infusion to maximal decrease in heart rate 4.3 min, mean rate decreased from 139 to 114 beats/min with diltiazem).[25] The RCT found no difference in response rate to diltiazem in people with atrial fibrillation versus those with atrial flutter. **Versus digoxin:** One RCT (30 consecutive people, 10 men, mean age 72 years, 26 with acute atrial fibrillation, 4 with atrial flutter, unspecified duration) compared intravenous diltiazem versus intravenous digoxin versus both given on admission to the Accident and Emergency Department.[26] Heart rate control was defined as a ventricular rate of less than 100 beats/minute. Intravenous digoxin (0.25 mg given as a bolus at 0 and 30 min) and intravenous diltiazem (initially 0.25 mg/kg over the first 2 min, followed by 0.35 mg/kg at 15 min and then a titratable infusion at a rate of 10–20 mg/h) were given to maintain heart rate control. The dosing regimens were the same whether the drugs were given alone or in combination. The RCT found that diltiazem versus digoxin significantly decreased ventricular heart rate within 5 minutes (P = 0.0006; mean rates 111 beats/min with diltiazem v 144 beats/min with digoxin). The decrease in heart rate achieved with digoxin did not reach statistical significance until 180 minutes (P = 0.01; mean rates 90 beats/min with diltiazem v 117 beats/min with digoxin). No additional benefit was found with the combination of digoxin and diltiazem. **Versus verapamil:** See text, p 7.

Harms: In one RCT, in the diltiazem treated group, seven people developed asymptomatic hypotension (systolic blood pressure < 90 mm Hg), three developed flushing, three developed itching, and one developed nausea and vomiting; these were not significantly different from placebo.[25] The second RCT was not large enough to adequately assess adverse effects, and none were apparent.[26] Rate limiting calcium channel blockers may exacerbate heart failure and hypotension.

Comment: The evidence suggests that rate limiting calcium channel blockers such as verapamil and diltiazem reduce ventricular rate in acute or recent onset atrial fibrillation, but they are probably no better than placebo in restoring sinus rhythm. We found no studies of the effect of rate limiting calcium channel blockers on exercise tolerance in people with acute or recent onset atrial fibrillation, but studies in people with chronic atrial fibrillation (see glossary, p 8) have found improved exercise tolerance.

OPTION   TIMOLOL

One small RCT found that timolol (a β blocker) versus placebo significantly reduced ventricular rate within 20 minutes and found a non-significant increase in conversion to sinus rhythm in people with atrial fibrillation of unspecified duration.

Benefits: We found no systematic review. **Versus placebo:** We found one RCT (61 people with atrial fibrillation of unspecified duration, ventricular rate > 120 beats/min) that compared intravenous timolol (a β blocker) (1 mg) versus intravenous placebo given immediately and repeated twice at 20 minute intervals if sinus rhythm was not achieved.[20] It found that 20 minutes after the last injection, intravenous timolol versus placebo significantly increased the proportion of people who had a ventricular rate below 100 beats/minute (41% with timolol v 3% with placebo; P < 0.01), and increased the proportion of people who converted to sinus rhythm, although the increase was not significant (5/29 [17%] v 2/32 [6%]; P = 0.18).

Harms: In the RCT, the most common adverse effects were bradycardia (2%) and hypotension (9%).[28] β Blockers may exacerbate heart failure and hypotension in acute atrial fibrillation. β Blockers plus rate limiting calcium channel blockers (diltiazem, verapamil) may increase the risk of asystole and sinus arrest.[29-31] β Blockers can precipitate bronchospasm.[32]

Comment: In addition to the evidence from people with acute atrial fibrillation, we found one systematic review of β blockers versus placebo in people with either acute or chronic atrial fibrillation (see glossary, p 8).[22] It found that in 7/12 comparisons at rest and in all during exercise, β blockers reduced ventricular rate compared with placebo. We found no RCTs that reported quality of life, functional capacity, or mortality.

OPTION   VERAPAMIL

Two RCTs found that intravenous verapamil (a calcium channel blocker) versus placebo significantly reduced heart rate at 10 or 30 minutes in people with atrial fibrillation or atrial flutter. One RCT found no significant difference with intravenous verapamil versus intravenous diltiazem (both calcium channel blockers) in rate control or measures of systolic function in people with atrial fibrillation or atrial flutter, but verapamil caused hypotension in some people.

Benefits: We found no systematic review in people with acute atrial fibrillation. **Versus placebo:** We found two RCTs.[33,34] The first RCT (21 men with atrial fibrillation and a rapid ventricular rate, age 37–70 years) was a crossover comparison of intravenous verapamil versus placebo (saline).[33] It found that intravenous verapamil versus placebo reduced ventricular rate within 10 minutes (reduction > 15% of the initial rate 17/20 [85%] with verapamil v 2/14 [14%] with saline). It also found that three people converted to sinus rhythm, but it is not clear from the results whether these effects can be attributed to verapamil or saline. The second RCT (double blind, crossover study of 20 people with atrial fibrillation or [atrial flutter — see glossary, p 8] for 2 h to 2 years) compared intravenous low dose verapamil (0.075 mg/kg) versus placebo.[34] A positive response was defined as conversion to sinus rhythm or a decrease of the ventricular response to less than 100 beats/minute, or by more than 20% of the initial rate. If a positive response did not occur within 10 minutes, then a second bolus injection was given (placebo for people who initially received verapamil, verapamil for people who initially received placebo). It found no significant difference between low dose verapamil (0.075 mg/kg) versus placebo. With the first bolus injection, verapamil versus placebo significantly reduced ventricular rate (mean heart rate 118 beats/min with verapamil *v* 138 beats/min with placebo), and more people converted to sinus rhythm within 30 minutes but the difference was not significant (3/20 [15%] with verapamil *v* 0/15 with placebo; P = 0.12). **Versus diltiazem:** We found one small double blind, crossover RCT (17 men, 5 with acute atrial fibrillation, 10 with atrial flutter, and 2 with combination of atrial fibrillation and atrial flutter; ventricular rate ≥ 120 beats/min, systolic blood pressure > 100 mm Hg) compared intravenous verapamil versus intravenous diltiazem.[27] It found no significant differences in rate control or measures of systolic function.

Harms: One RCT reported that intravenous verapamil caused a transient drop in systolic and diastolic blood pressure greater than with placebo (saline), which did not require treatment, but did not state the number of people affected.[33] The second RCT reported development of 1:1 flutter in one person with Wolff Parkinson White syndrome (see glossary, p 9) and 2:1 flutter.[34] In the third RCT, comparing verapamil versus diltiazem, 3/17 (18%) of people receiving verapamil as the first drug developed symptomatic hypotension and were withdrawn from the study before crossover.[27] Two people recovered, but the episode in the third person was considered to be life threatening. In people with Wolff Parkinson White syndrome, verapamil may increase the ventricular rate and can cause ventricular arrhythmias.[35] Rate limiting calcium channel blockers may exacerbate heart failure and hypotension.

Comment: See comment, p 6

GLOSSARY

Atrial flutter A similar arrhythmia to atrial fibrillation but the atrial electrical activity is less chaotic and has a characteristic saw tooth appearance on an electrocardiogram.

Chronic atrial fibrillation Refers to more sustained or recurrent forms of atrial fibrillation, which can be subdivided into paroxysmal, persistent, or permanent atrial fibrillation.

Paroxysmal atrial fibrillation If the atrial fibrillation recurs intermittently with sinus rhythm, with spontaneous recurrences/termination, it is designated as "paroxysmal", and the objective of management is suppression of paroxysms and maintenance of sinus rhythm.

Permanent atrial fibrillation If cardioversion is inappropriate, and has not been indicated or attempted, atrial fibrillation is designated as "permanent", where the objective of management is rate control and antithrombotic treatment.

Persistent atrial fibrillation When atrial fibrillation is more sustained, atrial fibrillation is designated "persistent", necessitating termination with pharmacological treatment or electrical cardioversion.

Wolff Parkinson White syndrome Occurs when an additional electrical pathway exists between the atria and ventricles as a result of anomalous embryonic development. The extra pathway may cause rapid arrhythmias. Worldwide it affects about 0.2% of the general population. In people with Wolff Parkinson White syndrome, β blockers, calcium channel blockers, and digoxin can increase the ventricular rate and cause ventricular arrhythmias.

REFERENCES

1 Benjamin EJ, Wolf PA, Kannel WA. The epidemiology of atrial fibrillation. In: Falk RH, Podrid P, eds. Atrial fibrillation: mechanisms and management. 2nd ed. Philadelphia: Lippincott-Raven Publishers, 1997:1–22.

2. Lip GYH, Tean KN, Dunn FG. Treatment of atrial fibrillation in a district general hospital. Br Heart J 1994;71:92–95.

3. Zarifis J, Beevers DG, Lip GYH. Acute admissions with atrial fibrillation in a British multiracial hospital population. Br J Clin Pract 1997;51:91–96.

4. Stewart FM, Singh Y, Persson S, Gamble GD, Braatvedt GD. Atrial fibrillation: prevalence and management in an acute general medical unit. Aust N Z J Med 1999;29:51–58.

5. Furlanello F, Bertoldi A, Dallago M, et al. Atrial fibrillation in elite athletes. J Cardiovasc Electrophysiol 1998;9(8 suppl):63–68.

6. Kannel WB, Wolf PA, Benjamin EJ, Levy D. Prevalence, incidence, prognosis, and predisposing conditions for atrial fibrillation: population-based estimates. Am J Cardiol 1998;82:2N–9N.

7. Pedersen OD, Bagger H, Kober L, Torp-Pedersen C. The occurrence and prognostic significance of atrial fibrillation/flutter following acute myocardial infarction. TRACE Study group. TRAndolapril Cardiac Evaluation. Eur Heart J 1999;20:748–754.

8. Clark DM, Plumb VJ, Epstein AE, Kay GN. Hemodynamic effects of an irregular sequence of ventricular cycle lengths during atrial fibrillation. J Am Coll Cardiol 1997;30:1039–1045.

9. Schumacher B, Luderitz B. Rate issues in atrial fibrillation: consequences of tachycardia and therapy for rate control. Am J Cardiol 1998;82:29N–36N.

10. Peterson P, Godfredson J. Embolic complications in paroxysmal atrial fibrillation. Stroke 1986;17:622–626.

11. Sherman DG, Goldman L, Whiting RB, Jurgensen K, Kaste M, Easton JD. Thromboembolism in patients with atrial fibrillation. Arch Neurol 1984;41:708–710.

12. Wolf PA, Kannel WB, McGee DL, Meeks SL, Bharucha NE, McNamara PM. Duration of atrial fibrillation and imminence of stroke: the Framingham study. Stroke 1983;14:664–667.

13. Corbalan R, Arriagada D, Braun S, et al. Risk factors for systemic embolism in patients with paroxysmal atrial fibrillation. Am Heart J 1992;124:149–153.

14. Stoddard ME, Dawkins PR, Prince CR, Ammash NM. Left atrial appendage thrombus is not uncommon in patients with acute atrial fibrillation and a recent embolic event: a transesophageal echocardiographic study. J Am Coll Cardiol 1995;25:452–459.

15. Lin HJ, Wolf PA, Kelly-Hayes M, et al. Stroke severity in atrial fibrillation. The Framingham Study. Stroke 1996;27:1760–1764.

16. Fuster V, Ryden LE, Asinger RW, et al. ACC/AHA/ESC Guidelines for the management of patients with atrial fibrillation: Executive summary. Circulation 2001;104:2118–2150.

17. Murray RD, Shah A, Jasper SE, et al. Transoesophageal echocardiography guided enoxaparin antithrombotic strategy for cardioversion of atrial fibrillation: the ACUTE II pilot study. Am Heart J 2000;139:1–7.

18. Lown B, Amarasingham R, Neuman J. Landmark article Nov 3, 1962: New method for terminating cardiac arrhythmias. Use of synchronised capacitator discharge. JAMA 1986:256;621–627.

19. DAAF trial group. Intravenous digoxin in acute atrial fibrillation. Results of a randomized, placebo-controlled multicentre trial in 239 patients. The Digitalis in Acute AF (DAAF) Trial Group. Eur Heart J 1997;18:649–654.

20. Jordaens L, Trouerbach J, Calle P, et al. Conversion of atrial fibrillation to sinus rhythm and rate control by digoxin in comparison to placebo. Eur Heart J 1997;18:643–648.

21. Falk RH, Knowlton AA, Bernard SA, Gotlieb NE, Battinelli NJ. Digoxin for converting recent-onset atrial fibrillation to sinus rhythm. Ann Intern Med 1987;106:503–506.

22. McNamara RL, Bass EB, Miller MR, et al. Management of new onset atrial fibrillation Evidence Report/Technology Assessment No. 12 (prepared by the John Hopkins University Evidence-based Practice centre in Baltimore, MD, under contract no. 290–97-0006). AHRQ publication number 01-E026. Rockville, MD: Agency for Healthcare Research and Quality. January 2001. Search date 1998; primary sources The Cochrane Library, Medline, Pubmed's "related links" feature, reviews of Cochrane hand search results, and handsearches of reference lists and scanning of tables of contents from relevant journals.

23. Farshi R, Kistner D, Sarma JS, Longmate JA, Singh BN. Ventricular rate control in chronic atrial fibrillation during daily activity and programmed exercise: a crossover open-label study of five drug regimens. J Am Coll Cardiol 1999;33:304–310.

24. Klein HO, Pauzner H, Di Segni E, David D, Kaplinsky E. The beneficial effects of verapamil in chronic atrial fibrillation. Arch Intern Med 1979;139:747–749.

25. Salerno DM, Dias VC, Kleiger RE, et al. Efficacy and safety of intravenous diltiazem for treatment of atrial fibrillation and atrial flutter: the Diltiazem-Atrial Fibrillation/Flutter Study Group. Am J Cardiol 1989;63:1046–1051.

26. Schreck DM, Rivera AR, Tricarico VJ. Emergency management of atrial fibrillation and flutter: intravenous diltiazem versus intravenous digoxin. Ann Emerg Med 1997;29:135–140.

27. Phillips BG, Gandhi AJ, Sanoski CA, Just VL, Bauman JL. Comparison of intravenous diltiazem

Cardiovascular disorders

and verapamil for the acute treatment of atrial fibrillation and atrial flutter. *Pharmacotherapy* 1997;17:1238–1245.

28. Sweany AE, Moncloa F, Vickers FF, Zupkis RV, Rahway NJ. Antiarrhythmic effects of intravenous timolol in supraventricular arrhythmias. *Clin Pharmacol Ther* 1985;37:124–127.

29. Lee TH, Salomon DR, Rayment CM, Antman EM. Hypotension and sinus arrest with exercise-induced hyperkalemia and combined verapamil/propranolol therapy. *Am J Med* 1986;80:1203–1204.

30. Misra M, Thakur R, Bhandari K. Sinus arrest caused by atenolol-verapamil combination. *Clin Cardiol* 1987;10:365–367.

31. Yeh SJ, Yamamoto T, Lin FC, Wang CC, Wu D. Repetitive sinoatrial exit block as the major mechanism of drug-provoked long sinus or atrial pause. *J Am Coll Cardiol* 1991;18:587–595.

32. Doshan HD, Rosenthal RR, Brown R, Slutsky A, Applin WJ, Caruso FS. Celiprolol, atenolol and propranolol: a comparison of pulmonary effects in asthmatic patients. *J Cardiovasc Pharmacol* 1986;8(suppl 4):105–108.

33. Aronow WS, Ferlinz J. Verapamil versus placebo in atrial fibrillation and atrial flutter. *Clin Invest Med* 1980;3:35–39.

34. Waxman HL, Myerburg RJ, Appel R, Sung RJ. Verapamil for control of ventricular rate in paroxysmal supraventricular tachycardia and atrial fibrillation or flutter: a double-blind randomized cross-over study. *Ann Intern Med* 1981;94:1–6.

35. Strasberg B, Sagie A, Rechavia E, et al. Deleterious effects of intravenous verapamil in Wolff-Parkinson-White patients and atrial fibrillation. *Cardiovasc Drugs Ther* 1989;2:801–806.

Bethan Freestone
Research Fellow
Haemostasis Thrombosis and Vascular Biology Unit University Department of Medicine City Hospital
Birmingham
UK

Sridhar Kamath
Research Fellow
Haemostasis Thrombosis and Vascular Biology Unit University Department of Medicine City Hospital
Birmingham
UK

Gregory Lip
Professor of Cardiovascular Medicine
Haemostasis Thrombosis and Vascular Biology Unit University Department of Medicine City Hospital
Birmingham
UK

Competing interests: GL is UK principal investigator for the ERAFT Trial (Knoll) and has been reimbursed by various pharmaceutical companies for attending several conferences, and running educational programmes and research projects. SK, none declared. BF, none declared.

QUESTIONS

INTERVENTIONS

Key Messages

Improving outcomes in acute myocardial infarction

■ **Angiotensin converting enzyme inhibitors** One overview and one systematic review in people within 36 hours of acute myocardial infarction have found that angiotensin converting enzyme inhibitors versus placebo significantly reduce mortality at 30 days. The overview also found that angiotensin converting enzyme inhibitors significantly increase persistent hypotension and renal dysfunction. The question of whether angiotensin converting enzyme inhibitors should be offered to everyone presenting with acute myocardial infarction or only to people with signs of heart failure remains unresolved.

■ **Aspirin** One systematic review in people with acute myocardial infarction has found that aspirin versus placebo significantly reduces mortality (NNT 41, 95% CI 31 to 62), non-fatal reinfarction (NNT 84, 95% CI 71 to 109), and non-fatal stroke (NNT 413, 95% CI 273 to 2025) at 1 month.

Acute myocardial infarction

- **β Blockers** Two systematic reviews and one subsequent RCT have found that β blockers versus control given within hours of infarction significantly reduce both mortality and reinfarction. One RCT in people receiving thrombolytic treatment found that immediate versus delayed treatment with metoprolol significantly reduced rates of reinfarction and recurrent chest pain at 6 days, but had no significant effect on mortality in the short term or at 1 year. One RCT comparing carvedilol versus placebo in people with recent myocardial infarction and left ejection fraction ≤ 40% receiving thrombolytic treatment found no significant difference in the combined endpoint of all cause mortality and hospital admission for any cardiovascular event after a median of 1.3 years, although mortality, and recurrent non fatal myocardial infarction were significantly lower with carvedilol.

- **Calcium channel blockers** RCTs in people within the first few days of an acute myocardial infarction have found that calcium channel blockers versus placebo do not reduce mortality, and in the subgroup of people with left ventricular dysfunction calcium channel blockers versus placebo may increase mortality.

- **Nitrates** One systematic review (prior to the introduction of thrombolysis) has found that nitrates versus placebo significantly reduced the risk of mortality. Two RCTs (after the introduction of thrombolysis) comparing nitrates versus placebo found no significant difference in mortality.

- **Primary percutaneous transluminal coronary angioplasty versus thrombolysis (performed in specialist centres)** Two systematic reviews have found that primary percutaneous transluminal coronary angioplasty versus primary thrombolysis significantly reduces mortality and reinfarction at 30 days. However, the trials were conducted mainly in specialist centres and the effectiveness of percutaneous transluminal coronary angioplasty versus thrombolysis in less specialist centres remains to be defined.

- **Thrombolysis** One overview of RCTs in people with acute myocardial infarction and ST elevation or bundle branch block on their initial electrocardiogram has found that prompt thrombolytic treatment (within 6 h and perhaps up to 12 h and longer after the onset of symptoms) versus placebo significantly reduces short term mortality. The overview found that thrombolytic treatment versus control significantly increased the risk of stroke or major bleeding. Meta-analysis of RCTs comparing different types of thrombolytic agents versus each other have found no significant difference in mortality.

Cardiogenic shock after acute myocardial infarction

- **Early invasive cardiac revascularisation** One RCT has found that early invasive cardiac revascularisation versus initial medical treatment alone significantly reduces mortality after 6 months (NNT 8, 95% CI 5 to 68) and 12 months (NNT 8, 95% CI 5 to 61). A second RCT found similar results, although the difference was not significant.

- **Intra-aortic balloon counterpulsation** One abstract of an RCT comparing intra-aortic balloon counterpulsation plus thrombolysis versus thrombolysis alone found no significant difference in mortality after 6 months.

- **Thrombolysis** Subgroup analysis of people with cardiogenic shock after acute myocardial infarction from one RCT comparing thrombolysis versus no thrombolysis found no significant difference in mortality after 21 days.

- **Early cardiac surgery; positive inotropes and vasodilators; pulmonary artery catheterisation; ventricular assistance devices and cardiac transplantation** We found no evidence from RCTs about the effects of these interventions.

DEFINITION **Acute myocardial infarction:** The sudden occlusion of a coronary artery leading to myocardial cell death. **Cardiogenic shock:** Defined clinically as a poor cardiac output plus evidence of tissue hypoxia that is not improved by correction of reduced intravascular volume.[1] When a pulmonary artery catheter is used, cardiogenic shock may be defined as a cardiac index (see glossary, p 27) below 2.2 litres/minute/m^2 despite an elevated pulmonary capillary wedge pressure ($\geq$ 15 mm Hg).[1-3]

INCIDENCE/ PREVALENCE **Acute myocardial infarction:** One of the most common causes of mortality in both developed and developing nations. In 1990, ischaemic heart disease was the leading cause of death worldwide, accounting for about 6.3 million deaths. The age standardised incidence varies among and within countries.[4] Each year, about 900 000 people in the USA experience an acute myocardial infarction and about 225 000 of them die. About half of these people die within 1 hour of symptoms and before reaching a hospital emergency room.[5] Event rates increase with age for both sexes and are higher in men than in women, and in poorer than richer people at all ages. The incidence of death from acute myocardial infarction has fallen in many Western countries over the past 20 years. **Cardiogenic shock:** Cardiogenic shock occurs in about 7% of people admitted to hospital with acute myocardial infarction.[6] Of these, about half have established cardiogenic shock at the time of admission to hospital, and most of the others develop it during the first 24–48 hours of their admission.[7]

AETIOLOGY/ RISK FACTORS **Acute myocardial infarction (AMI):** See aetiology/risk factors under primary prevention, p 155. The immediate mechanism of acute myocardial infarction is rupture of an atheromatous plaque causing thrombosis and occlusion of coronary arteries and myocardial cell death. Factors that may convert a stable plaque into an unstable plaque (the "active plaque") have yet to be fully elucidated; however, shear stresses, inflammation, and autoimmunity have been proposed. The changing rates of coronary heart disease in different populations are only partly explained by changes in the standard risk factors for ischaemic heart disease (particularly fall in blood pressure and smoking). **Cardiogenic shock:** Cardiogenic shock after acute myocardial infarction usually follows a reduction in functional ventricular myocardium, and is caused by left ventricular infarction (79% of people with cardiogenic shock) more often than by right ventricular infarction (3% of people with cardiogenic shock).[8] Cardiogenic shock after acute myocardial infarction may also be caused by cardiac structural defects, such as mitral valve regurgitation due to papillary muscle dysfunction (7% of people with cardiogenic shock), ventricular septal rupture (4% of people with cardiogenic shock), or cardiac tamponade following free cardiac wall rupture (1% of people with cardiogenic shock). Major risk factors for cardiogenic shock after acute myocardial infarction are previous myocardial infarction, diabetes mellitus, advanced age, hypotension, tachycardia or bradycardia, congestive heart failure with Killip class (see glossary, p 27) II–III, and low left ventricular ejection fraction (ejection fraction < 35%).[7,8]

PROGNOSIS	**Acute myocardial infarction:** May lead to a host of mechanical and cardiac electrical complications, including death, ventricular dysfunction, congestive heart failure, fatal and non-fatal arrhythmias, valvular dysfunction, myocardial rupture, and cardiogenic shock. **Cardiogenic shock:** Mortality rates for people in hospital with cardiogenic shock after acute myocardial infarction vary between 50–80%.[2,3,6,7] Most deaths occur within 48 hours of the onset of shock (see figure 1, p 34). People surviving until discharge from hospital have a reasonable long term prognosis (88% survival at 1 year).[10]
AIMS	To relieve pain; to restore blood supply to heart muscle; to reduce incidence of complications (such as congestive heart failure, myocardial rupture, valvular dysfunction, fatal and non-fatal arrhythmia); to prevent recurrent ischaemia and infarction; and to decrease mortality with minimal adverse effects of treatments.
OUTCOMES	**Efficacy outcomes:** Rates of major cardiovascular events, including death, recurrent acute myocardial infarction, refractory ischaemia, and stroke. **Safety outcomes:** Rates of major bleeding and intracranial haemorrhage.
METHODS	*Clinical Evidence* search and appraisal October 2001.

QUESTION **Which treatments improve outcomes in acute myocardial infarction?**

Nicolas Danchin

OPTION **ASPIRIN**

One systematic review in people with acute myocardial infarction has found that aspirin versus placebo significantly reduces mortality, reinfarction, and stroke at one month.

Benefits:	**Aspirin versus placebo:** We found one systematic review (search date 1990, 9 RCTs, 18 773 people), which compared antiplatelet agents versus placebo started soon after the onset of acute myocardial infarction (AMI) and for a period of at least 1 month afterwards.[11] The absolute and relative benefits found in the systematic review are shown in figure 2, p 35. The largest of the RCTs identified by the review (17 187 people with suspected AMI) compared placebo versus aspirin (162.6 mg) chewed and swallowed on the day of AMI and continued daily for 1 month.[12] In subsequent long term follow up, the mortality benefit was maintained for up to 4 years.[13] In the systematic review, the most widely tested aspirin regimens were 75–325 mg daily.[11] Doses throughout this range seemed similarly effective, with no evidence that "higher" doses were more effective (500–1500 mg aspirin daily *v* placebo; odds reduction 21%, 95% CI 14% to 27%) than "medium" doses (160–325 mg aspirin daily *v* placebo; odds reduction 28%, 95% CI 22% to 33%), or "lower" doses (75–160 mg aspirin daily *v* placebo; odds reduction 26%, 95% CI 5% to 42%). The review found insufficient evidence for efficacy of doses below 75 mg daily. One RCT identified by the review found that administering a loading dose of 160–325 mg daily achieved a prompt antiplatelet effect.[14]

Harms: The largest RCT identified by the review found no significant difference between aspirin versus placebo in rates of cerebral haemorrhage or bleeds requiring transfusion (0.4% on aspirin and placebo).[12] It also found a small absolute excess of "minor" bleeding
(ARI 0.6%, 95% CI not provided; P < 0.01).

Comment: None.

OPTION **THROMBOLYSIS**

**One overview of RCTs and one non-systematic review in people with acute
myocardial infarction and ST elevation or bundle branch block on their
initial electrocardiogram have found that prompt thrombolytic treatment
(within 6 h and perhaps up to 12 h and longer after the onset of
symptoms) versus placebo significantly reduces mortality. RCTs
comparing different types of thrombolytic agents versus each other have
found no significant difference in mortality. The overview found that
thrombolytic treatment versus control significantly increased the risk of
stroke or major bleeding. The overview and review have also found that
intracranial haemorrhage is more common in people of advanced age and
low body weight, those with hypertension on admission, and those given
tissue plasminogen activator rather than another thrombolytic agent. One
meta-analysis has found conflicting results of bolus treatment versus
infusion of thrombolytic agents on intracerebral haemorrhage.**

Benefits: **Versus placebo:** We found one overview (9 RCTs, 58 600 people
with suspected acute myocardial infarction [AMI]) comparing
thrombolysis versus placebo.[15] Baseline electrocardiograms
showed ST segment elevation in 68% of people, and ST segment
depression, T wave abnormalities, or no abnormality in the rest.
The overview found that thrombolysis versus placebo significantly
reduced short term mortality (9.6% with thrombolysis v 11.5%
with placebo; ARR 1.9%; RR 0.82, 95% CI 0.77 to 0.87; NNT 56).
The greatest benefit was found in the large subgroup of people
presenting with ST elevation (RR 0.79) or bundle branch block
(RR 0.75). Reduced rates of death were seen in people with all
types of infarction, but the benefit was several times greater in
those with anterior infarction (ARR 3.7%) compared with those
with inferior infarction (ARR 0.8%) or infarctions in other zones
(ARR 2.7%). One of the RCTs included in the overview found that
thrombolysis versus placebo significantly reduced mortality after
12 years (36/107 [34%] dead with thrombolysis v 55/112 [49%]
with placebo; ARR 15%, 95% CI 2.4% to 29%; RR 0.69, 95%
CI 0.49 to 0.95; NNT 7).[16] **Timing of treatment:** The overview
found that the earlier thrombolytic treatment was given (with
respect to the onset of symptoms), the greater the absolute
benefit of treatment (see figure 3, p 36).[15,17] For each hour of
delay in thrombolytic treatment, the absolute risk reduction for
death decreased by 0.16% (ARR for death if given within 6 h of
symptoms 3%; ARR for death if given 7–12 h after onset of
symptoms 2%).[15,17] Too few people in the overview received
treatment more than 12 hours after the onset of symptoms to
determine whether the benefits of thrombolytic treatment given
after 12 hours would outweigh the risks (see comment below).

Streptokinase versus tissue plasminogen activator: We found one non-systematic review (3 RCTs;[18–20] see table 1, p 31)[17] comparing streptokinase versus tissue plasminogen activator (tPA). The first RCT, in people with ST elevation and symptoms of AMI for less than 6 hours, was unblinded.[18] People were first randomised to intravenous tPA 100 mg over 3 hours or streptokinase 1.5 MU over 1 hour, and then further randomised to subcutaneous heparin 12 500 U twice daily beginning 12 hours later, or no heparin. It found no significant difference between thrombolysis plus heparin versus thrombolysis plus no heparin in mortality (AR of death in hospital 8.5% with thrombolysis plus heparin v 8.9% with thrombolysis plus no heparin; RRR 0.05, 95% CI −0.04 to +0.14). In the second RCT, people with suspected AMI presenting within 24 hours of symptoms were first randomised to receive either streptokinase 1.5 MU over 1 hour, tPA 0.6 MU/kg every 4 hours, or anisoylated plasminogen streptokinase activator complex (APSAC) 30 U every 3 minutes, and then further randomised to subcutaneous heparin 12 500 U starting at 7 hours and continued for 7 days, or no heparin.[19] All people received aspirin on admission. The RCT found no significant difference between thrombolytic agents in mortality (streptokinase 10.6%, APSAC 10.5%, tPA 10.3%), and no significant difference with thrombolysis plus heparin versus thrombolysis plus no heparin in mortality (AR of death 10.3% with thrombolysis plus heparin v 10.6% with thrombolysis plus no heparin) after 35 days. The third RCT was unblinded and in people with ST segment elevation presenting within 6 hours of symptom onset.[20] People were randomised to one of four regimens: streptokinase 1.5 MU over 1 hour plus subcutaneous heparin 12 500 U twice daily starting 4 hours after thrombolytic treatment; streptokinase 1.5 MU over 1 hour plus intravenous heparin 5000 U bolus followed by 1000 U every hour; accelerated tPA 15 mg bolus then 0.75 mg/kg over 30 minutes followed by 0.50 mg/kg over 60 minutes, plus intravenous heparin 5000 U bolus then 1000 U every hour; or tPA 1.0 mg/kg over 60 minutes, 10% given as a bolus, plus streptokinase 1.0 MU over 60 minutes.[20] Meta-analysis of the three trials, weighted by sample size, found no significant difference between treatments in the combined outcome of any stroke or death (ARs 9.4% for streptokinase only regimens v 9.2% for tPA based regimens, including the combined tPA and streptokinase arm in the third trial; ARR for tPA v streptokinase 0.2%, 95% CI −0.2% to +0.5%; RRR 2.1%).[17]

Comparison of other thrombolytic agents: We found two RCTs in people with AMI receiving concomitant treatment with aspirin and heparin, which compared tPA versus other thrombolytic agents.[21,22] The first RCT (15 059 people from 20 different countries with AMI evolving for < 6 h, with ST segment elevation or with the appearance of a new left bundle branch block on their electrocardiogram) compared tPA (accelerated iv administration according to the GUSTO regimen) versus reteplase (recombinant plasminogen activator; two 10 MU iv boluses, 30 min apart) and found no significant difference in mortality after 30 days (OR 1.03, 95% CI 0.91 to 1.18).[21] The second RCT (16 949 people; see comment below) compared tPA (accelerated iv administration) versus tenecteplase (a genetically engineered variant of tPA; 30–50 mg iv according to body weight as a single bolus).[22] It found no significant difference between treatments in total mortality after 30 days (6% with tenecteplase v 6% with tPA; RR 1.0, 95% CI 0.91 to 1.10).

Harms: **Stroke/intracerebral haemorrhage:** The overview found that thrombolytic treatment versus control significantly increased the risk of stroke (ARI 0.4%, 95% CI 0.2% to 0.5%; NNH 250).[15] In the third RCT comparing streptokinase versus tPA, the overall incidence of intracerebral haemorrhage was 0.7% and of stroke 1.4%, of which 31% were severely disabling and 50% were intracerebral haemorrhages.[20] The RCT also found that tPA versus streptokinase plus subcutaneous heparin or streptokinase plus intravenous heparin significantly increased the risk of haemorrhagic stroke (AR 0.54%; P = 0.03 for tPA compared with combined streptokinase arms). The RCT comparing reteplase versus tPA found that the incidence of stroke was similar with both treatments, and the odds ratio for the incidence of death or disabling stroke was 1.0.[21] The RCT comparing tenecteplase versus tPA found no significant difference between treatments in the rate of stroke or death (7% with tenecteplase v 7% with tPA; RR 1.01, 95% CI 0.91 to 1.13).[22] We found one meta-analysis which compared bolus thrombolytic treatment versus infusion treatment.[23] Meta-analysis of nine phase II trials (3956 people) found that bolus treatment significantly reduced the risk of intracerebral haemorrhage (OR 0.53, 95% CI 0.27 to 1.01). However, meta-analysis of six phase III trials (62 673 people) found that bolus treatment significantly increased the risk of intracerebral haemorrhage (OR 1.25, 95% CI 1.06 to 1.49). **Predictive factors for stroke/intracranial haemorrhage:** Multivariate analysis of data from a large database of people who experienced intracerebral haemorrhage after thrombolytic treatment identified four independent predictors of increased risk of intracerebral haemorrhage: age 65 years or older (OR 2.2, 95% CI 1.4 to 3.5); weight less than 70 kg (OR 2.1, 95% CI 1.3 to 3.2); hypertension on admission (OR 2.0, 95% CI 1.2 to 3.2); and use of tPA rather than another thrombolytic agent (OR 1.6, 95% CI 1.0 to 2.5).[21] Absolute risk of intracranial haemorrhage was 0.26% on streptokinase in the absence of risk factors, and 0.96%, 1.32%, and 2.17% in people with one, two, or three risk factors.[24] Analysis of 592 strokes in 41 021 people from the trials found seven factors to be predictors of intracerebral haemorrhage: advanced age, lower weight, history of cerebrovascular disease, history of hypertension, higher systolic or diastolic pressure on presentation, and use of tPA rather than streptokinase.[25,26] **Major bleeding:** The overview also found that thrombolytic treatment versus placebo significantly increased the risk of major bleeding (ARI 0.7%, 95% CI 0.6% to 0.9%; NNH 143).[15] Bleeding was most common in people undergoing procedures (coronary artery bypass grafting or percutaneous transluminal coronary angioplasty). Spontaneous bleeds were observed most often in the gastrointestinal tract.[20]

Comment: Extrapolation of the data from the overview (see figure 3, p 36) suggests that, at least for people suspected of having an acute myocardial infarction and with ST elevation on their electrocardiogram, there may be some net benefit of treatment between

12–18 hours after symptom onset (ARR for death 1%).[15] The evidence from the RCT comparing reteplase versus tPA is consistent with a similar efficacy for both treatments, although formal equivalence cannot be established because the trial was designed as a superiority trial.[21] Regarding this RCT's end point of overall mortality, the 95% confidence interval exceeded the 1% difference that might have been considered acceptable for defining equivalence; however, for the combined end point of mortality and disabling stroke (a secondary end point of the trial), the 95% confidence interval was less than 1%. The RCT comparing tPA versus tenecteplase was designed as an equivalence trial, accepting that tenecteplase would be equivalent to tPA if both the absolute risk of death with tenecteplase was not more than 1% higher than that with tPA and that the relative risk of mortality at 30 days would not exceed 14%.[22] The results confirmed equivalence between the two thrombolytics. The evidence suggests that it is far more important to administer prompt thrombolytic treatment than to debate which thrombolytic agent should be used. A strategy of rapid use of any thrombolytic in a broad population is likely to lead to the greatest impact on mortality. When the results of RCTs are taken together, tPA based regimens do not seem to confer a significant advantage over streptokinase in the combined outcome of any stroke and death (unrelated to stroke). The legitimacy of combining the results of the three trials can be questioned, as the selection criteria and protocols differed in important aspects (see review for arguments to justify combining the results of these trials despite their apparent differences).[17]

OPTION	β BLOCKERS

Two systematic reviews and one subsequent RCT have found that β blockers versus control given within hours of infarction significantly reduce both mortality and reinfarction. One RCT in people receiving thrombolytic treatment found that immediate versus delayed treatment with metoprolol significantly reduced rates of reinfarction and recurrent chest pain at 6 days, but had no significant effect on mortality in the short term or at 1 year. One RCT comparing carvedilol versus placebo in people with recent myocardial infarction and left ejection fraction ≤ 40% receiving thrombolytic treatment found no significant difference in the combined endpoint of all cause mortality and hospital admission for any cardiovascular event after a median of 1.3 years, although mortality, and recurrent non fatal myocardial infarction were significantly lower with carvedilol.

Benefits: **Given within hours of infarction:** We found two systematic reviews (search dates 1997[27] and not stated[28]) and one overview[29] investigating the early use of β blockers in people suffering acute myocardial infarction (AMI). The older reviews identified 27 RCTs and found that, within 1 week of treatment, β blockers significantly reduced the risk of death and major vascular events (for the combined outcome of death, non-fatal cardiac arrest, or non-fatal reinfarction: 1110 events *v* 1298 events; RR 0.84, 95% CI not provided; P < 0.001).[28,29] The largest of the RCTs identified by the review (16 027 people with AMI) compared atenolol (5–10 mg given iv immediately, followed by 100 mg orally given daily for 7 days) versus standard treatment (no β blocker).[30] The RCT found that atenolol significantly reduced vascular mortality after 7 days (3.9% with atenolol v 4.6% with standard treatment; ARR 0.7%; RR 0.85, 95% CI 0.73 to 0.88; NNT 147). The RCT found more benefit in people with electrocardiogram evidence of AMI at entry (in people with electrocardiogram suggesting anterior infarction, inferior infarction, both, or bundle branch block, AR of death: 5.33% with atenolol v 6.49% with control; ARR 1.16%; NNT 86, 95% CI not provided), and that people older than 65 years and those with large infarcts had the most benefit.[30] The more recent systematic review (82 RCTs, 54 234 people) separately analysed 51 short term RCTs (people with AMI up to 6 wk after the onset of pain) and 31 long term RCTs.[27] Most of the RCTs did not include thrombolysis. In the short term studies, seven RCTs reported no deaths and many reported only a few. Meta-analysis of the short term RCTs reporting at least one death found that β blockers versus placebo reduced mortality, but that the reduction was not significant (ARR 0.4%; OR 0.96, 95% CI 0.85 to 1.08). In the longer term RCTs, β blockers versus placebo significantly reduced mortality over 6 months to 4 years (OR 0.77, 95% CI 0.69 to 0.85). No significant difference in effectiveness was found between different types of β blocker (based on cardioselectivity or intrinsic sympathomimetic activity). Most evidence was obtained with propranolol, timolol, and metoprolol. **In people receiving thrombolytic treatment:** We found two RCTs.[31,32] The first RCT (1434 people with AMI who had received tissue plasminogen activator thrombolysis) compared early versus delayed metoprolol treatment.[31] Early treatment began on day 1 (iv then oral) and delayed treatment on day 6 (oral). It found that early treatment significantly reduced rates of reinfarction (AR 2.7% with early treatment v 5.1% with delayed treatment, 95% CI not provided; P = 0.02), and recurrent chest pain (AR 18.8% with early treatment v 24.1% with delayed treatment; P < 0.02) after 6 days. There were no early (6 days) or late (1 year) differences observed in mortality or left ventricular ejection fraction between the two groups. The second RCT (1959 people within 3–21 days of AMI and with left ventricular dysfunction; 46% of people had received thrombolysis or percutaneous transluminal coronary angioplasty at the acute stage of their infarction, and 97% of people received angiotensin converting enzyme inhibitors) compared carvedilol (6.25 mg increased to a maximum of 25 mg over 4–6 wk) versus placebo.[32] It found that carvedilol significantly reduced mortality (12% with carvedilol v 15% with placebo; HR 0.77, 95% CI 0.60 to 0.90) and non-fatal AMI (HR 0.59, 95% CI 0.39 to 0.90), but found no significant difference between treatments in the combined end point of total mortality and hospital admission for any cardiovascular event (HR 0.92, 95% CI 0.80 to 1.07) after a median of 1.3 years. **Long term use:** See β blockers under secondary prevention of ischaemic cardiac events, p 189.

Harms: People with asthma or severe congestive cardiac failure were excluded from most trials. One RCT found that in people given immediate versus delayed β blockers following tissue plasminogen activator, there was a non-significant increased frequency of heart failure during the initial admission to hospital (15.3% with immediate *v* 12.2% with delayed; P = 0.10).[31] The presence of first degree heart block and bundle branch block was associated with an increased frequency of adverse events.

Comment: Until recently trials involving the use of β blockers in AMI were mostly conducted in people considered to be of low risk (because of the supposed deleterious effect of β blockers on left ventricular function), and many of these trials took place in the prethrombolytic era. β Blockers may reduce rates of cardiac rupture and ventricular fibrillation. This may explain why people older than 65 years and those with large infarcts benefited most, as they also have higher rates of these complications. The trial comparing early versus delayed β blockade after thrombolysis was too small to rule out an effect on mortality of β blockers when added to thrombolysis.[31]

OPTION   **ANGIOTENSIN CONVERTING ENZYME INHIBITORS**

One overview and one systematic review in people within 36 hours of acute myocardial infarction have found that angiotensin converting enzyme inhibitors versus placebo significantly reduce mortality. The overview also found that angiotensin converting enzyme inhibitors versus control significantly increase persistent hypotension and renal dysfunction. The question of whether angiotensin converting enzyme inhibitors should be offered to everyone presenting with acute myocardial infarction or only to people with signs of heart failure remains unresolved.

Benefits: **In all people after an acute myocardial infarction (AMI):** We found one overview[33] and one systematic review (search date 1997)[34] of angiotensin converting enzyme (ACE) inhibitors versus placebo after AMI. The overview (4 large RCTs, 98 496 people irrespective of clinical heart failure or left ventricular dysfunction, within 36 h of the onset of symptoms of AMI) compared ACE inhibitors versus placebo.[33] It found that ACE inhibitors significantly reduced mortality after 30 days (7.1% with ACE inhibitors *v* 7.6% with placebo; RR 0.93, 95% CI 0.89 to 0.98; NNT 200). The absolute benefit was larger in some high risk subgroups: people in Killip class (see glossary, p 27) II–III (clinically moderate to severe heart failure at first presentation; RR 0.91; NNT 71, 99% CI 36 to 10 000), people with heart rates greater than 100 beats a minute at entry (RR 0.86; NNT 44, 99% CI 25 to 185), and people with an anterior AMI (RR 0.87; NNT 94, 99% CI 56 to 303). The overview also found that ACE inhibitors significantly reduced the incidence of non-fatal cardiac failure (AR 14.6% *v* 15.2%, 95% CI not provided; P = 0.01). The systematic review (search date 1997, 15 RCTs, 15 104 people) found similar results.[34] **In selected people after an AMI:** A selective strategy was tested in three RCTs.[35–37] Treatment was restricted to people with clinical heart failure, objective evidence of left ventricular dysfunction, or both, and was started a few days after AMI (about 6000 people). These RCTs found consistently that long term treatment with ACE inhibitors in this selected population significantly reduced mortality and reinfarction

(RRRs from 1 trial:[33] for cardiovascular death 21%, 95% CI 5% to 35%; for development of severe heart failure 37%, 95% CI 20% to 50%; for congestive heart failure requiring admission to hospital 22%, 95% CI 4% to 37%; and for recurrent AMI 25%, 95% CI 5% to 40%).

Harms: The overview found that ACE inhibitors versus control significantly increased persistent hypotension (AR 17.6% with ACE inhibitor v 9.3% with control, 95% CI for difference not provided; P < 0.01) and renal dysfunction (AR 1.3% v 0.6%; P < 0.01).[33] The relative and absolute risks of these adverse effects were uniformly distributed across both the high and lower cardiovascular risk groups.

Comment: The largest benefits of ACE inhibitors in people with AMI are seen when treatment is started within 24 hours. The evidence does not answer the question of which people with an AMI should be offered ACE inhibitors, and for how long after AMI it remains beneficial to start treatment with an ACE inhibitor. We found one systematic review (search date not stated; based on individual data from about 100 000 people in RCTs of ACE inhibitors), which found that people receiving both aspirin and ACE inhibitors had the same relative risk reduction as those receiving ACE inhibitors alone (i.e. there was no evidence of a clinically relevant interaction between ACE inhibitors and aspirin).[38]

OPTION   NITRATES

One systematic review (prior to the introduction of thrombolysis) has found that nitrates versus placebo significantly reduce the risk of mortality. Two RCTs (after the introduction of thrombolysis) compared nitrates versus placebo and found no significant difference in mortality.

Benefits: **Without thrombolysis:** We found one systematic review (search date not stated, 10 RCTs, 2000 people with acute myocardial infarction [AMI]), which compared intravenous glyceryl trinitrate or sodium nitroprusside versus placebo.[39] The trials were all conducted in the prethrombolytic era. The review found that nitrates significantly reduced mortality (RRR 35%, 95% CI 16% to 55%). **With aspirin/thrombolysis:** We found two large RCTs (58 050 people with AMI,[40] 17 817 people with AMI;[41] 90% received aspirin and about 70% received thrombolytic treatment), which compared nitrates (given acutely) versus placebo. In one RCT, people received oral controlled release isosorbide mononitrate 30–60 mg/day.[40] In the other RCT, people received intravenous glyceryl trinitrate for 24 hours followed by transdermal glyceryl trinitrate 10 mg daily.[41] Neither trial found a significant difference in mortality, either in the total sample or in subgroups of people at different risks of death. Nitrates were a useful adjunctive treatment to help control symptoms in people with AMI.

Harms: The systematic review and the large RCTs found no significant harm associated with routine use of nitrates.[39–41]

Comment: The two large RCTs had features that may have caused them not to find a benefit even if one exists: a large proportion of people took nitrates outside the study; there was a high rate of concurrent use of other hypotensive agents; people were relatively low risk; and nitrates were not titrated to blood pressure and heart rate.[40,41]

| OPTION | CALCIUM CHANNEL BLOCKERS |

RCTs in people within the first few days of an acute myocardial infarction have found that calcium channel blockers versus placebo do not reduce mortality, and in the subgroup of people with left ventricular dysfunction calcium channel blockers versus placebo may increase mortality.

Benefits: **Dihydropyridine calcium channel blockers:** We found one non-systematic review (2 large RCTs)[42] in people treated within the first few days of acute myocardial infarction (AMI), which compared short acting nifedipine versus placebo.[43,44] One RCT was terminated prematurely because of lack of efficacy.[44] It found that nifedipine versus placebo increased mortality by 33%, although the increase did not reach statistical significance. We found insufficient evidence about sustained release nifedipine, amlodipine, or felodipine in this setting. **Verapamil:** We found one systematic review (search date 1997, 7 RCTs, 6527 people with AMI),[45] which found that verapamil versus placebo had no significant effect on mortality (RR 0.86, 95% CI 0.71 to 1.04).

Harms: Two systematic reviews (search dates not stated; including both randomised and observational trials) in people with AMI investigating the use of calcium channel blockers found a non-significant increase in mortality of about 4% and 6%.[46,47] One RCT (2466 people with AMI) compared diltiazem (60 mg orally 4 times daily starting 3–15 days after AMI) versus placebo.[48] It found that overall there was no significant difference in total mortality or reinfarction. Subgroup analysis in people with congestive heart failure found that diltiazem significantly increased death or reinfarction (RRI 1.41, 95% CI 1.01 to 1.96).

Comment: None.

| OPTION | PRIMARY PERCUTANEOUS TRANSLUMINAL CORONARY ANGIOPLASTY VERSUS THROMBOLYSIS |

Two systematic reviews have found that primary percutaneous transluminal coronary angioplasty versus primary thrombolysis significantly reduces mortality and reinfarction. However, the trials were conducted mainly in specialist centres and the effectiveness of percutaneous transluminal coronary angioplasty versus thrombolysis in less specialist centres remains to be defined.

Benefits: We found two systematic reviews in people with acute myocardial infarction, which compared primary percutaneous transluminal coronary angioplasty (PTCA) versus primary thrombolysis.[49,50] The first systematic review (search date 1996, 10 RCTs, 2606 people) found that primary PTCA versus primary thrombolysis significantly reduced mortality at 30 days after intervention (4.4% with primary PTCA v 6.5% with primary thrombolysis; ARR 2.1%; OR 0.66, 95% CI 0.46 to 0.94; NNT 48).[49] It found that the effect was similar regardless of which thrombolysis regimen was used. The review also found that PTCA significantly reduced the combined end point of death and reinfarction (OR 0.58, 95% CI 0.44 to 0.76). The largest single RCT (1138 people, ST elevation on electrocardiogram within 12 h of symptom onset) included in the review found less favourable results. It compared primary PTCA versus thrombolysis with accelerated tissue plasminogen activator and found no significant difference in mortality after 30 days (5.7% with PTCA v 7.0% with thrombolysis).[51] It also found that primary PTCA significantly reduced the primary end point of death, non-fatal acute myocardial infarction, or non-fatal disabling stroke (9.6% with PTCA v 13.7% with thrombolysis; OR 0.67, 95% CI 0.47 to 0.97). The RCT found that this effect was substantially attenuated after 6 months. A second RCT included in the review has reported long term follow up; it found that primary PTCA versus primary thrombolysis significantly improves mortality after 5 years (25/194 [13%] with PCTA v 48/201 [24%] with streptokinase; RR 0.54, 95% CI 0.36 to 0.87).[52] The second systematic review (search date 1998, 10 RCTs, 2573 people) found overall similar results, with significant reductions in mortality and in reinfarction.[50]

Harms: **Stroke:** The review found that PTCA versus thrombolysis significantly reduced the risk of all types of stroke (0.7% with PTCA v 2.0% with thrombolysis) and haemorrhagic stroke (0.1% with PTCA v 1.1% with thrombolysis).[49]

Comment: Although collectively the trials found an overall short term reduction in deaths with PTCA compared with thrombolysis, there were several pitfalls common to individual RCTs, most of which may have inflated the benefit of PTCA.[53] RCTs comparing PTCA with thrombolysis could not be easily blinded, and ascertainment of end points that required some judgement, such as reinfarction or stroke, may have been influenced by the investigators' knowledge of the treatment allocation (only 1 trial had a blinded adjudication events committee). Also, people allocated to PTCA were discharged 1–2 days earlier than those allocated to thrombolysis, which favoured PTCA by reducing the time for detection of in hospital events. In addition, the RCTs conducted before the largest RCT in the first review[51] should be viewed as hypothesis generating, in that the composite outcome (death, reinfarction, and stroke) was not prospectively defined, and attention was only placed on these end points after there seemed to be some benefit on post hoc analysis. The results are also based on short term outcomes only and do not provide information on collective long term benefit. For example, in the largest RCT the composite end point was significant at 30 days but with a wide degree of uncertainty, and this was substantially attenuated to a non-significant difference by 6 months.[51] The lower mortality and reinfarction rates reported with primary PTCA are promising but not conclusive, and the real benefits may well be smaller. Only in a minority of centres that perform a high volume of PTCA, and in the hands of experienced interventionists, may primary PTCA be clearly superior to thrombolytic treatment. Elsewhere, primary PTCA may be of greatest benefit in people with contraindications to thrombolysis, in people in cardiogenic shock, or in people where the mortality reduction with thrombolysis is modest and the risk of intracranial haemorrhage is increased, for example, elderly people.[54] The value of PTCA over thrombolysis in people presenting to hospital more than 12 hours after onset of chest pain remains to be tested. In the largest RCT included in the first systematic review, the collective rate of haemorrhagic stroke in people given thrombolysis was 1.1%, substantially higher than that observed in trials

Acute myocardial infarction

comparing thrombolysis with placebo.[51] This may have been because the trials summarised above were in older people and used tissue plasminogen activator. However, the lower rates of haemorrhagic stroke with primary PTCA were consistent across almost all trials, and this may be the major advantage of PTCA over thrombolysis.

| QUESTION | Which treatments improve outcomes for cardiogenic shock after acute myocardial infarction |

Edoardo De Benedetti and Philip Urban

| OPTION | EARLY INVASIVE CARDIAC REVASCULARISATION |

One RCT found that early invasive cardiac revascularisation versus initial medical treatment alone significantly reduces mortality after 6 and 12 months. A second RCT found similar results, although the difference was not significant.

Benefits: We found no systematic review. We found two RCTs in people with cardiogenic shock within 48 hours of acute myocardial infarction comparing early invasive cardiac revascularisation (see glossary, p 27) versus initial medical treatment alone (see comment below).[2,3,55] The first RCT (302 people) found that early invasive cardiac revascularisation significantly reduced mortality after 6 and 12 months (see table 2, p 33).[2,55] The second RCT (55 people) found that early invasive cardiac revascularisation reduced mortality after 30 days and at 12 months, although the difference was not significant (see table 2, p 33). **Percutaneous transluminal coronary angioplasty versus coronary artery bypass graft:** We found no RCTs in people with cardiogenic shock after acute myocardial infarction comparing percutaneous transluminal coronary angioplasty versus coronary bypass grafting.

Harms: The first RCT (56 people aged ≥ 75 years) found that there was a non-significant increase in 30 day mortality with early invasive cardiac revascularisation (18/24 [75%] with early invasive cardiac revascularisation v 17/32 [53%] with medical treatment alone; RR 1.41, 95% CI 0.95 to 2.11).[2,55] The first RCT also found that acute renal failure (defined as a serum creatinine level > 265 μmol/L) was significantly more common in the medical treatment alone group versus the early cardiac revascularisation group (36/150 [24%] v 20/152 [13%]; RR 1.82, 95% CI 1.1 to 3.0; NNH 9, 95% CI 5 to 48). Other harms reported by the RCT included major haemorrhage, sepsis, and peripheral vascular occlusion, although comparative data between groups for these harms were not provided. The second RCT did not report harms.[3]

Comment: In the first RCT, medical treatment included intra-aortic balloon counterpulsation (see glossary, p 27) and thrombolytic treatment.[2,55] In the second RCT, medical treatment was not defined.[3] The second RCT was stopped prematurely because of difficulties with recruitment. Both RCTs were conducted in centres with expertise in early invasive cardiac revascularisation and their results may not be reproducible in other settings.[2,3,55]

OPTION   **THROMBOLYSIS**

Subgroup analysis of people with cardiogenic shock after acute myocardial infarction from one RCT comparing thrombolysis versus no thrombolysis found no significant difference in mortality after 21 days.

Benefits: We found no systematic review. We found one RCT (11 806 people within 12 h of acute myocardial infarction), which compared thrombolysis using streptokinase versus no thrombolysis (see comment below).[56] Subgroup analysis of people with cardiogenic shock found no significant difference in inpatient mortality after 21 days (280 people; 102/146 [69%] with thrombolysis v 94/134 [70%] with no thrombolysis; RR 1.0, 95% CI 0.85 to 1.16).

Harms: The RCT did not report harms specifically in the subgroup of people with cardiogenic shock.[56] Overall, adverse reactions attributed to streptokinase were found in 705/5860 (12%) people either during or after streptokinase infusion. These adverse reactions included minor and major bleeding (3.7%), allergic reactions (2.4%), hypotension (3.0%), anaphylactic shock (0.1%), shivering/fever (1.0%), ventricular arrhythmias (1.2%), and stroke (0.2%).

Comment: The RCT was not blinded.[56] Data presented are from a retrospective subgroup analysis and randomisation was not stratified by the presence of cardiogenic shock.

OPTION   **POSITIVE INOTROPES (DOBUTAMINE, DOPAMINE, ADRENALINE [EPINEPHRINE], NORADRENALINE [NOREPINEPHRINE], AMRINONE) AND VASODILATORS (ANGIOTENSIN CONVERTING ENZYME INHIBITORS, NITRATES)**

We found no RCTs comparing inotropes versus placebo or comparing vasodilators versus placebo.

Benefits: **Positive inotropes:** We found no systematic review or RCTs. We found three non-systematic reviews,[1,57,58] which identified no RCTs evaluating the use of positive inotropes in people with cardiogenic shock after acute myocardial infarction. **Vasodilators:** We found no systematic review or RCTs.

Harms: Positive inotropes may worsen cardiac ischaemia and induce ventricular arrhythmias.[1,57,58] We found no studies of harms specifically in people with cardiogenic shock after acute myocardial infarction (see harms of positive inotropic drugs and vasodilators under heart failure, p 106).

Comment: There is consensus that positive inotropes are beneficial in cardiogenic shock after acute myocardial infarction. We found no evidence to confirm or reject this view. The risk of worsening hypotension has led to concern about the use of any vasodilator to treat acute cardiogenic shock.[58]

| OPTION | PULMONARY ARTERY CATHETERISATION |

We found no RCTs comparing pulmonary artery catheterisation versus no catheterisation.

Benefits: We found no systematic review and no RCTs.

Harms: Observational studies have found an association between pulmonary artery catheterisation and increased morbidity and mortality, but it is unclear whether this arises from an adverse effect of the catheterisation or because people with a poor prognosis were selected for catheterisation.[59] Harms such as major arrhythmias, injury to the lung, thromboembolism (see thromboembolism, p 269), and sepsis occur in 0.1–0.5% of people undergoing pulmonary artery catheterisation.[59]

Comment: Pulmonary artery catheterisation helps to diagnose cardiogenic shock, guide correction of hypovolaemia, optimise filling pressures for both the left and right sides of the heart, and adjust doses of inotropic drugs.[1] There is consensus that pulmonary artery catheterisation is beneficial in patients with cardiogenic shock after acute myocardial infarction,[60,61] although we found no evidence to confirm or reject this view.

| OPTION | INTRA-AORTIC BALLOON COUNTERPULSATION |

One abstract of an RCT compared intra-aortic balloon counterpulsation plus thrombolysis versus thrombolysis alone and found no significant difference in mortality after 6 months.

Benefits: We found no systematic review. We found one abstract of an RCT (57 people), which compared intra-aortic balloon counterpulsation (see glossary, p 27) plus thrombolysis versus thrombolysis alone (see comment below).[62] The RCT found no significant difference in mortality after 6 months (22/57 [39%] with thrombolysis plus balloon counterpulsation v 25/57 [43%] with thrombolysis alone; RR 0.9, 95% CI 0.57 to 1.37; P = 0.3).

Harms: Harms were not reported in the abstract of the RCT.[62]

Comment: The abstract did not describe detailed methods for the trial, making interpretation of the results difficult.[58] We also found two additional small RCTs (30 people[63] and 20 people[64]), which compared intra-aortic balloon counterpulsation versus standard treatment in people after acute myocardial infarction. Neither RCT specifically recruited, or identified data from, people with cardiogenic shock after acute myocardial infarction. Neither RCT found a reduction in mortality with intra-aortic balloon counterpulsation. There is consensus that intra-aortic balloon counterpulsation is beneficial in people with cardiogenic shock after acute myocardial infarction. We found no evidence to confirm or reject this view.

| OPTION | VENTRICULAR ASSISTANCE DEVICES AND CARDIAC TRANSPLANTATION |

We found no RCTs evaluating either ventricular assistance devices or cardiac transplantation.

Benefits: We found no systematic review and no RCTs

Harms: We found no evidence of harms specifically associated with the use of ventricular assistance devices (see glossary, p 27) or cardiac transplantation in people with cardiogenic shock after acute myocardial infarction.

Comment: Reviews of observational studies[1,58,65] and retrospective reports,[66,67] have suggested that ventricular assistance devices may improve outcomes in selected people when used alone or as a bridge to cardiac transplantation. The availability of ventricular assistance devices and cardiac transplantation is limited to a few specialised centres, and results may not be applicable to other settings.

| OPTION | EARLY CARDIAC SURGERY |

We found no RCTs evaluating early surgical intervention for ventricular septal rupture, free wall rupture, or mitral valve regurgitation complicated by cardiogenic shock after acute myocardial infarction.

Benefits: We found no systematic review and no RCTs.

Harms: We found no evidence about the harms of surgery in people with cardiogenic shock caused by cardiac structural defects after acute myocardial infarction.

Comment: Non-systematic reviews of observational studies have suggested that death is inevitable following free wall rupture without early surgical intervention, and that surgery for both mitral valve regurgitation and ventricular septal rupture is more effective when carried out within 24–48 hours.[1,58]

GLOSSARY

Cardiac index A measure of cardiac output derived from the formula: cardiac output/unit time divided by body surface area (L/min/m^2).

Intra-aortic balloon counterpulsation A technique in which a balloon is placed in the aorta and inflated during diastole and deflated just before systole.

Invasive cardiac revascularisation A term used to describe either percutaneous transluminal coronary angioplasty or coronary artery bypass grafting.

Killip class A categorisation of the severity of heart failure based on easily obtained clinical signs. The main clinical features are Class I: no heart failure; Class II: crackles audible half way up the chest; Class III: crackles heard in all the lung fields; Class IV: cardiogenic shock.

Ventricular assistance device A mechanical device placed in parallel to a failing cardiac ventricle that pumps blood in an attempt to maintain cardiac output. Because of the risk of mechanical failure, thrombosis, and haemolysis they are normally used for short term support while preparing for a heart transplant.

REFERENCES

1. Califf RM, Bengtson JR. Cardiogenic shock. *N Engl J Med* 1994;330:1724–1730.

2. Hochman JS, Sleeper LA, Webb JG, et al, for the SHOCK investigators. Early revascularization in acute myocardial infarction complicated by cardiogenic shock. *N Engl J Med* 1999;341:625–634.

3. Urban P, Stauffer JC, Khatchatrian N, et al. A randomized evaluation of early revascularization to treat shock complicating acute myocardial infarction. The (Swiss) Multicenter Trial of Angioplasty SHOCK - (S)MASH. *Eur Heart Journal* 1999;20:1030–1038.

4. Murray C, Lopez A. Mortality by cause for eight regions of the world: global burden of disease study. *Lancet* 1997;349:1269–1276.

5. National Heart, Lung, and Blood Institute. *Morbidity and mortality: chartbook on cardiovascular, lung, and blood diseases.* Bethesda, Maryland: US Department of Health and Human Services, Public Health Service, National Institutes of Health; May 1992.

6. Goldberg RJ, Samad NA, Yarzebski J, Gurwitz J, Bigelow C, Gore JM. Temporal trends in cardiogenic shock complicating acute myocardial infarction. *N Engl J Med* 1999;340:1162–1168.

7. Hasdai D, Califf RM, Thompson TD, et al. Predictors of cardiogenic shock after thrombolytic therapy for acute myocardial infarction. *J Am Coll Cardiol* 2000;35:136–143.

8. Hochman JS, Buller CE, Sleeper LA, et al. Cardiogenic shock complicating acute myocardial infarction – etiology, management and outcome: a report from the SHOCK trial registry. *J Am Coll Cardiol* 2000;36:1063–1070.

9. Urban P, Bernstein M, Costanza M, Simon R, Frey R, Erne P. An internet-based registry of acute myocardial infarction in Switzerland. *Kardiovasculaäre Medizin* 2000;3:430–441.

10. Berger PB, Tuttle RH, Holmes DR, et al. One year survival among patients with acute myocardial infarction complicated by cardiogenic shock, and its relation to early revascularisation: results of the GUSTO-1 trial. *Circulation* 1999;99:873–878.

11. Antiplatelet Trialists' Collaboration. Collaborative overview of randomised trials of antiplatelet therapy I: prevention of death, myocardial infarction, and stroke by prolonged antiplatelet therapy in various categories of people. *BMJ* 1994;308:81–106. Search date 1990; primary sources Medline and Current Contents.

12. Second International Study of Infarct Survival (ISIS-2) Collaborative Group. Randomized trial of intravenous streptokinase, oral aspirin, both or neither among 17–187 cases of suspected acute myocardial infarction. *Lancet* 1988;ii:349–360.

13. Baigent BM, Collins R. ISIS-2: four year mortality of 17 187 patients after fibrinolytic and antiplatelet therapy in suspected acute myocardial infarction study [abstract]. *Circulation* 1993;88(suppl I):I–291–I–292.

14. Patrignani P, Filabozzi P, Patrono C. Selective cumulative inhibition of platelet thromboxane production by low-dose aspirin in healthy subjects. *J Clin Invest* 1982;69:1366–1372.

15. Fibrinolytic Therapy Trialists' (FTT) Collaborative Group. Indications for fibrinolytic therapy in suspected acute myocardial infarction: collaborative overview of early mortality and major morbidity results of all randomized trials of more than 1000 patients. *Lancet* 1994;343:311–322.

16. French JK, Hyde TA, Patel H, et al. Survival 12 years after randomization to streptokinase: the influence of thrombolysis in myocardial infarction flow at three to four weeks. *J Am Coll Cardiol* 1999;34:62–69.

17. Collins R, Peto R, Baigent BM, Sleight DM. Aspirin, heparin and fibrinolytic therapy in suspected acute myocardial infarction. *N Engl J Med* 1997;336:847–860.

18. Gruppo Italiano per lo studio della streptochinasi nell'infarto miocardico (GISSI). GISSI-2: a factorial randomised trial of alteplase versus streptokinase and heparin versus no heparin among 12–490 patients with acute myocardial infarction. *Lancet* 1990;336:65–71.

19. Third International Study of Infarct Survival (ISIS-3) Collaborative Group. ISIS-3: a randomised comparison of streptokinase vs tissue plasminogen activator vs anistreplase and of aspirin plus heparin vs aspirin alone among 41–299 cases of suspected acute myocardial infarction. *Lancet* 1992;339:753–770.

20. The GUSTO Investigators. An international randomized trial comparing four thrombolytic strategies for acute myocardial infarction. *N Engl J Med* 1993;329:673–682.

21. The Global Use of Strategies to Open Occluded Coronary Arteries (GUSTO III) investigators. A comparison of reteplase with alteplase for acute myocardial infarction. *N Engl J Med* 1997;337:1118–1123.

22. Assessment of the Safety and Efficacy of a New Thrombolytic (ASSENT-2) investigators. Single bolus tenecteplase compared to front-loaded alteplase in acute myocardial infarction: the ASSENT-2 double-blind randomised trial. *Lancet* 1999;354:716–722.

23. Eikelboom JW, Mehta SR, Pogue J, Yusuf S. Safety outcomes in meta-analyses of phase 2 vs phase 3 randomized trials: intracranial hemorrhage in trials of bolus fibrinolytic therapy. *JAMA* 2001;285:444–450.

24. Simoons MI, Maggioni AP, Knatterud G, et al. Individual risk assessment for intracranial hemorrhage during thrombolytic therapy. *Lancet* 1993;342:523–528.

25. Gore JM, Granger CB, Simoons MI, et al. Stroke after thrombolysis: mortality and functional outcomes in the GUSTO-1 trial. *Circulation* 1995;92:2811–2818.

26. Berkowitz SD, Granger CB, Pieper KS, et al. Incidence and predictors of bleeding after contemporary thrombolytic therapy for myocardial infarction. *Circulation* 1997;95:2508–2516.

27. Freemantle N, Cleland J, Young P, Mason J, Harrison J. Beta blockade after myocardial infarction: systematic review and meta regression analysis. *BMJ* 1999;318:1730–1737. Search date 1997; primary sources Medline, Embase, Biosis, Healthstar, Sigle, IHTA, Derwent drug file, dissertation abstracts, Pascal, international pharmaceutical abstracts, science citation index, and hand searches of reference lists.

28. Yusuf S, Peto R, Lewis S, et al. Beta-blockade during and after myocardial infarction: an overview of the randomized trials. *Prog Cardiovasc Dis* 1985;27:355–371. Search date not stated; primary sources computer-aided search of the literature, manual search of reference lists, and enquiries to colleagues about relevant papers.

29. Sleight P for the ISIS Study Group. Beta blockade early in acute myocardial infarction. *Am J Cardiol* 1987;60:6A–12A.

30. First International Study of Infarct Survival (ISIS-1) Collaborative Group. Randomised trial of

intravenous atenolol among 16 027 cases of suspected acute myocardial infarction. *Lancet.* 1986;2(8498):57–66.

31. Roberts R, Rogers WJ, Mueller HS, et al. Immediate versus deferred beta-blockade following thrombolytic therapy in patients with acute myocardial infarction: results of the thrombolysis in myocardial infarction (TIMI) II-B study. *Circulation* 1991;83:422–437.

32. The CAPRICORN investigators. Effect of carvedilol on outcome after myocardial infarction in patients with left-ventricular dysfunction: the CAPRICORN randomized trial. *Lancet* 2001;357:1385 1390.

33. ACE Inhibitor Myocardial Infarction Collaborative Group. Indications for ACE inhibitors in the early treatment of acute myocardial infarction: systematic overview of individual data from 100 000 patients in randomised trials. *Circulation* 1998;97:2202–2212. Search date not stated; primary source collaboration group of principal investigators of all randomised trials who collated individual patient data

34. Domanski MJ, Exner DV, Borkowf CB, Geller NL, Rosenberg Y, Pfeffer MA. Effect of angiotensin converting enzyme inhibition on sudden cardiac death in patients following acute myocardial infarction. A meta-analysis of randomized clinical trials. *J Am Coll Cardiol* 1999;33:598–604. Search date 1997; primary sources Medline and hand searches of reference lists.

35. Pfeffer MA, Braunwald E, Moye LA, et al. Effect of captopril on mortality and morbidity in patients with left ventricular dysfunction after myocardial infarction. *N Engl J Med* 1992;327:669–677.

36. The Acute Infarction Ramipril Efficacy (AIRE) Study Investigators. Effect of ramipril on mortality and morbidity of survivors of acute myocardial infarction with clinical evidence of heart failure. *Lancet* 1993;342:821–828.

37. The Trandolapril Cardiac Evaluation (TRACE) Study Group. A clinical trial of the angiotensin-converting-enzyme inhibitor trandolapril in patients with left ventricular dysfunction after myocardial infarction. *N Engl J Med* 1995;333:1670 1676.

38. Latini R, Tognoni G, Maggioni AP, et al. Clinical effects of early angiotensin-converting enzyme inhibitor treatment for acute myocardial infarction are similar in the presence and absence of aspirin. Systematic overview of individual data from 96 712 randomized patients. *J Am Coll Cardiol* 2000;35:1801–1807. Search date not stated; primary source individual patient data on all trials involving more than 1000 patients.

39. Yusuf S, Collins R, MacMahon S, Peto R. Effect of intravenous nitrates on mortality in acute myocardial infarction: an overview of the randomised trials. *Lancet* 1988;1:1088–1092. Search date not stated; primary sources literature, colleagues, investigators, and pharmaceutical companies.

40. Fourth International Study of Infarct Survival (ISIS-4) Collaborative Group. ISIS-4: a randomised factorial trial assessing early oral captopril, oral mononitrate, and intravenous magnesium sulphate in 58 050 patients with suspected acute myocardial infarction. *Lancet* 1995;345:669–685.

41. Gruppo Italiano per lo studio della streptochinasi nell'infarto miocardico (GISSI). GISSI-3: effects of lisinopril and transdermal glyceryl trinitrate singly and together on 6-week mortality and ventricular function after acute myocardial infarction. *Lancet* 1994;343:1115–1122.

42. Opie LH, Yusuf S, Kubler W. Current status of safety and efficacy of calcium channel blockers in cardiovascular disease: a critical analysis based on 100 studies. *Prog Cardiovasc Dis* 2000;43.171–196.

43. Wilcox RG, Hampton JR, Banks DC, et al. Early nifedipine in acute myocardial infarction: the TRENT study. *BMJ* 1986;293:1204–1208.

44. Goldbourt U, Behar S, Reicher-Reiss H, et al. Early administration of nifedipine in suspected acute myocardial infarction: the secondary prevention reinfarction Israel nifedipine trial 2 study. *Arch Intern Med* 1993;153:345–353.

45. Pepine CJ, Faich G, Makuch R, Verapamil use in patients with cardiovascular disease: an overview of randomized trials. *Clin Cardiol* 1998;21:633 641. Search date 1997; primary sources Medline, Science Citation Index, Current Contents, and hand searches of reference lists.

46. Yusuf S, Furberg CD. Effects of calcium channel blockers on survival after myocardial infarction. *Cardiovasc Drugs Ther* 1987;1:343–344. Search dates not stated and primary sources not stated.

47. Teo KK, Yusuf S, Furberg CD. Effects of prophylactic antiarrhythmic drug therapy in acute myocardial infarction: an overview of results from randomized controlled trials. *JAMA* 1993;270:1589 1595. Search date not stated; primary sources Medline and correspondence with investigators and pharmaceutical companies.

48. The Multicenter Diltiazem Post Infarction Trial Research Group. The effect of diltiazem on mortality and reinfarction after myocardial infarction. *N Engl J Med* 1988;319:385–392.

49. Weaver WD, Simes RJ, Betriu A, et al. Comparison of primary coronary angioplasty and intravenous thrombolytic therapy for acute myocardial infarction: a quantitative review. *JAMA* 1997;278:2093–2098. Search date 1996; primary sources Medline and scientific session abstracts of stated journals.

50. Cucherat M, Bonnefoy E, Tremeau G. Primary angioplasty versus intravenous thrombolysis for acute myocardial infarction. In: The Cochrane Library, Issue 1, 2001. Oxford: Update Software. Search date 1998; primary sources The Cochrane Library, Medline, and references from reviews and experts.

51. The GUSTO IIb Angioplasty Substudy Investigators. A clinical trial comparing primary coronary angioplasty with tissue plasminogen activator for acute myocardial infarction. *N Engl J Med* 1997;336:1621–1628.

52. Zijlstra F, Hoorntje JC, de Boer MJ, et al. Long-term benefit of primary angioplasty as compared with thrombolytic therapy for acute myocardial infarction. *N Engl J Med* 1999 341:1413–1419.

53. Yusuf S, Pogue J. Primary angioplasty compared to thrombolytic therapy for acute myocardial infarction [editorial]. *JAMA* 1997;278:2110–2111.

54. Van de Werf F, Topol EJ, Lee KL, et al. Variations in patient management and outcomes for acute myocardial infarction in the United States and other countries: results from the GUSTO trial. *JAMA* 1995;273:1586–1591.

55. Hochman JS, Sleeper LA, White HD et al. One year survival following early revascularization for cardiogenic shock. *JAMA* 2001;285:190–192.

56. GISSI-1. Effectiveness of intravenous thrombolytic treatment in acute myocardial infarction. *Lancet* 1986;1:397–401.

57. Herbert P, Tinker J. Inotropic drugs in acute circulatory failure. *Intensive Care Med* 1980;6:101–111.

58. Hollenberg SM, Kavinsky CJ, Parrillo JE. Cardiogenic shock. *Ann Int Med*

1999;131:47–59. Search date 1998; primary sources Medline and hand searches of bibliographies of relevant papers.

59. Bernard GR, Sopko G, Cerra F, et al. Pulmonary artery catheterization and clinical outcomes. *JAMA* 2000;283:2568–2562.

60. Hollenberg SM, Hoyt J. Pulmonary artery catheters in cardiovascular disease. *New Horiz* 1977;5:207–213. Search date 1996; primary sources not stated.

61. Participants. Pulmonary artery catheter consensus conference: consensus statement. *Crit Care Med* 1997;25:910–925.

62. Ohman EM, Nanas J, Stomel R, et al. Thrombolysis and counterpulsation to improve cardiogenic shock survival (Tactics): results of a prospective randomized trial [abstract]. *Circulation* 2000;102(suppl II):II-600.

63. O'Rourke, MF, Norris RM, Campbell TJ, Chang VP, Sammel NL. Randomized controlled trial of intraaortic balloon counterpulsation in early myocardial infarction with acute heart failure. *Am J Cardiol* 1981;47:815–820.

64. Flaherty JT, Becker LC, Weiss JL, et al. Results of a randomized prospective trial of intraaortic balloon counterpulsation and intravenous nitroglycerin in patients with acute myocardial infarction. *J Am Coll Cardiol* 1985;6:434–446.

65. Frazier OH. Future directions of cardiac assistance. *Semin Thorac Cardiovasc Surg* 2000;12:251–258.

66. Pagani FD, Lynch W, Swaniker F, et al. Extracorporal life support to left ventricular assist device bridge to cardiac transplantation. *Circulation* 1999;100(suppl 19):II206–210.

67. Mavroidis D, Sun BC, Pae WE. Bridge to transplantation: the Penn State experience. *Ann Thorac Surg* 1999;68:684–687.

Nicolas Danchin
Professor of Medicine Université Paris VI
Hôpital Européen Georges Pompidou
Paris
France

Philip Urban
Director, Interventional Cardiology
Hôpital de la Tour
Meyrin-Geneva
Switzerland

Edoardo De Benedetti
Cardiologist
C.H.U.V.
Lausanne
Switzerland

Competing interests: PU has received funds for research and public speaking from a variety of pharmaceutical and device companies, both related and unrelated to products discussed here. EdB and ND none declared.

TABLE 1 Direct randomised comparisons of the standard streptokinase regimen with various tPA based fibrinolytic regimens in patients with suspected AMI in the GISSI-2, ISIS-3, and GUSTO-1 trials (see text, p 15).[18-20]

Trial and treatment	Number of participants randomised	Any stroke Absolute number (%)	Any death Absolute number (%)	Death not related to stroke* Absolute number (%)	Stroke or death Absolute number (%)
GISSI-2†[18]					
Streptokinase	10 396	98 (0.9)	958 (9.2)	916 (8.8)	1014 (9.8)
t-PA	10 372	136 (1.3)	993 (9.6)	931 (9.0)	1067 (10.3)
Effect/1000 people treated with t-PA instead of streptokinase		3.7 ± 1.5 more	3.6 ± 4.0 more	1.7 ± 4.0 more	5.3 ± 4.2 more
ISIS-3‡[19]					
Streptokinase	13 780	141 (1.0)	1455 (10.6)	1389 (10.1)	1530 (11.1)
t-PA	13 746	188 (1.4)	1418 (10.3)	1325 (9.6)	1513 (11.0)
Effect/1000 people treated with t-PA instead of streptokinase		3.5 ± 1.3 more	2.4 ± 3.7 fewer	4.4 ± 3.6 fewer	1.0 ± 3.8 fewer
GUSTO-1§[20]					
Streptokinase (sc heparin)	9841	117 (1.2)	712 (7.3)	666 (6.8)	783 (8.0)
Streptokinase (iv heparin)	10 410	144 (1.4)	763 (7.4)	709 (6.8)	853 (8.2)
t-PA alone	10 396	161 (1.6)	653 (6.3)	585 (5.6)	746 (7.2)
t-PA plus streptokinase	10 374	170 (1.6)	723 (7.0)	647 (6.2)	817 (7.9)
Effect/1000 people treated with t-PA-based regimens instead of streptinokinase		3.0 ± 1.2 more	6.6 ± 2.5 fewer	8.6 ± 2.4 fewer	5.5 ± 2.6 fewer

TABLE 1 continued

χ²/2 heterogeneity of effects between 3 trials	0.7	5.6	7.0	5.4
P value	0.3	0.06	0.03	0.07
Weighted average of all 3 trials¶				
Effect/1000 patient treated with t-PA-based regimens instead of streptokinase	3.3 ± 0.8 more	2.9 ± 1.9 fewer	4.9 ± 1.8 fewer	1.6 ± 1.9 fewer
P value	< 0.001	> 0.1	< 0.01	0.4

Values are numbers (%). This table should not be used to make direct non-randomised comparisons between the absolute event rates in different trials, because the patient populations may have differed substantially in age and other characteristics. Deaths recorded throughout the first 35 days are included for GISSI-2 and ISIS-3 and throughout the first 30 days for GUSTO-1. Numbers randomised and numbers with follow up are from the ISIS-3 report[19] and GUSTO-1[20] (supplemented with revised GUSTO-1 data from the National Auxiliary Publications Service), and numbers with events and the percentages (based on participants with follow up) are from the ISIS-3 report[19] and Van de Werf, et al.[54] Plus-minus values are ± standard deviation. In all three trials, streptokinase was given in intravenous infusions of 1.5 MU over a period of 1 hour. AMI, acute myocardial infarction; iv, intravenous; t-PA, tissue plasminogen activator; sc, subcutaneous.

*Death not related to stroke was defined as death without recorded stroke.

†In the GISSI-2 trial, the t-PA regimen involved an initial bolus of 10 mg, followed by 50 mg in the first hour and 20 mg in each of the second and third hours.

‡In the ISIS-3 trial, the t-PA regimen involved 40 000 clot-lysis units/kg of body weight as an initial bolus, followed by 360 000 units/kg in the first hour and 67 000 units/kg in each of the next 3 hours.

§In the GUSTO-1 trial, the t-PA alone regimen involved an initial bolus of 15 mg, followed by 0.75 mg/kg (up to 50 mg) in the first 30 minutes and 0.5 mg/kg (up to 35 mg) in the next hour; in the GUSTO-1 trial the other t-PA based regimen involved 0.1 mg of t-PA/kg (up to 9 mg) as an initial bolus and 0.9 mg/kg (up to 81 mg) in the remainder of the first hour, plus 1 MU of streptokinase in the first hour.

¶The weights are proportional to the sample sizes of the trials, so this average gives most weight to the GUSTO-1 trial and least to the GISSI-2 trials.[17]

TABLE 2 Comparison of early invasive cardiac revascularisation versus initial medical treatment on mortality at 30 days, 6 months, and 12 months (see text, p 24).[2,3,55]

Time after AMI	Mortality in early invasive cardiac revascularisation group Number dead/total number (%)	Mortality in medical treatment alone group Number dead/total number (%)	ARR (95% CI)	RR (95% CI)	NNT (95% CI)
SHOCK study[2,55]					
30 days	71/152 (47)	84/150 (56)	9.3% (−2 to +20.2)	0.83 (0.67 to 1.04)	NA
6 months	76/152 (50)	94/150 (63)	12.7% (1.5 to 23.4)	0.80 (0.65 to 0.93)	8 (5 to 68)
12 months	81/152 (53)	99/150 (66)	12.7% (1.6 to 23.3)	0.80 (0.67 to 0.97)	8 (5 to 61)
SMASH study[3]					
30 days	22/32 (69)	18/23 (78)	9.5% (−14.6 to +30.6)	0.88 (0.64 to 1.2)	NA
12 months	23/32 (74)	19/23 (83)	10.7% (−12.7 to +30.9)	0.87 (0.65 to 1.16)	NA

AMI, acute myocardial infarction; NA, not applicable.

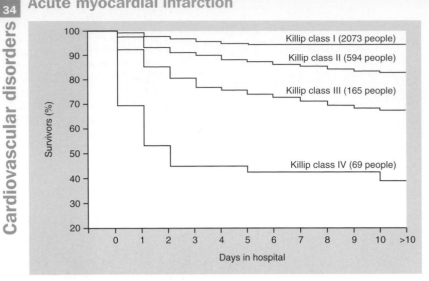

FIGURE 1 The AMIS registry Kaplan–Meier survival curves as a function of Killip class at hospital admission for 3138 people admitted in 50 Swiss hospitals between 1977 and 1998. Published with permission (see text, p 14).[9]

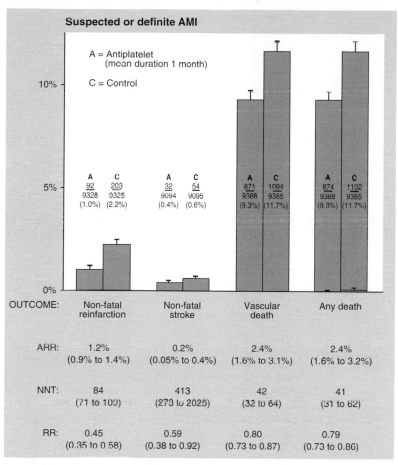

OUTCOME:	Non-fatal reinfarction	Non-fatal stroke	Vascular death	Any death
	A: 92 / 9328 (1.0%) C: 203 / 9325 (2.2%)	A: 32 / 9094 (0.4%) C: 54 / 9095 (0.6%)	A: 871 / 9388 (9.3%) C: 1094 / 9385 (11.7%)	A: 874 / 9388 (9.3%) C: 1102 / 9385 (11.7%)
ARR:	1.2% (0.9% to 1.4%)	0.2% (0.05% to 0.4%)	2.4% (1.6% to 3.1%)	2.4% (1.6% to 3.2%)
NNT:	84 (71 to 109)	413 (273 to 2025)	42 (32 to 64)	41 (31 to 62)
RR:	0.45 (0.35 to 0.58)	0.59 (0.38 to 0.92)	0.80 (0.73 to 0.87)	0.79 (0.73 to 0.86)

A = Antiplatelet (mean duration 1 month)

C = Control

FIGURE 2 Absolute effects of antiplatelet treatment on various outcomes in people with a prior suspected or definite acute myocardial infarction (AMI).[11] The columns show the absolute risks over 1 month for each category; the error bars are the upper 95% confidence interval. In "any death" column, non-vascular deaths are represented by lower horizontal lines. The table displays for each outcome the absolute risk reduction (ARR), the number of people needing treatment for 1 month to avoid one additional event (NNT), and the relative risk reduction (RRR), with their 95% CIs (see text, p 14). Published with permission.[11]

Cardiovascular disorders

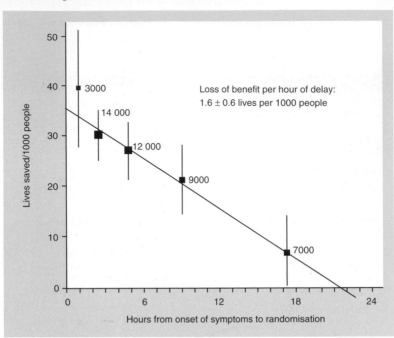

Search date February 2002

Kate Ackerman and David Creery

INTERVENTIONS

*Although we found no direct
evidence to support their use,
widespread consensus holds that
these interventions should be
universally applied to children
who have arrested on the basis
of indirect evidence and
extrapolation from adult data.
Placebo controlled trials would
be considered unethical.

See glossary, p 43

Key Messages

- **Bystander cardiopulmonary resuscitation** It is widely accepted that cardiopulmonary resuscitation should be undertaken in children who have arrested.
  Placebo controlled trials would be considered unethical. One systematic review
  of observational studies has found that children who received bystander
  cardiopulmonary resuscitation versus no bystander cardiopulmonary resuscitation were more likely to survive to hospital discharge.

- **Intubation versus bag-mask ventilation** One controlled clinical trial, in
  children requiring airway management in the community, found no significant
  difference with endotracheal intubation versus bag-mask ventilation in survival
  or neurological outcome.

- **Airway management and ventilation; direct current cardiac shock;
  standard dose intravenous adrenaline (epinephrine)** Although we found
  no direct evidence to support their use, widespread consensus based on
  indirect evidence and extrapolation from adult data holds that these interventions should be universally applied to children who have arrested. Placebo
  controlled trials would be considered unethical.

- **High dose intravenous adrenaline (epinephrine); intravenous bicarbonate; intravenous calcium; training parents to perform cardiopulmonary
  resuscitation** We found no RCTs or prospective cohort studies on the effects
  of these interventions in children who have arrested in the community.

Cardiorespiratory arrest in children

DEFINITION Non-submersion out of hospital cardiorespiratory arrest in children is a state of pulselessness and apnoea occurring outside of a medical facility and not caused by submersion in water.[1]

INCIDENCE/ PREVALENCE We found 12 studies (3 prospective, 9 retrospective) reporting the incidence of non-submersion out of hospital cardiorespiratory arrest in children (see table 1, p 44).[2–13] Eleven studies reported the incidence in both adults and children, and eight reported the incidence in children.[2–9,11-13] Incidence of arrests in the general population ranged from 2.2–5.7/100 000 people a year (mean 3.1, 95% CI 2.1 to 4.1). Incidence of arrests in children ranged from 6.9–18.0/100 000 children a year (mean 10.6, 95% CI 7.1 to 14.1).[8] One prospective study (300 children) found that about 50% of out of hospital cardiorespiratory arrests occurred in children under 12 months, and about two thirds occurred in children under 18 months.[11]

AETIOLOGY/ RISK FACTORS We found 26 studies reporting the causes of non-submersion pulseless arrests (see glossary, p 43) in a total of 1574 children. The commonest causes of arrest were undetermined causes as in sudden infant death syndrome (see glossary, p 43) (39%), trauma (18%), chronic disease (7%), and pneumonia (4%) (see table 2, p 45).[1,3-12,14-28]

PROGNOSIS We found no systematic review that investigated non-submersion arrests alone. We found 27 studies (5 prospective, 22 retrospective; total of 1754 children) that reported only on out of hospital arrest.[1–12,14-28] The overall survival rate following out of hospital arrest was 5% (87 children). Nineteen of these studies (1140 children) found that of the 48 surviving children, 12 (25%) had no or mild neurological disability and 36 (75%) had moderate or severe neurological disability. We found one systematic review (search date 1997), which reported outcomes after cardiopulmonary resuscitation for both in hospital and out of hospital arrests of any cause, including submersion in children.[29] Studies were excluded if they did not report survival. The review found evidence from prospective and retrospective observational studies that out of hospital arrest of any cause in children carries a poorer prognosis than arrest within hospital (132/1568 children [8%] survived to hospital discharge after out of hospital arrest v 129/544 children [24%] after in hospital arrests). About half of the survivors were involved in studies that reported neurological outcome. Of these, survival with "good neurological outcome" (i.e. normal or mild neurological deficit) was higher in children who arrested in hospital compared with those who arrested elsewhere (60/77 surviving children [78%] in hospital v 28/68 [41%] elsewhere).[29]

AIMS To improve survival and minimise neurological sequelae in children suffering non-submersion out of hospital cardiorespiratory arrest.

OUTCOMES Out of hospital death rate; rate of death in hospital without return of spontaneous circulation; return of spontaneous circulation with subsequent death in hospital; and return of spontaneous circulation with successful hospital discharge with mild, moderate, severe, or no neurological sequelae; adverse effects of treatment.

METHODS   Clinical Evidence search and appraisal February 2002. In addition, we searched citation lists of retrieved articles and relevant review articles. Studies reporting out of hospital arrest in adults that listed "adolescent" as a MeSH heading were also reviewed. Both authors reviewed the retrieved studies independently and differences were resolved by discussion. We selected studies reporting out of hospital cardiorespiratory arrests in children. Studies were excluded if data relating to submersion could not be differentiated from non-submersion data (except where we found no data relating exclusively to non-submersion arrest; in such cases we have included studies that did not differentiate these types of arrest, and have made it clear that such evidence is limited by this fact). Some features of cardiorespiratory arrest in adults appear to be different from arrest in children, so studies were excluded if data for adults could not be differentiated from data for children.

| QUESTION | What are the effects of treatments for non-submersion out of hospital cardiorespiratory arrest? |

| OPTION | AIRWAY MANAGEMENT AND VENTILATION |

It is widely accepted that good airway management and rapid ventilation should be undertaken in a child who has arrested, and it would be considered unethical to test its role in a placebo controlled trial.

Benefits: We found no studies comparing airway management and ventilation versus no intervention.

Harms: We found insufficient information.

Comment: It would be considered unethical to test the role of airway management and ventilation in a placebo controlled trial.

| OPTION | INTUBATION VERSUS BAG-MASK VENTILATION |

One controlled trial found no evidence of a difference in survival or neurological outcome between bag-mask ventilation and endotracheal intubation in children requiring airway management in the community.

Benefits: We found no systematic review. We found one high quality controlled trial (830 children requiring airway management in the community, including 98 children who had arrested after submersion) comparing (using alternate day allocation) bag-mask ventilation versus endotracheal intubation (given by paramedic staff trained in these techniques).[30] Treatments were not randomised; each was allocated on alternate days. Analysis was by intention to treat (see comment below). The trial found no significant difference in rates of survival or good neurological outcome (normal, mild deficit, or no change from baseline function) between the two treatment groups (105/349 [30%] survived after bag-mask ventilation v 90/373 [24%] after intubation; OR 1.36, 95% CI 0.97 to 1.89; good neurological outcome achieved in 80/349 [23%] of children after bag-mask ventilation v 70/373 [19%] after intubation; OR 1.27, 95% CI 0.89 to 1.83; OR for non-submersion cardiorespiratory arrest calculated by author).

Harms: The trial found that time spent at the scene of the arrest was longer when intubation was intended, and this was the only significant determinant of a longer total time from dispatch of paramedic team to arrival at hospital (mean time at scene 9 min with bag-mask v 11 min with intubation; P < 0.001; mean total time 20 min with bag-mask v 23 min with intubation; P < 0.001).[30] However, the trial found no significant difference between bag-mask ventilation and intubation for complications common to both treatments (complications in 727 children for whom data were available, bag-mask v intubation: gastric distension 31% v 7%; P = 0.20; vomiting 14% v 14%; P = 0.82; aspiration 14% v 15%; P = 0.84; oral or airway trauma 1% v 2%; P = 0.24). A total of 186 children across both treatment groups were thought by paramedical staff to be successfully intubated. Of these, oesophageal intubation occurred in three children (2%); the tube became dislodged in 27 children (14%; unrecognised in 12 children, recognised in 15); right main bronchus intubation occurred in 33 children (18%); and an incorrect size of tube was used in 44 children (24%). Death occurred in all but one of the children with oesophageal intubation or unrecognised dislodging of the tube.[30]

Comment: **Population characteristics:** The baseline characteristics of children did not differ significantly between groups in age, sex, ethnicity, or cause of arrest. The trial did not report the frequency of pulseless arrest (see glossary, p 43) versus respiratory arrest (see glossary, p 43). **Intention to treat:** Intubation and bag-mask ventilation are not mutually exclusive. The study protocol allowed bag-mask ventilation before intubation and after unsuccessful intubation. Of 420 children allocated to intubation, 115 received bag-mask ventilation before intubation, 128 received bag-mask ventilation after attempted intubation, four were lost to follow up, and the remainder received intubation that was believed to be successful. Of 410 children allocated to bag-mask ventilation, 10 children were intubated successfully (although in violation of study protocol), nine received bag-mask ventilation after attempted intubation, six were lost to follow up, and the remainder received bag-mask ventilation in accordance with study protocol.[30]

| OPTION | INTRAVENOUS ADRENALINE (EPINEPHRINE) |

Intravenous adrenaline (epinephrine) at "standard dose" (0.01 mg/kg) is a widely accepted treatment for establishing return of spontaneous circulation. We found no prospective evidence comparing adrenaline (epinephrine) versus placebo, or comparing standard or single doses versus high or multiple doses of adrenaline (epinephrine), in children who have arrested in the community.

Benefits: We found no systematic review, no RCTs, and no prospective observational studies.

Harms: We found no prospective data in this context.

Comment: **Versus placebo:** Standard dose adrenaline (epinephrine) is a widely accepted treatment for arrests in children. Placebo controlled trials would be considered unethical. **High versus low dose:** Two small retrospective studies (128 people) found no evidence of a difference in survival to hospital discharge between low or single dose and high or multiple dose adrenaline (epinephrine), although the studies were too small to rule out an effect.[8,12]

OPTION   INTRAVENOUS BICARBONATE

We found no RCTs on the effects of intravenous bicarbonate in out of hospital cardiorespiratory arrest in children.

Benefits: We found no RCTs.

Harms: We found insufficient evidence.

Comment: Bicarbonate is widely believed to be effective in arrest associated with hyperkalaemic ventricular tachycardia or fibrillation, but we found no prospective evidence supporting this.

OPTION   INTRAVENOUS CALCIUM

We found no RCTs on the effects of intravenous calcium in out of hospital cardiorespiratory arrest in children.

Benefits: We found no RCTs.

Harms: We found insufficient evidence.

Comment: Calcium is widely believed to be effective in arrest associated with hyperkalaemic ventricular tachycardia or fibrillation, but we found no prospective evidence supporting this.

OPTION   BYSTANDER CARDIOPULMONARY RESUSCITATION

It is widely accepted that cardiopulmonary resuscitation and ventilation should be undertaken in children who have arrested. Placebo controlled trials would be considered unethical. We found no RCTs on the effects of training parents to perform cardiopulmonary resuscitation. One systematic review of observational studies has found that children who were witnessed having an arrest and who received bystander cardiopulmonary resuscitation were more likely to survive to hospital discharge.

Benefits: We found no RCTs. We found one systematic review (search date 1997) of prospective and retrospective studies.[29] This concluded that survival was improved in children who were witnessed to arrest and received cardiopulmonary resuscitation from a bystander. Of 150 witnessed arrests outside hospital, 28/150 (19%) survived to hospital discharge. Of those children who received bystander cardiopulmonary resuscitation, 20/76 (26%) survived to discharge.[29] The review did not report survival rates in children whose arrests were not witnessed, but the overall survival rate for out of hospital cardiac arrest was 8%. **Training parents to perform cardiopulmonary resuscitation:** We found no systematic review and no RCTs examining the effects of training parents to perform cardiopulmonary resuscitation in children who have arrested outside hospital.

Harms: Potential harms include those resulting from unnecessary chest compression after respiratory arrest with intact circulation.

Comment: The review of observational studies found that children who received bystander cardiopulmonary resuscitation had a hospital discharge rate of 20/76 (26%) versus 8/74 (11%) for children who also had their arrests witnessed but had not received cardiopulmonary resuscitation. Cardiopulmonary resuscitation was not randomly allocated and children resuscitated may be systematically different from those who did not receive resuscitation. The apparent survival rates for witnessed arrests and arrests with bystander initiated cardiopulmonary resuscitation may be artificially high because of inappropriate evaluation of true arrest. However, assuming confounding variables were evenly distributed between groups, then the best estimate of the benefit of cardiopulmonary resuscitation is a 15% absolute increase in the probability that children will be discharged alive from hospital.

OPTION   DIRECT CURRENT CARDIAC SHOCK

It is widely accepted that children who arrest outside hospital and are found to have ventricular fibrillation or pulseless ventricular tachycardia should receive direct current cardiac shock treatment. Placebo controlled trials would be considered unethical. We found no RCTs on the effects of direct current cardiac shock in children who have arrested in the community, regardless of the heart rhythm.

Benefits: We found no systematic review and no RCTs.

Harms: We found insufficient evidence.

Comment: **In children with ventricular fibrillation:** One retrospective study (29 children with ventricular fibrillation who had arrested out of hospital from a variety of causes, including submersion) found that of 27 children who were defibrillated, 11 survived (5 with no sequelae, 6 with severe disability). The five children with good outcome all received defibrillation within 10 minutes of arrest (time to defibrillation not given for those who died). Data on the two children who were not defibrillated were not presented.[31] **In children with asystole:** One retrospective study in 90 children with asystole (see glossary, p 43) (including those who had arrested after submersion) found that 49 (54%) had received direct current cardiac shock treatment. None of the children survived to hospital discharge, regardless of whether or not direct current cardiac shock was given.[32] We found one systematic review (search date 1997) of observational studies (1420 children who had arrested outside hospital) that recorded electrocardiogram rhythm.[29] Bradyasystole or pulseless electrical activity (see glossary, p 43) were found in 73%, whereas ventricular fibrillation or pulseless ventricular tachycardia (see glossary, p 43) were found in 10%.[29] The review found that survival after ventricular fibrillation or ventricular tachycardia arrest was higher than after asystolic arrest in children. Survival to discharge reported in the systematic review was 39/802 (5%) for children with initial rhythm asystole (see glossary, p 43) and 30% (29/97) with initial rhythm ventricular fibrillation (see glossary, p 43) or ventricular tachycardia.[29]

GLOSSARY

Asystole The absence of cardiac electrical activity
Bradyasystole Bradycardia clinically indistinguishable from asystole
Initial rhythm asystole The absence of cardiac electrical activity at initial determination
Initial rhythm ventricular fibrillation Electrical rhythm is ventricular fibrillation at initial determination
Pulseless arrest Absence of palpable pulse
Pulseless electrical activity The presence of cardiac electrical activity in absence of a palpable pulse
Pulseless ventricular tachycardia Electrical rhythm of ventricular tachycardia in absence of a palpable pulse
Respiratory arrest Absence of respiratory activity
Sudden infant death syndrome The sudden unexpected death of a child, usually between the ages of 1 month and 1 year, for which a thorough postmortem examination does not define an adequate cause of death. Near miss sudden infant death syndrome refers to survival of a child after an unexpected arrest of unknown cause

REFERENCES

1. Schindler MB, Bohn D, Cox PN, et al. Outcome of out of hospital cardiac or respiratory arrest in children. *N Engl J Med* 1996;335:1473–1479.

2. Broides A, Sofer S, Press J. Outcome of out of hospital cardiopulmonary arrest in children admitted to the emergency room. *Isr Med Assoc J* 2000;2:672–674.

3. Eisenberg M, Bergner L, Hallstrom A. Epidemiology of cardiac arrest and resuscitation in children. *Ann Emerg Med* 1983;12:672–674.

4. Applebaum D, Slater PE. Should the Mobile Intensive Care Unit respond to pediatric emergencies? *Clin Pediatr (Phila)* 1986;25:620–623.

5. Tsai A, Kallsen G. Epidemiology of pediatric prehospital care. *Ann Emerg Med* 1987;16:284–292.

6. Thompson JE, Bonner B, Lower GM. Pediatric cardiopulmonary arrests in rural populations. *Pediatrics* 1990;86:302–306.

7. Safranek DJ, Eisenberg MS, Larsen MP. The epidemiology of cardiac arrest in young adults. *Ann Emerg Med* 1992;21:1102–1106.

8. Dieckmann RA, Vardis R. High-dose epinephrine in pediatric out of hospital cardiopulmonary arrest. *Pediatrics* 1995;95:901–913.

9. Kuisma M, Suominen P, Korpela R. Paediatric out of hospital cardiac arrests — epidemiology and outcome. *Resuscitation* 1995;30:141–150.

10. Ronco R, King W, Donley DK, Tilden SJ. Outcome and cost at a children's hospital following resuscitation for out of hospital cardiopulmonary arrest. *Arch Pediatr Adolesc Med* 1995;149:210–214.

11. Sirbaugh PE, Pepe PE, Shook JE, et al. A prospective, population-based study of the demographics, epidemiology, management, and outcome of out of hospital pediatric cardiopulmonary arrest. *Ann Emerg Med* 1999;33:174–184.

12. Friesen RM, Duncan P, Tweed WA, Bristow G. Appraisal of pediatric cardiopulmonary resuscitation. *Can Med Assoc J* 1982;126:1055–1058.

13. Hu OO. Out of hospital cardiac arrest in an Oriental metropolitan city. *Am J Emerg Med* 1994;12:491–494.

14. Barzilay Z, Somekh E, Sagy M, Boichis H. Pediatric cardiopulmonary resuscitation outcome. *J Med* 1988;19:229–241.

15. Bhende MS, Thompson AE. Evaluation of an end-tidal CO_2 detector during pediatric cardiopulmonary resuscitation. *Pediatrics* 1995;95:395–399.

16. Brunette DD, Fischer R. Intravascular access in pediatric cardiac arrest. *Am J Emerg Med* 1988;6:577–579.

17. Clinton JE, McGill J, Irwin G, Peterson G, Lilja GP, Ruiz E. Cardiac arrest under age 40: etiology and prognosis. *Ann Emerg Med* 1984;13:1011–1015.

18. Hazinski MF, Chahine AA, Holcomb GW, Morris JA. Outcome of cardiovascular collapse in pediatric blunt trauma. *Ann Emerg Med* 1994;23:1229–1235.

19. Losek JD, Hennes H, Glaeser P, Hendley G, Nelson DB. Prehospital care of the pulseless, nonbreathing pediatric patient. *Am J Emerg Med* 1987;5:370–374.

20. Ludwig S, Kettrick RG, Parker M. Pediatric cardiopulmonary resuscitation. A review of 130 cases. *Clin Pediatr (Phila)* 1984;23:71–75.

21. Nichols DG, Kettrick RG, Swedlow DB, Lee S, Passman R, Ludwig S. Factors influencing outcome of cardiopulmonary resuscitation in children. *Pediatr Emerg Care* 1986;2:1–5.

Cardiorespiratory arrest in children

22. O'Rourke PP. Outcome of children who are apneic and pulseless in the emergency room. *Crit Care Med* 1986;14:466–468.

23. Rosenberg NM. Pediatric cardiopulmonary arrest in the emergency department. *Am J Emerg Med* 1984;2:497–499.

24. Sheikh A, Brogan T. Outcome and cost of open- and closed-chest cardiopulmonary resuscitation in pediatric cardiac arrests. *Pediatrics* 1994;93:392–398.

25. Suominen P, Rasanen J, Kivioja A. Efficacy of cardiopulmonary resuscitation in pulseless paediatric trauma patients. *Resuscitation* 1998;36:9–13.

26. Suominen P, Korpela R, Kuisma M, Silfvast T, Olkkola KT. Paediatric cardiac arrest and resuscitation provided by physician-staffed emergency care units. *Acta Anaesthesiol Scand* 1997;41:260–265.

27. Torphy DE, Minter MG, Thompson BM. Cardiorespiratory arrest and resuscitation of children. *Am J Dis Child* 1984;138:1099–1102.

28. Walsh R. Outcome of pre-hospital CPR in the pediatric trauma patient [abstract]. *Crit Care Med* 1994;22:A162.

29. Young KD, Seidel JS. Pediatric cardiopulmonary resuscitation: a collective review. *Ann Emerg Med* 1999;33:195–205. Search date 1997; primary sources Medline and bibliographic search.

30. Gausche M, Lewis RJ, Stratton SJ, et al. Effect of out of hospital pediatric endotracheal intubation on survival and neurological outcome. *JAMA* 2000;283:783–790.

31. Mogayzel C, Quan L, Graves JR, Tiedeman D, Fahrenbruch C, Herndon P. Out of hospital ventricular fibrillation in children and adolescents: causes and outcomes. *Ann Emerg Med* 1995;25:484–491.

32. Losek JD, Hennes H, Glaeser PW, Smith DS, Hendley G. Prehospital countershock treatment of pediatric asystole. *Am J Emerg Med* 1989;7:571–575.

Kate Ackerman
The Children's Hospital
Boston
USA

David Creery
Children's Hospital of Eastern Ontario
Ottawa
Canada

Competing interests: None declared.

| TABLE 1 | Incidence of non-submersion out of hospital cardiorespiratory arrest in children* (see text, p 38). |

Reference	Location	Year	Incidence per 100 000 people in total population	Incidence per 100 000 children
12	Manitoba, Canada	1982	2.9	ND
3	King County, USA	1983	2.4	9.9
4	Jerusalem, Israel	1986	2.5	6.9
5	Fresno, USA	1987	5.7	ND
6	Midwestern USA	1990	4.7	ND
7	King County, USA	1992	2.4	10.1
13	Taipei, Taiwan	1994	1.3	ND
8	San Francisco, USA	1995	2.2	16.1
9	Helsinki, Finland	1995	1.4	9.1
10	Birmingham, USA	1995	ND	6.9
11	Houston, USA	1999	4.9	18.0
2	Southern Israel	2000	3.5	7.8

* Incidence represents arrests per 100 000 population per year. ND, no data.

| TABLE 2 | Causes of non-submersion out of hospital cardiorespiratory arrest in children* (see text, p 38). |

Cause	Number of arrests (%)	Number of survivors (%)
Undetermined	691 (43.9)	1 (0.1)
Trauma	311 (19.8)	10 (3.2)
Chronic disease	126 (8.0)	9 (7.1)
Pneumonia	75 (4.8)	6 (8.0)
Non-accidental injury	23 (1.5)	2 (8.7)
Aspiration	20 (1.3)	0 (0)
Overdose	19 (1.2)	3 (15.8)
Other	309 (19.6)	28 (9.1)
Total	**1574 (100)**	**59 (3.7)**

*Figures represent the numbers of arrests/survivors in children with each diagnosis.

Cardiovascular disease in diabetes

Search date April 2002

Janine Malcolm, Hilary Meggison, and Ronald Sigal

Key Messages

■ **Angiotensin converting enzyme (ACE) inhibitor versus β blockers (as initial treatment in hypertension)** One RCT found that an ACE inhibitor captopril versus β blockers or diuretic significantly reduced myocardial infarction, stroke, or death (NNT 15, 95% CI 8 to 105). One large RCT found no significant difference with the ACE inhibitor captopril versus the β blocker atenolol in the number of cardiovascular events over about 8 years.

- **ACE inhibitor versus calcium channel blocker (as initial treatment in hypertension)** One systematic review in people with type 2 diabetes has found that ACE inhibitors versus calcium channel blockers as initial treatment for hypertension significantly reduce cardiovascular events (NNT 13, 95% CI 7 to 25).

- **Angiotensin II receptor antagonist versus β blocker** Subgroup analysis of one RCT in people with diabetes and left ventricular hypertrophy found that after 4 years, losartan versus atenolol significantly reduced primary cardiovascular composite outcomes (cardiovascular mortality, stroke, myocardial infarction) (NNT 19, 95% CI 11 to 142)

- **Antihypertensive treatment** One RCT in people with diabetes and high blood pressure (BP 165–220/ < 95 mm Hg) found that hypertensive treatment (nitrendipine or enalapril with or without hydrochlorothiazide) versus placebo significantly reduced all cardiovascular events over a median of 2 years (NNT 13, 95% CI 10 to 31) but found no significant reduction in overall mortality. One RCT in people aged 55–80 years with diabetic nephropathy and hypertension found no significant difference with amlodipine versus placebo and with irbesartan versus placebo or amlodipine in cardiovascular composite end points (non-fatal myocardial infarction, heart failure). One RCT in people with diabetes, hypertension, and microalbuminuria found no significant reduction in non-fatal cardiovascular events with irbesartan versus placebo. One systematic review in people aged over 50 years has found that blood pressure lowering in people with diabetes significantly reduces mortality and stroke but had no significant effect on myocardial infarction. One RCT in people with diabetes aged over 55 years with additional cardiac risk factors, previously diagnosed coronary vascular disease, or both, has found that the ACE inhibitor ramipril versus placebo significantly reduces major cardiovascular events (NNT 22, 95% CI 14 to 43) and overall mortality (NNT 32, 95% CI 19 to 98) within 4.5 years. One RCT in people with diabetes and baseline blood pressure less than 140/90 mm Hg found that intensive (target diastolic BP 10 mm Hg below baseline) versus moderate (diastolic BP 80–89 mm Hg) blood pressure lowering significantly reduces cerebral vascular accidents (NNT 27, 95% CI 14 to 255) but found no significant difference for cardiovascular death, myocardial infarction, congestive heart failure, or all cause mortality.

- **Antiplatelet treatment** One RCT in men aged 40–80 years with diabetes has found that aspirin versus placebo significantly reduces the risk of first acute myocardial infarction within 5 years (NNT 16, 95% CI 12 to 47). Another RCT in people with diabetes and prior cardiovascular disease found no significant difference with aspirin versus placebo in the risk of acute myocardial infarction or overall mortality within 5 years. Subgroup analysis in one RCT of people presenting with unstable angina or acute myocardial infarction without ST elevation found that the addition of a glycoprotein IIb/IIIa inhibitor (tirofiban) to heparin significantly reduced the risk of death or myocardial infarction at 180 days (NNT 13, 95% CI 7 to 146). One systematic review has found that aspirin versus placebo significantly reduces the risk of morbidity and death from cardiovascular disease within 2 years (NNT 26, 95% CI 17 to 66) in people with diabetes and other risk factors for a cardiovascular event.

- **Blood glucose control** RCTs found that glucose lowering with insulin, sulphonylureas, or metformin may reduce the risk of first acute myocardial infarction. One large RCT in people with acute myocardial infarction found that intensive insulin treatment versus standard treatment significantly reduced mortality at 3.4 years.

Cardiovascular disease in diabetes

- **Coronary artery bypass graft (CABG) versus percutaneous transluminal coronary angioplasty (PTCA)** One large RCT in people with diabetes and multivessel coronary artery disease has found that CABG versus PTCA significantly reduces mortality or myocardial infarction within 8 years (NNT 7, 95% CI 4 to 20). Another RCT found a non-significant reduction in mortality with CABG versus PTCA at 4 years. A third RCT in people with diabetes and multivessel coronary artery disease found no significant difference between CABG and PTCA with stent in short term outcome (to time of discharge) but at 1 year after the procedure there was significantly greater cumulative incidence of combined death, myocardial infarction, or repeat CABG or PTCA.

- **Lipid regulating agents (statins and fibrates)** One systematic review found that in people with diabetes, lovastatin or gemfibrozil versus placebo did not significantly reduce non-fatal myocardial infarction and death from coronary artery disease. One RCT in people aged 35–65 years with type 2 diabetes and hyperlipidaemia found that bezafibrate versus placebo significantly reduced myocardial infarction or new ischaemic changes on electrocardiogram within 3 years (NNT 6, 95% CI 5 to 20). Another RCT in people with diabetes aged 40–80 years found a significant decrease in all cause mortalilty, non-fatal myocardial infarction, coronary heart disease death, total stroke, or any revascularisation with simvastatin versus placebo. It found significant risk reduction in people with diabetes and previous coronary heart disease (NNT 23, 95% CI 12 to 897) and in people with diabetes and no prior coronary heart disease (NNT 21, 95% CI 14 to 40). Three RCTs identified by a systematic review found that statins versus placebo significantly decreased cardiovascular event rates (person years needed to treat 120, 95% CI 61 to 4856). One RCT including people with diabetes found a borderline significant difference in relative risk of coronary heart disease death or non-fatal acute myocardial infarction with gemfibrozil versus placebo. One RCT found that in people with type 2 diabetes, dyslipidaemia and at least one coronary lesion, fenofibrate versus placebo did not significantly reduce myocardial infarction or death. One RCT found that in people aged 21–74 years with diabetes who had previously undergone coronary artery bypass grafting, aggressive versus moderate lipid lowering did not significantly reduce the four year life event rate relative risk for myocardial infarction or death.

- **Lower target blood pressures** Large RCTs including people with diabetes and hypertension have found that tighter control of blood pressure with target diastolic blood pressures of less than or equal to 80 mm Hg reduces the risk of major cardiovascular events.

- **PTCA versus thrombolysis** One RCT in people with diabetes and prior acute myocardial infarction found that at 30 days there was a lower rate of composite endpoint (death, reinfarction or disabling stroke) but the difference was not significant.

- **Screening for high cardiovascular risk** We found no RCTs on screening people with diabetes for cardiovascular risk.

- **Smoking cessation** We found no RCTs on promotion of smoking cessation. Observational evidence and extrapolation from people without diabetes suggest that promotion of smoking cessation is likely to reduce cardiovascular events.

- **Stent plus glycoprotein IIb/IIIa inhibitors in people undergoing PTCA** RCTs in people with diabetes undergoing PTCA have found that the combination of stent and a glycoprotein IIb/IIIa inhibitor (abciximab) significantly reduces restenosis rates and serious morbidity.

DEFINITION **Diabetes mellitus:** See definition under glycaemic control in diabetes, p 97. **Cardiovascular disease:** Atherosclerotic disease of the heart and/or the coronary, cerebral, or peripheral vessels leading to clinical events such as acute myocardial infarction (see glossary, p 66), congestive heart failure, sudden cardiac death, stroke, gangrene, and/or need for revascularisation procedures.

INCIDENCE/ Diabetes mellitus is a major risk factor for cardiovascular disease. In
PREVALENCE the USA, 60–75% of people with diabetes die from cardiovascular causes.[1] The annual incidence of cardiovascular disease is increased in people with diabetes (men: RR 2–3; women: RR 3–4, adjusted for age and other cardiovascular risk factors).[2] About 45% of middle aged and older white people with diabetes have evidence of coronary artery disease compared with about 25% of people without diabetes in the same populations.[2] In a Finnish population based cohort study (1059 people with diabetes and 1373 people without diabetes, aged 45–64 years), the 7 year risk of acute myocardial infarction was as high in adults with diabetes without previous cardiac disease (20.2/100 person years) as it was in people without diabetes with previous cardiac disease (18.8/100 person years).[3]

AETIOLOGY/ Diabetes mellitus increases the risk of cardiovascular disease.
RISK FACTORS Cardiovascular risk factors in people with diabetes include conventional risk factors (age, prior cardiovascular disease, cigarette smoking, hypertension, dyslipidaemia, sedentary lifestyle, family history of premature cardiovascular disease) and more diabetes specific risk factors (elevated urinary protein excretion, poor glycaemic control). Conventional risk factors for cardiovascular disease contribute to increasing the relative risk of cardiovascular disease in people with diabetes to about the same extent as in those without diabetes (see aetiology under primary prevention, p 155). One prospective cohort study (164 women and 235 men with diabetes, mean age 65 years; 437 women and 1099 men without diabetes, mean age 61 years followed for mortality for a mean 3.7 years following acute myocardial infarction) found that more people with diabetes died compared with people without diabetes (116/399 [29%] v 204/1536 [13%]; RR 2.2, 95% CI 1.8 to 2.7).[4] It also found that the mortality risk after myocardial infarction associated with diabetes was higher for women than for men (adjusted HR 2.7, 95% CI 1.8 to 4.2 for women v 1.3, 95% CI 1 to 1.8 for men). Physical inactivity is a significant risk factor for cardiovascular events in both men and women. One cohort study of women with diabetes found that participation in little (< 1 h/wk) or no physical activity compared with physical activity for at least 7 hours a week was associated with doubling of the risk of a cardiovascular event.[5] Another cohort study (1263 men with diabetes, mean follow up 12 years) found that low baseline cardiorespiratory fitness compared with moderate or high fitness increased overall mortality (RR 2.9, 95% CI 2.1 to 3.6); and overall mortality was higher in those reporting no recreational exercise in the previous 3 months compared with those reporting any recreational physical activity in the same period (RR 1.8, 95% CI 1.3 to 2.5).[6] The absolute risk of cardiovascular disease is almost the same in women as in men with diabetes. Diabetes specific cardiovascular risk factors include the duration of diabetes during adulthood (the years of exposure to

diabetes before age 20 years add little to the risk of cardiovascular disease); raised blood glucose concentrations (reflected in fasting blood glucose or HbA1c [see glossary, p 66]); and any degree of microalbuminuria (albuminuria 30–299 mg/24 h).[7] People with diabetes and microalbuminuria have a higher risk of coronary morbidity and mortality than people with normal levels of urinary albumin and a similar duration of diabetes (RR 2–3).[8,9] Clinical proteinuria increases the risk of major cardiac events in type 2 diabetes (RR 3)[10] and in type 1 diabetes (RR 9)[7,11,12] compared with individuals with the same type of diabetes having normal albumin excretion. An epidemiological analysis of people with diabetes enrolled in the Heart Outcomes Prevention Evaluation (HOPE) clinical trial (3498 people with diabetes and at least 1 other cardiovascular risk factor; age > 55 years, of whom 1140 [32%] had microalbuminuria at baseline; 5 years' follow up) found higher risk for major cardiovascular events in those with microalbuminuria (albumin : creatinine ratio [ACR] ≥ 2.0 mg/mmol) compared with those without microalbuminuria (adjusted RR 1.97, 95% CI 1.68 to 2.31); and for all cause mortality (RR 2.15, 95% CI 1.78 to 2.60). It also found an association between ACR and the risk of major cardiovascular events (ACR 0.22 to 0.57 mg/mmol: RR 0.85, 95% CI 0.63 to 1.14; ACR 0.58 to 1.62 mg/mmol: RR 1.11, 95% CI 0.86 to 1.43; ACR 1.62 to 1.99 mg/mmol: RR 1.89, 95% CI 1.52 to 2.36).[13]

PROGNOSIS Diabetes mellitus increases the risk of mortality or serious morbidity after a coronary event (RR 1.5–3).[2,3,14,15] This excess risk is partly accounted for by increased prevalence of other cardiovascular risk factors in people with diabetes. A systematic review (search date 1998) found that, in people with diabetes admitted to hospital for acute myocardial infarction, "stress hyperglycaemia" versus lower blood glucose levels was associated with increased mortality in hospital (RR 1.7, 95% CI 1.2 to 2.4).[16] One large prospective cohort study (91 285 men aged 40–84 years, 5 years' follow up) found higher all cause and coronary heart disease mortality in men with diabetes versus men without coronary artery disease or diabetes (age adjusted RR 3.3, 95% CI 2.6 to 4.1 in men with diabetes and without coronary artery disease v RR 2.3, 95% CI 2.0 to 2.6 in healthy people; RR 5.6, 95% CI 4.9 to 6.3 in men with coronary artery disease but without diabetes v RR 2.2, 95% CI 2.0 to 2.4 in healthy people; RR 12.0, 95% CI 9.9 to 14.6 in men with both risk factors v RR 4.7, 95% CI 4.0 to 5.4 in healthy people). Multivariate analysis did not materially alter these associations.[17] These findings support previous studies. Diabetes mellitus alone is associated with a twofold increase in risk for all cause death, a threefold increase in risk of death from coronary heart disease and, in people with pre-existing coronary heart disease, a 12-fold increase in risk of death from coronary heart disease compared with people with neither risk factor.[17]

AIMS To reduce mortality and morbidity from cardiovascular disease, with minimum adverse effects.

OUTCOMES Incidence of fatal or non-fatal acute myocardial infarction; congestive heart failure; sudden cardiac death; coronary revascularisation; stroke; gangrene; angiographic evidence of coronary, cerebral, vascular, or peripheral arterial stenosis.

METHODS   *Clinical Evidence* update search and appraisal April 2002. We searched for systematic reviews and RCTs with at least 10 confirmed clinical cardiovascular events among people with diabetes. Studies reporting only intermediate end points (e.g. regression of plaque on angiography, lipid changes) were not included. Most of the evidence comes from subgroup analyses of large RCTs that included people with diabetes. As with all subgroup analyses, and studies with small numbers, these results must be interpreted as suggestive rather than definitive.

QUESTION	What are the effects of screening for high cardiovascular risk in people with diabetes?

We found no large RCTs on screening people with diabetes for cardiovascular risk.

Benefits: We found no systematic review and no large RCTs.

Harms: We found no RCTs.

Comment: Screening for conventional risk factors as well as regular determination of HbA1c (see glossary, p 66), lipid profile, and urinary albumin excretion will identify people at high risk.[18,19] Consensus opinion in the USA recommends screening for cardiovascular disease with exercise stress testing in previously sedentary adults with diabetes who are planning to undertake vigorous exercise programmes.[18,20] We found no evidence that such testing prevents cardiac events.

QUESTION	What are the effects of promoting smoking cessation in people with diabetes?

We found no RCTs on promotion of smoking cessation specifically in people with diabetes. Observational evidence and extrapolation from people without diabetes suggest that promotion of smoking cessation is likely to reduce cardiovascular events.

Benefits: We found no systematic review or RCTs on promotion of smoking cessation specifically in people with diabetes.

Harms: We found no RCTs.

Comment: Observational studies have found that cigarette smoking is associated with increased cardiovascular death in people with diabetes. In people without diabetes, smoking cessation has been found to be associated with reduced risk. People with diabetes are likely to benefit from smoking cessation at least as much as people who do not have diabetes but have other risk factors for cardiovascular events (see smoking cessation under secondary prevention of ischaemic cardiac events, p 189).

Cardiovascular disease in diabetes

QUESTION What are the effects of controlling blood pressure in people with diabetes?

OPTION ANTIHYPERTENSIVE TREATMENT VERSUS NO ANTIHYPERTENSIVE TREATMENT

One RCT in people with diabetes and high blood pressure (BP 165–220/< 95 mm Hg) found that hypertensive treatment (nitrendipine or enalapril with or without hydrochlorothiazide) versus placebo significantly reduced all cardiovascular events over a median of 2 years but found no significant reduction in overall mortality. One RCT in people aged 30–70 years with diabetic nephropathy and hypertension found no significant difference in cardiovascular composite end points (non-fatal myocardial infarction, heart failure) with amlodipine versus placebo and with irbesartan versus placebo or amlodipine. The RCT found a higher incidence of hyperkalemia resulting in discontinuation of treatment with irbesartan versus placebo, or amlodipine. One RCT in people with diabetes, hypertension, and microalbuminuria found no significant reduction in non-fatal cardiovascular events with irbesartan versus placebo. One systematic review found that lowering blood pressure significantly reduced mortality and stroke but found no significant effect of blood pressure lowering on myocardial infarction. One RCT in people with diabetes aged over 55 years with additional cardiac risk factors, previously diagnosed coronary vascular disease, or both, has found that the angiotensin converting enzyme inhibitor ramipril versus placebo significantly reduces major cardiovascular events and overall mortality within 4.5 years. One RCT in people with diabetes and baseline blood pressure less than 140/90 mm Hg found that intensive (target diastolic BP 10 mm Hg below baseline) versus moderate (diastolic BP 80–89 mm Hg) blood pressure lowering significantly reduces cerebral vascular accidents but found no significant difference for cardiovascular death, myocardial infarction, congestive heart failure, or all cause mortality.

Benefits: **Primary prevention:** See table 1, p 70. We found one systematic review (published 1997, but withdrawn from the Cochrane Library and currently being updated)[21] and three subsequent RCTs.[22–24] The first subsequent RCT (4695 people, 495 with diabetes, aged ≥ 60 years with blood pressure 165–220/< 95 mm Hg) found that antihypertensive treatment (nitrendipine or enalapril with or without hydrochlorothiazide) versus placebo reduced all cardiovascular events over a median of 2 years (13/252 [5.2%] with antihypertensive treatment v 31/240 [12.9%] with placebo; ARR 8%, 95% CI 3% to 10%; RR 0.4, 95% CI 0.21 to 0.75; NNT 13, 95% CI 10 to 31), but had no significant effect on overall mortality (16/252 [6.3%] for antihypertensive treatment v 26/240 [10.8%] for controls; ARR +4.5%, 95% CI –0.7% to +7.4%; RR 0.59, 95% CI 0.32 to 1.06).[22] The second subsequent RCT (1715 people with nephropathy due to type 2 diabetes and hypertension, aged 30–70 years) found no significant difference in cardiovascular composite end points (non-fatal myocardial infarction, heart failure) with irbesartan versus placebo (NNT 68, 95% CI –29 to +16; NS), amlodipine versus placebo (NNT 37, 95% CI –45 to +13; NS), or irbesartan versus amlodipine (NNT 79, 95% CI –28 to +17; NS).[23]

The third subsequent RCT (590 people with type 2 diabetes, microalbuminuria, and hypertension, mean age 58 years) found a non-significant reduction in non-fatal cardiovascular events with irbesartan (300 mg) versus placebo (8/194 [4.1%] v 17/201 [8.5%]; NNT 23, 95% CI −236 to +11).[24] **Primary and secondary prevention:** See table 3, p 73. We found one systematic review (search date not stated, 6 RCTs, 7572 people with diabetes out of 15 367 people aged > 50 years)[25] and two subsequent RCTs.[26,27] The systematic review found that lowering blood pressure significantly reduced mortality (10 deaths/1000 person-years in treatment arms v 19 deaths/1000 person years in control arms; RR 0.51 95% CI 0.38 to 0.69) and stroke (8/1000 person years in treatment arms v 14/1000 person years in control arms; RR 0.61, 95% CI 0.46 to 0.83), but found no significant effect of blood pressure lowering on myocardial infarction (14/1000 person years in treatment arms v 16/1000 person years in control arms; rate ratio 0.76, 96% CI 0.51 to 1.01).[25] The first subsequent RCT (3577 people with diabetes out of 9541 people aged ≥ 55 years with at least 1 of the following risk factors: diagnosed coronary vascular disease, current smoker, hypercholesterolaemia, hypertension, or microalbuminuria) compared ramipril (10 mg) versus placebo and vitamin E versus placebo over 4.5 years in a 2 x 2 factorial design (see table 3, p 73).[26] It found that ramipril versus placebo significantly reduced major cardiovascular events (coronary vascular disease death, acute myocardial infarction, or stroke 277/1808 [15.3%] with ramipril v 351/1769 [19.8%] with placebo; RR 0.75, 95% CI 0.64 to 0.88; ARR 4.5%; NNT 22 meaning that 22 older people with diabetes and additional risk factors need to be treated for 4.5 years to prevent 1 major cardiovascular event, 95% CI 14 to 43), and death from any cause (196/1808 v 248/1769; RR 0.76, 95% CI 0.67 to 0.92; ARR 3.2%; NNT 32, 95% CI 19 to 98). The relative effect of ramipril was present in all subgroups regardless of hypertensive status, microalbuminuria, type of diabetes, and nature of diabetes treatment (diet, oral agents, or insulin). Vitamin E versus placebo had no significant effect on morbidity or mortality.[26] The second subsequent RCT compared intensive (target diastolic BP 10 mm Hg below baseline) versus moderate diastolic blood pressure control (diastolic BP 80–89 mm Hg) in normotensive (BP < 140/90) people with diabetes (480 people, 243 randomised to placebo, mean age 58.5 years; 118 to nisoldipine, mean age 59.1 years; and 119 to enalapril, mean age 59.4 years) over 5.3 years.[27] It found that people randomised to intensive treatment had a significantly lower incidence of cerebral vascular accidents compared to people receiving moderate treatment (4/237 [1.7%] v 13/243 [5.4%]; OR 3.29, CI 1.06 to 10.25; NNT 27, 95% CI 14 to 255). It found no significant differences in cardiovascular death, myocardial infarction, congestive heart failure, or all cause mortality.[27] **Secondary prevention:** We found one systematic review (search date 1997, but withdrawn from the Cochrane Library and currently being updated).[21]

Harms: **Primary prevention:** One RCT did not report any adverse effect.[22] The second RCT reported that participants (15.4 % with treatment v 22.8% with placebo) had serious adverse effects but did not state what they were.[24] The third RCT reported a higher incidence of hyperkalemia resulting in discontinuation of treatment with irbesartan versus amlodipine or placebo (11/579 [1.9%] with irbesartan v 3/567 [0.5%] with amlodipine v 2/569 [0.4%] with placebo; P = 0.01 for both comparisons).[23] **Primary and secondary prevention:** One RCT found that cough was 5% more frequent with angiotensin converting enzyme inhibitor (ramipril) versus placebo.[26] One systematic review and one RCT did not report on adverse effects.[25,27]

Comment: None.

| OPTION | DIFFERENT ANTIHYPERTENSIVE DRUGS |

One systematic review in people with type 2 diabetes has found that angiotensin converting enzyme inhibitors versus calcium channel blockers as initial treatment for hypertension significantly reduces cardiovascular events. Subgroup analysis of one RCT in people with a mean age of 76 years with diabetes and hypertension found no significant difference in major cardiovascular events over 4 years with angiotensin converting enzyme inhibitors versus calcium channel blockers versus β blockers or diuretics. One RCT found that an angiotensin converting enzyme inhibitor captopril versus diuretics or β blockers significantly reduced myocardial infarction, stroke, or death (NNT 15, 95% CI 8 to 105). One large RCT found no significant difference with the angiotensin converting enzyme inhibitor captopril versus the β blocker atenolol in the number of cardiovascular events over about 8 years. Subgroup analysis of one RCT in people aged 55–80 years with diabetes and left ventricular hypertrophy found that after 4 years, losartan versus atenolol significantly reduced primary cardiovascular composite outcomes (cardiovascular mortality, stroke, myocardial infarction).

Benefits: We found one systematic review (search date 2000, 4 RCTs, 2180 people with diabetes aged 51–68 years)[28] and two subsequent RCTs.[29,30] The systematic review compared angiotensin converting enzyme (ACE) inhibitors (captopril, enalapril, fosinopril) versus other antihypertensive drugs (diuretics, β blockers, or calcium channel blockers; 1047 people).[28] **ACE inhibitors versus calcium channel blockers:** We found one systematic review,[28] which found two RCTs[31,32] comparing ACE inhibitors (enalapril, fosinopril) versus calcium channel blockers (amlodipine, nisoldipine) in people with diabetes, and one subsequent RCT[29] comparing ACE inhibitors (enalapril, lisinopril) versus calcium channel blockers (felodipine, isradipine) versus conventional treatment (β blockers [atenolol, metoprolol, pindolol] or hydrochlorothiazide plus amiloride). The two RCTs in the systematic review found that ACE inhibitors versus calcium channel blockers significantly reduced combined cardiovascular events (cardiovascular death, acute myocardial infarction, congestive heart failure, stroke, pulmonary infarction, angina) (34/424 [8%] with ACE inhibitors v 70/426 [16%] with calcium channel blockers; ARR 8%, 95% CI 4% to 13%; RR 0.49, 95% CI 0.33 to 0.72; NNT 13, 95% CI 7 to 25). ACE inhibitors versus calcium channel blockers also reduced the three outcomes of death, acute myocardial infarction, and stroke, but the reductions were not significant. The subsequent RCT (6614 people, 719 with diabetes, mean age 76 years, mean blood pressure 190/99 mm Hg) found (among the subgroup of people with diabetes) no significant difference in the incidence of major cardiovascular events over 4 years (64.2 events/1000 person years with ACE inhibitors v 67.7 with calcium channel blockers v 75.0 with the conventional agents — β blockers or diuretics).[29] **ACE inhibitors versus diuretics:** We found one systematic review,[28] which found no RCIs specifically comparing ACE inhibitors versus diuretics in people with diabetes, but found one RCT (572 people, 6.1 years) comparing ACE inhibitors versus alternative treatment that included β blockers, combination β blockers and diuretics, and diuretics in people with and without diabetes.[33] It found that captopril versus diuretics or β blockers reduced the number of people who experienced acute myocardial infarction, stroke, or death (43/263 [18%] with diuretics/β blockers v 30/309 [10%] with captopril; ARR 6.6%, 95% CI 1.1% to 12.2%; NNT 15, 95% CI 8 to 105).[28] **ACE inhibitors versus β blockers:** We found one systematic review,[28] which included one RCT (758 people, 456 cardiovascular events) comparing an ACE inhibitor (captopril) versus a β blocker (atenolol) over 8.4 years.[34] The RCT found no significant difference between captopril versus atenolol in the number of cardiovascular events (102/400 [25.5%] with captopril v 75/358 [20.9%] with atenolol; ARI +5%, 95% CI −1% to +11%; RR 1.22, 95% CI 0.94 to 1.58). **Angiotensin II receptor antagonists versus β blockers:** Subgroup analysis of the results of the third RCT (1195 people with diabetes out of 9193 people, aged 55–80 years)[35] comparing losartan (586 people) versus atenolol (609 people) in people with left ventricular hypertrophy showed that after a 4 year follow up, losartan versus atenolol significantly reduced the primary cardiovascular composite end points (cardiovascular mortality, stroke, and myocardial infarction occurred in 103/586 [17.6%] with losartan group v 139/609 [22.8%] with atenolol; NNT 19, 95% CI 11 to 142).[35] **Other comparisons:** We found no systematic review but found one RCT.[30] The RCT (people aged ≥ 55 years, with hypertension and either previous coronary vascular disease or at least 1 additional coronary vascular disease risk factor) compared chlortalidone (chlorthalidone), doxazosin, amlodipine, and lisinopril.[30] After 3.3 years' follow up, the RCT found no significant difference between doxazosin (3183 people with diabetes) and chlortalidone (5481 people) in the primary outcome (fatal coronary heart disease or non-fatal acute myocardial infarction), but the doxazosin arm was terminated because of an excess risk of combined coronary vascular disease events (coronary heart disease death, non-fatal acute myocardial infarction, stroke, revascularisation procedures, angina, congestive heart failure, and peripheral vascular disease) compared with chlortalidone (OR 1.24, 95% CI 1.12 to 1.38). The RCT is still in progress.[30]

Harms: **ACE inhibitors versus calcium channel blockers:** The systematic review gave no information on adverse effects.[28] In one RCT, people taking atenolol gained more weight than those taking captopril (3.4 kg with atenolol v 1.6 kg with captopril; P = 0.02).[34] Over the first 4 years of the trial, people allocated to atenolol had higher mean HbA1c (see glossary, p 66) (7.5% v 7.0%; P = 0.004), but no significant difference was found between groups over the subsequent 4 years. There was no difference between atenolol and captopril in rates of hypoglycaemia, lipid concentrations, tolerability, blood pressure lowering, or prevention of disease events. **Angiotensin II receptor antagonists versus β blockers:** The RCT found that discontinuation of treatment because of adverse effects was less common with losartan versus atenolol (2/586 v 9/609). Adverse events occurring with significantly different frequency in losartan versus atenolol were bradycardia (1% v 9%; P < 0.0001), cold extremities (4% v 6%; P < 0.0001), albuminuria (5% v 6%; P = 0.0002), hyperglycaemia (5% v 7%; P = 0.007), asthenia/fatigue (15% v 17%; P = 0.001), back pain (12% v 10%; P = 0.004), dyspnoea (10% v 14%; P = 0.002).[35]

Comment: We found evidence that ACE inhibitors are superior to calcium channel blockers as initial treatment. We found no clear evidence directly comparing ACE inhibitors and diuretics. It is unclear whether ACE inhibitors and β blockers are equivalent. In most RCTs, combination treatment with more than one agent was required to achieve target blood pressures. One large RCT found that the ACE inhibitor ramipril, which reduces urinary protein excretion, also reduced cardiovascular morbidity and mortality in older diabetic people with other cardiac risk factors.[26] However, the relative cardioprotective effect was present to the same extent in people with or without microalbuminuria. The evidence suggests that thiazide diuretics, β blockers, and ACE inhibitors significantly reduce cardiovascular events in people with diabetes and are probably superior to calcium channel blockers as initial treatment for hypertension.

| OPTION | TARGET BLOOD PRESSURE |

Large RCTs including people with diabetes and hypertension have found that tighter control of blood pressure with target diastolic blood pressures of less than or equal to 80 mm Hg reduces the risk of major cardiovascular events.

Benefits: We found no systematic review but found several RCTs with large numbers of participants with diabetes (see table 1, p 70 and table 2, p 72).[34,36,37] One large RCT (1148 people with type 2 diabetes and with hypertension managed with atenolol or captopril) found that tight blood pressure control (≤ 150/≤ 85 mm Hg) versus less tight control (≤ 180/≤105 mm Hg) reduced incidence of any diabetes related end points and diabetes related deaths (see glossary, p 66) (primarily cardiovascular deaths, stroke, and microvascular disease).[34,37] See UKPDS hypertension study in table 1, p 70. Another RCT found half the risk of major cardiovascular events with a target diastolic blood pressure of 80 mm Hg or less versus 90 mm Hg or less.[36] See HOT study in table 1, p 70.

Harms: We found no good evidence of a threshold below which it is harmful to lower blood pressure.

Comment: Aggressive lowering of blood pressure in people with diabetes and hypertension reduces cardiovascular morbidity and mortality. In most trials, combination treatment with more than one agent was required to achieve target blood pressures.

QUESTION | What are the effects of treating hyperlipidaemias in people with diabetes?

OPTION | LIPID REGULATING AGENTS

A systematic review found that in people with diabetes, lovastatin or gemfibrozil versus placebo did not significantly reduce non-fatal myocardial infarction and death from coronary artery disease. One RCT in people aged 35–65 years with type 2 diabetes and hyperlipidaemia found that bezafibrate versus placebo significantly reduced myocardial infarction or new ischaemic changes on electrocardiogram within 3 years. Another RCT in people with diabetes aged 40–80 years found a significant decrease in all cause mortality, non-fatal myocardial infarction, coronary heart disease death, total stroke, or any revascularisation with simvastatin versus placebo. It found significant risk reduction in people with diabetes and previous coronary heart disease and in people with diabetes and no prior coronary heart disease. Three RCTs identified by a systematic review found that statins versus placebo significantly decreased cardiovascular event rates. One RCT including people with diabetes found a borderline significant difference in relative risk of coronary heart disease death or non-fatal acute myocardial infarction with gemfibrozil versus placebo. One RCT found that in people with type 2 diabetes, dyslipidaemia and at least one coronary lesion, fenofibrate versus placebo did not significantly reduce myocardial infarction or death. One RCT found that in people aged 21–74 years with diabetes who had previously undergone coronary artery bypass grafting, aggressive versus moderate lipid lowering did not significantly reduce the 4 year life event rate relative risk for myocardial infarction or death.

Benefits: | **Primary prevention:** We found one systematic review (search date 2000,[25] 2 RCTs[38,39]), one additional RCT,[40] and one subsequent RCT[41] comparing lipid lowering agents versus placebo (see table 1, p 70). The systematic review pooled the results from two RCTs (290 people with diabetes, mean age 49 and 58 years) comparing lovastatin or gemfibrozil versus placebo for 5 years.[41] The review found that lovastatin or gemfibrozil versus placebo decreased non-fatal myocardial infarction and death from coronary artery disease by 11 events per 1000 person years, but this decrease was not statistically significant (8 v 19 events/1000 person years; summary rate ratio 0.44, 95% CI 0.17 to 1.20, person years needed to treat 97, 95% CI 45 to not meaningful).[25] The additional RCT (164 men and women with type 2 diabetes, aged 35–65 years; baseline lipids included one or more of the following: total cholesterol 5.2–8.0 mmol/L, serum triglyceride 1.8–8.0 mmol/L, high density lipoprotein cholesterol ≤ 1.1 mmol/L, or total to high density lipoprotein cholesterol ratio ≥ 4.7 mmol/L) compared bezafibrate versus placebo for 3 years.[40] The RCT found that bezafibrate versus placebo significantly reduced myocardial infarction or new ischaemic changes on electocardiogram (5/64 [7.8%] v 16/64 [25%]; NNT 6, 95% CI 5 to 20). The subsequent RCT (5963 men and women with diabetes, aged 40–80 years, among whom 3982 had no previous coronary heart disease) compared simvastatin versus placebo for the primary prevention of coronary heart disease, stroke, and revascularisation over 5 years.[41] The RCT found a significant decrease in outcomes (all cause mortalilty, non-fatal myocardial infarction, coronary heart disease death, total stroke, or any revascularisation) with simvastatin versus placebo, even though by the end of the study 38% of those allocated placebo were taking a non-study statin. The risk reduction was similar for people with diabetes and previous coronary heart disease (325/972 [33.4%] with simvastatin v 381/1009 [37.8%] with placebo; ARR 4.3%, NNT 23, 95% CI 12 to 897) and people with diabetes and no prior coronary heart disease (276/2006 [13.8%] with simvastatin v 367/1976 [18.6%] with placebo; ARR 4.8%, NNT 21, 95% CI 14 to 40; see comment below).[41] **Secondary prevention:** See table 2, p 72. We found one systematic review (search date 2000, 2313 people with diabetes, mean age 58 years, 5 RCTs[42-46]).[25] Three RCTs[42,43,45] included in the review found that statins (pravastatin, simvastatin) versus placebo significantly decreased cardiovascular event rates (34 events with statins v 44 events with placebo per 1000 person years; RR 0.77 95% CI 0.62 to 0.96; person years needed to treat 120, 95% CI 61 to 4856).[25] One RCT included in the systematic review (4444 men and women aged 35–70 years with previous acute myocardial infarction [see glossary, p 66] or angina pectoris, total cholesterol concentrations of 5.5–8.0 mmol/L, and triglycerides ≤ 2.5 mmol/L) compared simvastatin versus placebo over a median of 5.4 years.[42] Simvastatin dosage was initially 20 mg daily, with blinded dosage titration up to 40 mg daily, according to cholesterol response during the first 6–18 weeks. The relative risk of main end points in people with diabetes treated with simvastatin were as follows: total mortality 0.57 (95% CI 0.30 to 1.08); major cardiovascular events 0.45 (95% CI 0.27 to 0.74); and any atherosclerotic event 0.63 (95% CI 0.43 to 0.92).[26] The second RCT included in the review (4159 men and women aged 21–75 years, 3–20 months after acute myocardial infarction and with total cholesterol < 6.2 mmol/L, triglycerides < 3.92 mmol/L, and low density lipoprotein cholesterol 3.0–4.5 mmol/L) compared pravastatin 40 mg daily versus placebo over a median of 5 years.[45] Among the people with diabetes, the relative risk of major coronary events (death from coronary disease, non-fatal acute myocardial infarction, coronary artery bypass graft, or percutaneous transluminal coronary angioplasty) was 0.75 (95% CI 0.57 to 1.0). The third RCT included in the review (9014 men and women aged 31–75 years with acute myocardial infarction or unstable angina, plasma total cholesterol 4.0–7.0 mmol/L, and plasma triglycerides < 5.0 mmol/L) compared pravastatin 40 mg daily versus placebo for a mean of 6.1 years.[43] Among the 782 participants with diabetes, the relative risk of coronary heart disease death or non-fatal acute myocardial infarction was 0.84 (95% CI 0.59 to 1.10). The fourth RCT included in the review (2531 men aged < 74 years with previous coronary vascular disease, acute myocardial infarction, angina, revascularisation, or angiographically documented coronary stenosis; high density lipoprotein cholesterol ≤ 1.0 mmol/L, low density lipoprotein cholesterol ≤ 3.6 mmol/L, and triglycerides ≤ 3.4 mmol/L) compared gemfibrozil 1200 mg daily with placebo for a median of 5.1 years (treatment was intended to raise high density lipoprotein cholesterol levels rather than reduce low density lipoprotein cholesterol).[44] Among the 627 participants with diabetes, the relative risk of coronary heart disease death or non-fatal acute myocardial infarction was 0.76 (95% CI 0.57 to 1.0). **Mixed primary and secondary prevention:** See table 3, p 73. We found three RCTs.[41,46,47] The first RCT (305 men and 113 women; mean age 57 years; with type 2 diabetes; HbA1c [see glossary, p 66] ≤ 170% of the upper limit of normal; at least 1 visible coronary lesion on angiogram; high density lipoprotein cholesterol/cholesterol ratio ≥ 4 plus either an low density lipoprotein cholesterol of 3.5–4.5 mmol/L and triglycerides ≤ 5.2 mmol/L, or triglycerides 1.7–5.2 mmol/L and low density lipoprotein cholesterol of 4.5 mmol/L; 50% had no previous clinical history of coronary artery disease) that compared the effect of fenofibrate 200 mg daily versus placebo on progression of coronary artery disease in type 2 diabetes for a minimum of 3 years.[47] The RCT found that, after 39 months on treatment and 6 additional months' follow up, fenofibrate versus placebo did not significantly reduce the number of people who either had myocardial infarction or died (15/207 [7.2%] with fenofibrate v 21/211 [9.9%] with placebo; ARR 2.7%, 95% CI −2.8% to +8.3%; RR 0.73, 95% CI 0.39 to 1.37).[47] The second RCT (1351 people, 116 with type 2 diabetes, aged 21–74 years, mean age 63.1 years) compared the effects of aggressive lipid lowering (lovastatin and cholestyramine as necessary to achieve and low density lipoprotein cholesterol of 1.55–2.20 mmol, 60–85 mg/dL) versus moderate lipid lowering (the same medication to achieve and low density lipoprotein cholesterol of 3.36–3.62 mmol/L, 130–140 mg/dL), in people who had undergone coronary artery bypass grafting 1–11 years previously (mean 4.3 years post coronary artery bypass grafting).[46] The RCT found a reduction in the 4 year event rate for death in those randomised to aggressive cholesterol lowering treatment versus moderate treatment (6.5 v 9.6; RR 0.67, 99% CI 0.12 to 3.75) and a reduction in the 4 year event rate for myocardial infarction in those allocated to aggressive versus moderate treatment groups (4.8 v 11.6; RR 0.40, 99% CI 0.07 to 2.47). None of these findings were statistically significant.[46]

Harms: The RCTs found no significant differences in adverse outcomes between placebo and treatment groups.

Comment: We found one RCT that is of major importance.[41] This study is interesting as it was not necessary to have an abnormal lipid profile or prior vascular disease to be enrolled in the study and provides the first clear evidence that statin treatment is effective for primary prevention of cardiovascular disease.[41] The RCT comparing aggressive versus moderate lipid lowering had limited power because of the small number of patients enrolled with diabetes.[46] Most published clinical trials with sufficient power to detect effects on cardiovascular events have enrolled comparatively few people with diabetes or have excluded them altogether. The available evidence is therefore based almost entirely on subgroup analyses of larger trials. Several large ongoing trials are evaluating the effects of fibrates in people with diabetes.

Cardiovascular disorders

| OPTION | PROPHYLACTIC ASPIRIN |

One RCT in men aged 40 to 80 years with diabetes has found that aspirin versus placebo significantly reduces the risk of first acute myocardial infarction within 5 years. Another RCT in people with diabetes and prior cardiovascular disease found no significant difference with aspirin versus placebo in the risk of acute myocardial infarction or overall mortality within 5 years. One systematic review has found that aspirin versus placebo significantly reduces the risk of morbidity and death from cardiovascular disease within 2 years in people with diabetes and other risk factors for a cardiovascular event.

Benefits: **Primary prevention:** We found no systematic review but found two RCTs. In the only large primary prevention RCT, comparing aspirin versus placebo and reporting results for people with diabetes, 22 701 US male physicians aged 40–80 years were assigned to aspirin 325 mg every other day or to placebo, and followed for an average of 5 years.[48] The trial found that, after 5 years, among the 533 physicians with diabetes, aspirin versus placebo reduced the risk of acute myocardial infarction (see glossary, p 66) (11/275 [4%] with aspirin v 26/258 [10.1%] with placebo; RR 0.39, 95% CI 0.20 to 0.79; NNT 16, 95% CI 12 to 47). A second RCT comparing aspirin with placebo did not specify the number of people with diabetes, but it did report that aspirin reduced acute myocardial infarction to a similar degree in the subgroup of people with diabetes and in the overall trial population (RR 0.85).[36] **Primary and early secondary prevention:** We found one RCT (3711 people with diabetes, 30% with type 1 diabetes, 48% with prior cardiovascular disease).[49] It compared aspirin (650 mg daily) versus placebo and followed the participants for a mean of 5 years. It found a non-significant reduction in overall mortality in those treated with aspirin (RR 0.91, 95% CI 0.75 to 1.11). Acute myocardial infarction occurred in 289 people (16%) in the aspirin group and 336 (18%) in the placebo group (ARR 2%, 95% CI 0.1% to 4.9%). Fifty people would need to be treated for 5 years with aspirin 650 mg daily to prevent one additional acute myocardial infarction. **Secondary prevention:** We found one systematic review (search date 1990, 145 RCTs of antiplatelet treatment, primarily aspirin).[50] Results for people with diabetes are tabulated (see table 2, p 72).

Harms: In the large trial comparing aspirin versus placebo for primary and secondary prevention, fatal or non-fatal stroke occurred in 5% on aspirin and 4.2% on placebo (P = NS).[35] There was no significant increase with aspirin in the risks of vitreous, retinal, gastrointestinal, or cerebral haemorrhage. In the systematic review, doses of aspirin ranged from 75–1500 mg daily. Most trials used aspirin 75–325 mg daily. Doses higher than 325 mg daily increased the risk of haemorrhagic adverse effects without improving preventive efficacy. No difference in efficacy or adverse effects was found in the dose range 75–325 mg.[50]

Comment: We found insufficient evidence to define precisely which people with diabetes should be treated with aspirin. The risk of cardiovascular disease is very low before age 30 years; most white adults with diabetes aged over 30 years are at increased risk of cardiovascular disease. Widely accepted contraindications to aspirin treatment include aspirin allergy, bleeding tendency, anticoagulant treatment, recent gastrointestinal bleeding, and clinically active liver disease.[18,51]

OPTION   GLYCOPROTEIN IIB/IIIA INHIBITORS

Subgroup analysis in one RCT of people presenting with unstable angina or acute myocardial infarction without ST elevation found that the addition of a glycoprotein IIb/IIIa inhibitor (tirofiban) to heparin significantly reduced the risk of death or myocardial infarction at 180 days.

Benefits: We found one RCT (1570 people, including 228 men and 134 women with diabetes, mean age 65 years, presenting with unstable angina or acute myocardial infarction [see glossary, p 66] without ST elevation, all started on aspirin at time of randomisation) comparing addition of a glycoprotein IIb/IIIa inhibitor (tirofiban) to heparin versus heparin alone.[68] Subgroup analysis at 180 days in people with diabetes found that addition of tirofiban to heparin versus heparin alone reduced the number of deaths or myocardial infarctions (19/169 [11.2%] with tirofiban plus heparin v 37/193 [19.2%] with heparin alone; ARR 8.0%, 95% CI 0.7% to 15.3%; NNT 13, 95% CI 7 to 146). **Adjunct to percutaneous coronary revascularisation:** See benefits of intracoronary stenting plus glycoprotein IIb/IIIa inhibitors, p 65.

Harms: The RCT found no significant difference between tirofiban plus heparin and aspirin versus heparin and aspirin alone in risk of bleeding (9.5% with tirofiban plus heparin and aspirin v 8.3% with heparin and aspirin alone).[68]

Comment: None.

QUESTION   What are the effects of blood glucose control in prevention of cardiovascular disease in people with diabetes?

RCTs found that glucose lowering with insulin, sulphonylureas, or metformin may reduce the risk of first acute myocardial infarction. One large RCT in people with acute myocardial infarction found that intensive insulin treatment versus standard insulin treatment significantly reduced mortality at 3.4 years

Benefits: **Primary prevention:** See table 1, p 70. We found no systematic review but found three RCTs of intensive versus conventional treatment of hyperglycaemia and the microvascular and macrovascular complications of diabetes.[53,54,66,67] One RCT (3867 people, newly diagnosed with type 2 diabetes, median age 54 years, fasting blood glucose 6.1 to 15 mmol/L after 3 months dietary treatment) compared conventional treatment (1138 people treated with diet only, drugs added if fasting blood glucose > 15.0 mmol/L or hyperglycaemic symptoms occurred) versus intensive treatment (1573 people treated with sulphonylureas, 1156 people treated with insulin).[66] It found that intensive treatment reduced the risk of acute myocardial infarction (14.7/1000 person years for intensive v 17.4/1000 person years for conventional; RR 0.84, 95% CI 0.71 to 1.0), diabetes related outcomes (see glossary, p 66) (RR 0.88, 95% CI 0.80 to 0.99; NNT 39 for 5 years to prevent 1 additional diabetes related outcome), and improved glycaemic control (HbA1c [see glossary, p 66] 7% with intensive treatment v 7.9% with conventional treatment), but found no significant difference for risks of stroke and amputation.[66] The second RCT (753 people with newly diagnosed type 2 diabetes, > 120% of ideal body weight) compared intensive treatment with metformin (aiming for fasting blood glucose < 6 mmol/L) versus conventional treatment (mainly diet alone).[67] It found that metformin versus conventional treatment significantly reduced the risk of a diabetes related outcome (32%, 95% CI 13 to 47; P = 0.002) and diabetes related death (see glossary, p 66) (42%, 95% CI 0 to 63; P = 0.017).[67] The third RCT (1441 people with type 1 diabetes aged 13–39 years and free of cardiovascular disease, hypertension, hypercholesterolaemia, and obesity at baseline) compared conventional versus intensive treatment, followed for a mean of 6.5 years (3.5–9 years) for atherosclerosis related events.[53] It found that major macrovascular events were almost twice as frequent in the conventionally treated group (40 events) as in the intensive treatment group (23 events), although the differences were not significant (ARR 2.2%; RR 0.59, 95% CI 0.32 to 1.1). **Secondary prevention:** See table 2, p 72. We found no systematic review but found two RCTs.[55–57] One small RCT (153 men with type 2 diabetes, mean age 60 years, many of whom had previous cardiovascular events) compared standard insulin (once daily) with intensive treatment with a stepped plan designed to achieve near normal blood sugar levels.[55] After 27 months, the rate of new cardiovascular events was not significantly different between the groups (24/75 [32%] with intensive treatment v 16/80 [20%] with standard insulin; RR 1.6, 95% CI 0.92 to 2.5). In the second RCT (620 people, mean age 68 years, 63% men, 84% with type 2 diabetes) with random blood glucose greater than or equal to 11 mmol/L were randomised within 24 hours of an acute myocardial infarction to either standard treatment or intensive insulin treatment.[56,57] The intensive insulin group received an insulin-glucose infusion for 24 hours followed by subcutaneous insulin four times daily for at least 3 months. The standard treatment group received insulin only when it was clinically indicated. HbA1c fell significantly with intensive insulin treatment (absolute fall of 1.1% with intensive treatment v 0.4% with standard treatment at 3 months and 0.9% v 0.4% at 12 months). Intensive treatment lowered mortality (ARs 19% v 26% at 1 year and 33% v 44% at a mean of 3.4 years; RR 0.72, 95% CI 0.55 to 0.92; NNT 9 treated for 3.4 years to prevent 1 additional premature death). The absolute reduction in the risk of mortality was particularly striking in people who were not previously using insulin and had no more than one of the following risk factors before the acute myocardial infarction that preceded randomisation: age 70 years or over, history of previous acute myocardial infarction, history of congestive heart failure, current treatment with digitalis. In this low risk subgroup, the ARR was 15% (NNT 7 for 3.4 years).

Harms: Sulphonylureas and insulin, but not metformin, increased the risks of weight gain and hypoglycaemia. On an intention to treat basis, the proportions of people per year with severe hypoglycaemic episodes were 0.7%, 1.2%, 1%, 2%, and 0.6% for the conventional chlorpropamide, glibenclamide, insulin, and metformin groups, respectively. These frequencies of hypoglycaemia were much lower than those observed with intensive treatment in people with type 1 diabetes.[53,54] One RCT found no evidence that any specific treatment (insulin, sulphonylurea, or metformin) increased overall risk of cardiovascular disease.[66,67]

Comment: The role of intensive glucose lowering in primary prevention of cardiovascular events remains unclear. However, such treatment clearly reduces the risk of microvascular disease and does not increase the risk of cardiovascular disease. The potential of the larger primary prevention RCT to demonstrate an effect of tighter glycaemic control was limited by the small difference achieved in median HbA1c between intensive and conventional treatment.[53,54] In contrast, in another primary prevention trial, a larger 1.9% difference in median HbA1c was achieved between groups, but the young age of the participants and consequent low incidence of cardiovascular events limited the power of the study to detect an effect of treatment on incidence of cardiovascular disease.[53,54] The study of insulin in type 2 diabetes[55] included men with a high baseline risk of cardiovascular events and achieved a 2.1% absolute difference in HbA1c. The RCT was small and the observed difference between groups could have arisen by chance. The design of the trial of intensive versus standard glycaemic control following acute myocardial infarction does not distinguish whether the early insulin infusion or the later intensive subcutaneous insulin treatment was the more important determinant of improved survival in the intensively treated group.[57] The possibility that oral hypoglycaemics may be harmful after acute myocardial infarction cannot be ruled out. The larger primary prevention trial found no evidence that oral hypoglycaemics increase cardiovascular mortality.[66,67]

QUESTION What are the effects of revascularisation procedures in people with diabetes

---

OPTION CORONARY ARTERY BYPASS VERSUS PERCUTANEOUS TRANSLUMINAL ANGIOPLASTY

One large RCT in people with diabetes and multivessel coronary artery disease has found that coronary artery bypass graft (CABG) versus percutaneous transluminal coronary angioplasty (PTCA) significantly reduces mortality or myocardial infarction within 8 years. Another RCT found a non-significant reduction in mortality with CABG versus PTCA at 4 years. A third RCT in people with diabetes and multivessel coronary artery disease found no significant difference between CABG and PTCA with

Cardiovascular disorders

stent in short term outcome (to time of discharge), but at 1 year after the procedure there was significantly greater cumulative incidence of combined death, myocardial infarction, or repeat CABG or PTCA.

Benefits: We found no systematic review but found three RCTs (see table 2, p 72).[52,58,59] Two RCTs compared CABG versus PTCA, without stenting or a glycoprotein IIb/IIIa inhibitor,[52,58] and one RCT compared CABG versus PTCA with stenting.[59] The first RCT (1829 people with 2 or 3 vessel coronary disease, 353 with diabetes, mean age 62 years) found that, after a mean of 7.7 years, CABG versus PTCA significantly reduced the number of people who died or suffered Q-wave myocardial infarction (60/173 [34.7%] with CABG v 85/170 [50%] with PTCA; ARR 15%, 95% CI 5% to 26%; RR 0.69, 95% CI 0.54 to 0.89; NNT 7, 95% CI 4 to 20). This survival benefit was confined to those receiving at least one internal mammary graft. The second RCT (1054 people, 125 with diabetes, 94 men and 31 women, mean age 61 years) found a non-significant reduction in number of people who had died at 4 years' follow up with CABG versus PTCA (8/63 [12.5%] v 14/62 [22.6%]; ARR 9.9%, 95% CI −3.4% to +23.1%; NNT 10; NS).[58] The third RCT (1205 people with 2 or 3 vessel coronary disease, 208 with diabetes 112 randomised to PTCA with stent, 96 to CABG, mean age 62 years) found no significant difference in people with diabetes treated with CABG or PTCA in short term risks (up to discharge) of composite end point of death, myocardial infarction, repeat CABG, and repeat PTCA (11/112 [9.8%] with PTCA v 9/96 [9.4%] with CABG; NNT 224; NS). However at 1 year, the RCT found significantly higher incidence of the composite end point with PTCA/stent versus CABG (41/112 [36%] with PTCA/stent v 15 /96 [15.6%] with CABG, NNT 5, 95% CI 4 to 11).[59]

Harms: In the first RCT, in-hospital mortality among people with diabetes was 1.2% after CABG versus 0.6% after PTCA. Myocardial infarction during the initial hospitalisation was three times more common after CABG than after PTCA (5.8% v 1.8%). None of these differences were found to be significant.[52] The third RCT found a significant increase in risk of stroke with CABG versus PTCA with stent in people with diabetes (4 v 0; P = 0.04).[59]

Comment: None.

| OPTION | PERCUTANEOUS TRANSLUMINAL CORONARY ANGIOPLASTY VERSUS THROMBOLYSIS |

One RCT in people with diabetes and prior acute myocardial infarction found that at 30 days there was a lower rate of composite end point (death, reinfarction, or disabling stroke) but the difference was not significant.

Benefits: We found no systematic review but found one RCT.[69] The RCT (1138 people with acute myocardial infarction presenting within 12 h of chest pain onset, 177 with diabetes mean age of 65 years) compared percutaneous transluminal coronary angioplasty (PTCA) versus thrombolysis (alteplase).[69] At 30 days, fewer people with diabetes assigned to PTCA experienced the composite end point of death, reinfarction, or disabling stroke, but the difference was not significant (11/99 [11%] with PTCA v 13/78 [17%] with alteplase; ARR +5.6%, 95% CI −4.8 to +15.9%). The RCT found no significant difference in 30 day mortality among people with diabetes (8/99 [8.1%] after PTCA v 5/78 [6.4%] after alteplase) (see table 2, p 72).[69]

Harms: See harms of coronary artery bypass versus PTCA, p 64.

Comment: None.

OPTION | **INTRACORONARY STENTING PLUS GLYCOPROTEIN IIB/IIIA INHIBITORS**

RCTs in people with diabetes undergoing percutaneous transluminal coronary angioplasty have found that the combination of stent and a glycoprotein IIb/IIIa inhibitor (abciximab) significantly reduces restenosis rates and serious morbidity.

Benefits: We found no systematic review but found two RCTs (see table 2, p 72).[60–63] The first RCT (2792 people, 638 with diabetes, mean age 61 years, 38% female, all undergoing percutaneous transluminal coronary angioplasty or directional atherectomy without stenting) compared placebo plus standard dose heparin versus abciximab plus standard dose heparin versus abciximab plus low dose heparin. Abciximab was given as a bolus with 12 hour infusion. The primary indications for intervention were unstable angina (51%), stable ischaemia (33%), and recent acute myocardial infarction (16%). A total of 44% had a prior coronary intervention, 56% had multivessel disease, and 74% a history of hypertension. Abciximab versus placebo reduced the combined end point of death or acute myocardial infarction (see glossary, p 66) in both standard dose and low dose heparin arms (at 30 days by > 60% and at 6 months by > 50%). Abciximab reduced the rate of restenosis in people without diabetes (HR 0.78), but not in people with diabetes. The second RCT (2401 people; 491 with diabetes; mean age 60 years; 29% female, 69% hypertensive, 30% recent smokers, 48% prior acute myocardial infarction, 10% prior coronary artery bypass) compared stent plus placebo (173 people) versus stent plus abciximab (162 people) versus balloon angioplasty plus abciximab (156 people). The RCT found significant differences between stent plus abciximab versus the other two groups for death or large acute myocardial infarction at 12 months (4.9% with stent plus abciximab v 8.3% with percutaneous transluminal coronary angioplasty plus abciximab v 13.9% with stent plus placebo), and for subsequent revascularisation rates (13.7% with stent and abciximab v 25.3% with percutaneous transluminal coronary angioplasty plus abciximab v 22.4% with stent plus placebo).[61–63] We found an analysis of individual people results (1462 people with diabetes) of these two trials and a third, earlier trial.[64] It found that abciximab reduced overall mortality (26/540 [4.8%] v 21/844 [2.5%]; ARR 2.3%; NNT 43, 95% CI 23 to 421).

Cardiovascular disease in diabetes

Harms: There was slightly greater bleeding in people given abciximab than in those given placebo (4.3% v 3.0% for major bleeding; 6.9% v 6.3% for minor bleeding; 0% v 0.17% for intracranial haemorrhage). None of these differences were significant.[65]

Comment: For people with diabetes undergoing percutaneous procedures, the combination of stent and glycoprotein IIb/IIIa inhibitor reduces restenosis rates and serious morbidity. It is unclear whether these adjunctive treatments would reduce morbidity, mortality, and restenosis associated with percutaneous revascularisation procedures to the levels seen with coronary artery bypass. There was imbalance of the baseline characteristics among the study groups of the second RCT.[61] However, in a multivariate analysis, the treatment effects remained after adjusting for baseline differences.

GLOSSARY

Acute myocardial infarction is infarction that occurs when circulation to a region of the heart is obstructed and necrosis is occurring; clinical symptoms include severe pain, pallor, perspiration, nausea, dyspnoea, and dizziness. Myocardial infarction is gross necrosis of the myocardium as a result of interruption of blood supply usually caused by atherosclerosis of the coronary arteries; myocardial infarction without pain or other symptoms (silent infarction) is common in people with diabetes

Diabetes related death includes fatal acute myocardial infarction or sudden death; fatal stroke; death from peripheral vascular disease; death from renal disease; death from hypoglycaemia or hyperglycaemia.

Diabetes related outcomes include the first occurrence of non-fatal acute myocardial infarction, heart failure, or angina; non-fatal stroke, amputation, renal failure, retinal photocoagulation or vitreous haemorrhage; cataract extraction or blindness in one eye.

HbA1c The haemoglobin A1c test is the most common laboratory test of glycated haemoglobin (haemoglobin that has glucose irreversibly bound to it). HbA1c provides an indication of the "average" blood glucose over the last 3 months. The HbA1c is a weighted average over time of the blood glucose level; many different glucose profiles can produce the same level of HbA1c.

REFERENCES

1. Geiss LS, Herman WH, Smith PJ. Mortality in non-insulin-dependent diabetes. In: Harris MI, ed. *Diabetes in America.* 2nd ed. Bethesda, MD: National Institutes of Health, 1995:233–255.

2. Wingard DL, Barrett-Connor E. Heart disease and diabetes. In: Harris MI, ed. *Diabetes in America.* 2nd ed. Bethesda, MD: National Institutes of Health, 1995:429–448.

3. Haffner SM, Lehto S, Ronnemaa T, et al. Mortality from coronary heart disease in subjects with type 2 diabetes and in nondiabetic subjects with and without prior myocardial infarction. *N Engl J Med* 1998;339:229–234.

4. Mukamai KJ, Nesto RW, Cohen MC, et al. Impact of diabetes on long-term survival after acute myocardial infarction. *Diabetes Care* 2001;24:1422–1427.

5. Hu FB, Stampfer MJ, Solomon C, et al. Physical activity and risk for cardiovascular events in diabetic women. *Ann Intern Med* 2001;134:96–105.

6. Wei M, Gibbons LW, Kampert JB, Nichaman MZ, Blair SN. Low cardiorespiratory fitness and physical inactivity as predictors of mortality in men with type 2 diabetes. *Ann Intern Med* 2000;132:605–611.

7. Krolewski AS, Warram JH, Freire MB. Epidemiology of late diabetic complications. A basis for the development and evaluation of preventive programs. *Endocrinol Metab Clin North Am* 1996;25:217–242.

8. Messent JW, Elliott TG, Hill RD, et al. Prognostic significance of microalbuminuria in insulin-dependent diabetes mellitus: a twenty-three year follow-up study. *Kidney Int* 1992;41:836–839.

9. Dinneen SF, Gerstein HC. The association of microalbuminuria and mortality in non-insulin-dependent diabetes mellitus: a systematic overview of the literature. *Arch Intern Med* 1997;157:1413–1418. Search date 1995; primary sources Medline, SciSearch, and hand searching of bibliographies.

10. Valmadrid CT, Klein R, Moss SE, Klein BE. The risk of cardiovascular disease mortality associated with microalbuminuria and gross proteinuria in persons with older-onset diabetes mellitus. *Arch Intern Med* 2000;160:1093–1100.

11. Borch Johnsen K, Andersen PK, Deckert T. The
    effect of proteinuria on relative mortality in type 1
    (insulin-dependent) diabetes mellitus.
    Diabetologia 1985;28:590–596.
12. Warram JH, Laffel LM, Ganda OP, et al. Coronary
    artery disease is the major determinant of excess
    mortality in patients with insulin-dependent
    diabetes mellitus and persistent proteinuria. *J Am
    Soc Nephrol* 1992;3(suppl 4):104–110.
13. Gerstein Hertzel C, Johannes FE, Qilong Yi, et al.
    Albuminuria and risk of cardiovascular events,
    death and heart failure in diabetic and nondiabetic
    individuals. *JAMA* 2001;286:421–426.
14. Behar S, Boyko V, Reicher-Reiss H, et al. Ten-year
    survival after acute myocardial infarction:
    comparison of patients with and without diabetes.
    SPRINT Study Group. Secondary Prevention
    Reinfarction Israeli Nifedipine Trial. *Am Heart J*
    1997;133:290–296.
15. Mak KH, Moliterno DJ, Granger CB, et al.
    Influence of diabetes mellitus on clinical outcome
    in the thrombolytic era of acute myocardial
    infarction: GUSTO I Investigators: global utilization
    of streptokinase and tissue plasminogen activator
    for occluded coronary arteries. *J Am Coll Cardiol*
    1997;30:171–179.
16. Capes SE, Hunt D, Malmberg K, et al. Stress
    hyperglycaemia and increased risk of death after
    myocardial infarction in patients with and without
    diabetes: a systematic overview. *Lancet*
    2000;355:773–778. Search date 1998; primary
    sources Medline, Science Citation Index, hand
    searches of bibliographies of relevant articles, and
    contact with experts in the field.
17. Lotufo PA, Gazziano M, Chae CU, et al. Diabetes
    and all-cause coronary heart disease mortality
    among US male physicians. *Arch Intern Med*
    2001;161:242–247.
18. Meltzer S, Leiter L, Daneman D, et al. Clinical
    practice guidelines for the management of
    diabetes in Canada. *Can Med Assoc J*
    1998;159(suppl 8):1–29.
19. American Diabetes Association. Clinical practice
    recommendations 2000. *Diabetes Care*
    2000;23(suppl 1):1–116.
20. American Diabetes Association. Diabetes mellitus
    and exercise. *Diabetes Care* 2000;23(suppl
    1):50–54.
21. Fuller J, Stevens LK, Chaturvedi N, et al.
    Antihypertensive therapy in preventing
    cardiovascular complications in people with
    diabetes mellitus. In: The Cochrane Library, Issue
    3, 2001. Oxford, Update Software. Search date
    not stated; primary sources Medline, Embase, and
    hand searches of specialist journals in
    cardiovascular disease, stroke, renal disease, and
    hypertension. Review subsequently withdrawn by
    The Cochrane Library and is currently being
    updated.
22. Tuomilehto J, Rastenyte D, Birkenhäger WH, et al.
    Effects of calcium-channel blockade in older
    patients with diabetes and systolic hypertension. *N
    Engl J Med* 1999;340:677–684.
23. Lewis EJ, Hunsicker LG, et al. Renoprotective
    effect of the angiotensin receptor antagonist
    irbesartan in patients wit nephropathy due to type
    2 diabetes. *NEJM* 2001;345:851–860.
24. Parving HH, Lehnert H, et al. The effect of
    irbesartan on the development of diabetic
    nephropathy in patients with type 2 diabetes.
    NEJM 2001;345:870–878.
25. Huang ES, Meigs JB, Singer DE. The effect of
    interventions to prevent cardiovascular disease in
    patients with type 2 diabetes mellitus. *American J
    Med* 2001;111:633–642.
26. Heart Outcomes Prevention Evaluation (HOPE)
    Study Investigators. Effects of ramipril on
    cardiovascular and microvascular outcomes in
    people with diabetes mellitus: results of the HOPE
    study and the MICRO-HOPE substudy. *Lancet*
    2000;355:253–259.
27. Schrier RW, Estacio RO, et al. Effects of aggressive
    blood pressure control in normotensive type 2
    diabetic patients on albuminuria, retinopathy and
    strokes. *Kidney International* 2002;6:1086–1097.
28. Pahor M, Psaty BM, Alderman MH, et al.
    Therapeutic benefits of ACE inhibitors and other
    antihypertensive drugs in patients with type 2
    diabetes. *Diabetes Care* 2000;23:888–892.
    Search date 2000; primary source Medline.
29. Lindholm LH, Hansson L, Ekbom T, et al.
    Comparison of antihypertensive treatment in
    preventing cardiovascular events in elderly diabetic
    patients: results from the Swedish trial in old
    patients with hypertension-2. *J Hypertens*
    2000;18:1671–1675.
30. ALLHAT Collaborative Research Group. Major
    cardiovascular events in hypertensive patients
    randomised to doxazosin vs chlorthalidone: the
    antihypertensive and lipid-lowering treatment to
    prevent heart attack trial (ALLHAT). *JAMA*
    2000;283:1967–1975.
31. Tatti P, Pahor M, Byington RP, et al. Outcome
    results of the Fosinopril versus Amlodipine
    Cardiovascular Events randomised Trial (FACET) in
    patients with hypertension and NIDDM. *Diabetes
    Care* 1998;21:597–603.
32. Estacio RO, Jeffers BW, Hiatt WR, et al. The effect
    of nisoldipine as compared with enalapril on
    cardiovascular events in patients with
    non-insulin-dependent diabetes and hypertension.
    N Engl J Med 1998;338:645–652.
33. Niskanen L, Hedner T, et al. Reduced
    cardiovascular morbidity and mortality in
    hypertensive diabetic patients on first line therapy
    with an ACE inhibitor compared with diuretic beta
    blocker based treatment regiment, a sub analysis
    of the captopril prevention project. *Diabetes Care*
    2001;24:2091–2096.
34. UK Prospective Diabetes Study Group. Efficacy of
    atenolol and captopril in reducing risk of
    macrovascular and microvascular complications in
    type 2 diabetes: UKPDS 39. *BMJ*
    1998;317:713–720.
35. Dahlof B, Devereux RB, et al. Cardiovascular
    morbidity and mortality in the losartan intervention
    for endpoint reduction in hypertension study
    (LIFE): a randomized trial against atenolol. *Lancet*
    2002;359:995–1003.
36. Hansson L, Zanchetti A, Carruthers SG, et al.
    Effects of intensive blood-pressure lowering and
    low-dose aspirin in patients with hypertension:
    principal results of the Hypertension Optimal
    Treatment (HOT) randomised trial. *Lancet*
    1998;351:1755–1762.
37. UK Prospective Diabetes Study Group. Tight blood
    pressure control and risk of macrovascular and
    microvascular complications in type 2 diabetes:
    UKPDS 38. *BMJ* 1998;317:703–713.
38. Downs JR, Clearfield M, Weis S, et al. Primary
    prevention of acute coronary events with lovastatin
    in men and women with average cholesterol
    levels: results of AFCAPS/TexCAPS. Air Force/Texas
    Coronary Atherosclerosis Prevention Study. *JAMA*
    1998;279:1615–1622.
39. Koskinen P, Manttari M, Manninen V, et al.
    Coronary heart disease incidence in NIDDM
    patients in the Helsinki Heart Study. *Diabetes Care*
    1992;15:820–825.
40. Elkeles RS, Diamond JR, Poulter C, et al.
    Cardiovascular outcomes in type 2 diabetes. A
    double-blind placebo-controlled study of
    bezafibrate: the St Mary's, Ealing, Northwick Park

Diabetes Cardiovascular Disease Prevention (SENDCAP) Study. *Diabetes Care* 1998;21:641–648.

41. Heart Protection Study Collaborative Group. MRC/BHF Heart Protection Study of cholesterol lowering with simvastatin in 20 536 high-risk individuals: a randomised placebo-controlled trial. *Lancet* 2002;360:7–22.

42. Pyorala K, Pedersen TR, Kjekshus J, et al. Cholesterol lowering with simvastatin improves prognosis of diabetic patients with coronary heart disease. A subgroup analysis of the Scandinavian Simvastatin Survival Study (4S). *Diabetes Care* 1997;20:614–620.

43. The Long-term Intervention with Pravastatin in Ischemic Disease (LIPID) Study Program. Prevention of cardiovascular events and death with pravastatin in patients with coronary heart disease and a broad range of initial cholesterol levels. *N Engl J Med* 1998;339:1349–1357.

44. Rubins HB, Robins SJ, Collins D, et al. Gemfibrozil for the secondary prevention of coronary heart disease in men with low levels of high-density lipoprotein cholesterol. Veterans Affairs High-Density Lipoprotein Cholesterol Intervention Trial Study Group. *N Engl J Med* 1999;341:410–418.

45. Sacks FM, Pfeffer MA, Moye LA, et al. The effect of pravastatin on coronary events after myocardial infarction in patients with average cholesterol levels. Cholesterol and Recurrent Events Trial investigators. *N Engl J Med* 1996;335:1001–1009.

46. Hoogwerf BJ, Waness A, et al. Effects of aggressive cholesterol lowering and low dose anticoagulation on clinical and angiographic outcomes in patients with diabetes. *Diabetes* 1999;48:1289–1294.

47. Anonymous. Effect of fenofibrate on progression of coronary-artery disease in type 2 diabetes: The Diabetes Atherosclerosis Interventions Study, a Randomized Study. *Lancet* 2001;357:905–910.

48. Steering Committee of the Physicians' Health Study Research Group. Final report on the aspirin component of the ongoing Physicians' Health Study. *N Engl J Med* 1989;321:129–135.

49. ETDRS Investigators. Aspirin effects on mortality and morbidity in patients with diabetes mellitus. *JAMA* 1992;268:1292–1300.

50. Collaborative overview of randomised trials of antiplatelet therapy–I: Prevention of death, myocardial infarction, and stroke by prolonged antiplatelet therapy in various categories of patients. Antiplatelet Trialists' Collaboration. *BMJ* 1994;308:81–106. Search date 1990; primary sources Medline, Current Contents, manual searches of journals, reference lists from clinical trials and review articles, and enquiry among colleagues and manufacturers of antiplatelet agents for unpublished studies.

51. American Diabetes Association. Aspirin therapy in diabetes. *Diabetes Care* 1997;20:1772–1773.

52. The BARI Investigators. Seven-year outcome in the Bypass Angioplasty Revascularization Investigation (BARI) by treatment and diabetic status. *J Am Coll Cardiol* 2000;35:1122–1129.

53. DCCT Research Group. Effect of intensive diabetes management on macrovascular events and risk factors in the Diabetes Control and Complications Trial. *Am J Cardiol* 1995;75:894–903.

54. DCCT Research Group. The effect of intensive treatment of diabetes on the development and progression of long-term complications in insulin-dependent diabetes mellitus. *N Engl J Med* 1993;329:977–986.

55. Abraira C, Colwell J, Nuttall F, et al. Cardiovascular events and correlates in the Veterans Affairs

Diabetes Feasibility Trial: Veterans Affairs Cooperative Study on glycemic control and complications in type II diabetes. *Arch Intern Med* 1997;157:181–188.

56. Malmberg K, Ryden L, Efendic S, et al. Randomised trial of insulin-glucose infusion followed by subcutaneous insulin treatment in diabetic patients with acute myocardial infarction (DIGAMI study): effects on mortality at 1 year. *J Am Coll Cardiol* 1995;26:57–65.

57. Malmberg K. Prospective randomised study of intensive insulin treatment on long term survival after acute myocardial infarction in patients with diabetes mellitus. DIGAMI (Diabetes Mellitus, Insulin Glucose Infusion in Acute Myocardial Infarction) Study Group. *BMJ* 1997;314:1512–1515.

58. Kurbaan AS, Bowker TJ, Ilsley CD, et al. Difference in the mortality of the CABRI diabetic and nondiabetic populations and its relation to coronary artery disease and the revascularization mode. *Am J Cardiol* 2001;87:947–950.

59. Abizaid A, Costa MA, et al. Clinical and economic impact of diabetes mellitus on percutaneous and surgical treatment of multivessel coronary disease patients indights form the arterial revascularization therapy study (ARTS) trial. Circulation 2001;104:533–538.

60. Kleiman NS, Lincoff AM, Kereiakes DJ, et al. Diabetes mellitus, glycoprotein IIb/IIIa blockade, and heparin: evidence for a complex interaction in a multicenter trial. EPILOG Investigators. *Circulation* 1998;97:1912–1920.

61. Marso SP, Lincoff AM, Ellis SG, et al. Optimizing the percutaneous interventional outcomes for patients with diabetes mellitus: results of the EPISTENT (Evaluation of platelet IIb/IIIa inhibitor for stenting trial) diabetic substudy. *Circulation* 1999;100:2477–2484.

62. The EPISTENT Investigators. Randomised placebo-controlled and balloon-angioplasty-controlled trial to assess safety of coronary stenting with use of platelet glycoprotein-IIb/IIIa blockade. The EPISTENT Investigators. Evaluation of platelet IIb/IIIa inhibitor for stenting. *Lancet* 1998;352:87–92.

63. Topol EJ, Mark DB, Lincoff AM, et al. Outcomes at 1 year and economic implications of platelet glycoprotein IIb/IIIa blockade in patients undergoing coronary stenting: results from a multicentre randomised trial. EPISTENT Investigators. Evaluation of Platelet IIb/IIIa Inhibitor for Stenting. *Lancet* 1999;354:2019–2024. [Published erratum appears in *Lancet* 2000;355:1104].

64. The EPIC Investigation. Use of a monoclonal antibody directed against the platelet glycoprotein IIb/IIIa receptor in high-risk coronary angioplasty. *N Engl J Med* 1994;330:956–961.

65. Bhatt DL, Marso SP, Lincoff AM, et al. Abciximab reduces mortality in diabetics following percutaneous coronary intervention. *J Am Coll Cardiol* 2000;35:922–928.

66. UK Prospective Diabetes Study Group. Intensive blood-glucose control with sulphonylureas or insulin compared with conventional treatment and risk of complications in patients with type 2 diabetes (UKPDS 33). *Lancet* 1998;352:837–853.

67. UK Prospective Diabetes Study Group. Effect of intensive blood-glucose control with metformin on complications in overweight patients with type 2 diabetes (UKPDS 34). *Lancet* 1998;352:854–865.

68. Theroux P, Alexander J, Pharand C, et al. Glycoprotein IIb/IIIa receptor blockade improves outcomes in diabetic patients presenting with unstable angina/Non-ST-elevation myocardial

Cardiovascular disorders

infarction results from the platelet receptor inhibitor in ischemic syndrome management in patients limited by unstable signs and symptoms. *Circulation* 2000;102:2466–2472.

69. Hasdai D, Granger CB, Srivatsa S, et al. Diabetes mellitus and outcome after primary coronary angioplasty for acute myocardial infarction: lessons from the GUSTO-IIb angioplasty study. *J Am Coll Cardiol* 2000;35:1502–1512.

Janine Malcolm
Fellow, Endocrinology and Metabolism

Hilary Meggison
Fellow, Endocrinology and Metabolism

Ottawa Hospital
Ottawa
Canada

Ronald Sigal
Assistant Professor of Medicine and Human Kinetics
University of Ottawa
Ottawa
Canada

Competing interests: RS has received speaker's fees from Aventis (manufacturer of glyburide, metformin, glimepiride, ramipril, and insulin glargine), Novo Nordisk (manufacturer of insulin and repaglinide), and Pfizer (manufacturer of atorvastatin). He has received reimbursement for travel expenses from Bristol-Myers Squibb (manufacturer of pravastatin), Aventis, and Pfizer, and has received consulting fees from Pfizer. HM and JM none declared.

TABLE 1 Primary prevention of cardiovascular events in people with diabetes: evidence from systematic reviews and randomised trials (see text, p 52).

Study	Interventions	Study type	Duration (years)	Outcome	Events / Sample size (%)*		NNT	95% CI for NNT
					Intervention	Control		
Antihypertensive medication								
UKPDS Hypertension Study[34,37]	"Tight" target BP (≤ 150/≤ 85) with captopril or atenolol v "less tight" target (≤ 180/≤ 105)	RCT	8.4	AMI (fatal or non-fatal) Stroke Peripheral vascular events	107/758 (14%) 38/758 (5.0%) 8/758 (1.1%)	83/390 (21%) 34/390 (8.7%) 8/390 (2.1%)	14 27 ND	9 to 35 18 to 116 ND
HOT[36]	Felodipine and ACE inhibitor, or β blocker, with 3 distinct target BPs	RCT	3.8	AMI (fatal or non-fatal), stroke (fatal or non-fatal), or other cardiovascular death	22/499 (4.4%) Target diastolic BP 80 mmHg	45/501 (9.0%) Target diastolic BP 90 mmHg	22	16 to 57
FACET[31]	Fosinopril v amlodipine	RCT	2.9	AMI, stroke, or admission to hospital for angina	14/189 (7.4%) Fosinopril	27/191 (14%) Amlodipine	15	10 to 199
ABCD[32]	Enalapril v nisoldipine	RCT	5	AMI (fatal or non-fatal)	5/235 (2.1%) Enalapril	25/235 (11%) Nisoldipine	12	10 to 19
Syst-Eur[22]	Nitrendipine; enalapril ± hydrochlorothiazide (20 mm Hg BP lowering) v placebo	RCT	2	MI, CHF, or sudden cardiac death	13/252 (5%)	31/240 (13%)	13	10 to 31

TABLE 1 continued

					Treatment	Control	NNT	CI
Lipid-regulating agents								
AFCAPS/TexCAPS[38]	Lovastatin	RCT	5	MI, unstable angina, or sudden cardiac death	4/84 (4.8%)	6/71 (8.5%)	27	NS
SENDCAP[40]	Bezafibrate	RCT	3	MI or new ischaemic changes on ECG	5/64 (7.8%)	16/64 (25%)	6	5 to 20
Helsinki[39]	Gemfibrozil	RCT	5	MI or cardiac death	2/59 (3.4%)	8/76 (10.5%)	14	NS
HPS[41]	Simvastatin v placebo	RCT	5	CHD, stroke, revascularisation	133/1455 (9.1%)	197/1457 (13.5%)	23	15 to 48
Blood glucose control								
UKPDS[65]	Intensive treatment with insulin and/or sulphonylurea v conventional treatment	RCT	5	MI (fatal or non-fatal)	387/2729 (14.2%)	186/1138 (16.3%)	46	NS
UKPDS[67]	Intensive treatment with metformin v conventional treatment	RCT	5	MI (fatal or non-fatal)	39/342 (11%)	73/411 (18%)	16	10 to 71
DCCT[53,54]	Intensive insulin treatment in type 1 diabetes	RCT	6.5	Major macrovascular events‡	23/711 (3.2%)	40/730 (5.5%)	45	28 to 728
Aspirin								
Physicians' Health Study[48]	Aspirin	RCT	5	MI (fatal or non-fatal)	11/275 (4.0%)	26/258 (10%)	16	12 to 47
ETDRS (mixed primary and secondary prevention)[49]	Aspirin	RCT	5	MI (fatal or non-fatal)	289/1856 (15.6%)	335/1855 (18.1%)	39	21 to 716

*People with diabetes only. ‡Combined MI (fatal or non-fatal), sudden cardiac death, revascularisation procedure, angina with coronary artery disease confirmed by angiography or by non-invasive testing, stroke, lower limb amputation, peripheral arterial events requiring revascularisation, claudication with angiographic evidence of peripheral vascular disease. ACE, angiotensin converting enzyme; AMI, acute myocardial infarction; BP, blood pressure; CHD, coronary heart disease; CHF, chronic heart failure; CVD, cardiovascular disease; ECG, electrocardiogram; MI, myocardial infarction; ND, no data; NNT, number needed to treat; NS, not significant; RCT, randomised

TABLE 2 Secondary prevention of cardiovascular events in people with diabetes (see text, p 57).

Study	Interventions	Study Type	Duration (years)	Outcome	Events / sample size (%)*		NNT	95% CI for NNT
					Intervention	Control		
Lipid-regulating agents								
4S[42]	Simvastatin	RCT	5.4	CHD death or non-fatal MI	24/105 (23%)	44/97 (45%)	5	3 to 10
CARE[45]	Pravastatin	RCT	5	Coronary disease death, non-fatal MI, or revascularisation	81/282 (29%)	112/304 (37%)	12	7 to 194
LIPID[43]	Pravastatin	RCT	6.1	CHD death or non-fatal MI	76/396 (19%)	88/386 (23%)	28	NS
Veterans[44]	Gemfibrozil	RCT	5.1	CHD death or non-fatal MI	88/309 (29%)	116/318 (37%)	13	7 to 144
Blood glucose control								
DIGAMI[56,57]	Insulin infusion followed by intensive insulin treatment v usual care	RCT	3.4	Overall mortality	102/306 (33%)	138/314 (44%)	9	6 to 33
Antiplatelet treatments								
Antiplatelet trialists[50]	Aspirin v placebo	SR	Median 2 years	CVD mortality and morbidity	415/2248 (19%)	502/2254 (22%)	26	17 to 66
PRISM-PLUS[68]	Tirofiban plus heparin v heparin alone	RCT	180 days	Death or MI	Tirofiban plus heparin 16/169 (11.2%)	Heparin alone 37/193 (19.2%)	13	7 to 146
Revascularisation								
ARTS[59]	CABG v PTCA and stent	RCT	1	Death, MI, revascularisation	CABG 15/96 (15.6%)	PTCA and stent 41/112 (36.6%)	5	3 to 11
GUSTO IIb[69]	PTCA v alteplase	RCT	2	Death, non-fatal reinfarction, or disabling stroke	PTCA 11/99 (11%)	Alteplase 13/78 (16%)	18	NS
BARI[52]	CABG v PTCA	RCT	7.7	Death or non-fatal Q wave MI	CABG 60/173 (35%)	PTCA 85/170 (50%)	7	4 to 21
CABRI[58]	CABG v PTCA	RCT	4	Death	CABG 8/63 (12.7%)	PTCA 14/62 (22.6%)	10	NS
EPIC[64]/EPILOG[60]/EPISTENT[61-63]	Abciximab v control	Pooled	1	Overall death rate	26/540 (4.8%)	21/844 (2.5%)	43	23 to 422
EPIC[64]/EPILOG[60]/EPISTENT[61-63]	Abciximab v control	Pooled	1	Death or non-fatal MI	185/540 (34%)	246/844 (29%)	20	9 to 1423

*People with diabetes only. CABG, coronary artery bypass grafting; CHD, coronary heart disease; CVD, cardiovascular disease; MI, myocardial infarction;

TABLE 3 Mixed primary and secondary prevention of cardiovascular events in people with diabetes (see text, p 52).

Interventions	Study type	Duration (years)	Outcome	Events / sample size (%) (people with diabetes only)		NNT	95% CI for NNT
				Intervention	Control		
Antihypertensive medication							
ACE inhibitors v diuretics or calcium channel blockers[28]	Meta-analysis	2.8 to 6.2	CVD death, MI, CHF, angina, or stroke.	ACE inhibitor 158/733	Diuretics or calcium channel blockers 266/789	6	4 to 8
Captopril v diuretics and/or β blockers[33]	RCT	6	Fatal and non-fatal MI, stroke, CV deaths	39/309 (13%)	67/263 (26%)	15	9 to 93
Enalapril or nisoldipine v placebo[27]	RCT	5	AMI (fatal or non-fatal)	68/237 (29%)	66/243 (27%)	65	11 to 16
Enalapril v placebo[27]	RCT	5	AMI (fatal or non-fatal)	67/237 (28%)	67/234 (29%)	72	21 to 15
Losartan v atenolol[35]	RCT	4	CV death, stroke, MI	39/586 (7%)	53/609 (9%)	47	20 to 109
Ramipril 10 mg daily versus placebo[26]	RCT	4.5	MI, stroke, or CVD. Overall mortality	277/1808 (15%) 196/1808 (11%)	351/1769 (20%) 240/1769 (14%)	22 32	14 to 43 19 to 98
Lipid-regulating agents							
Micronised fenofibrate v placebo[47]	RCT	3.8 (including 6 months' follow up)	Death or MI	15/207 (7.2%)	21/111(10%)	37	NS

*People with diabetes only. ACE, angiotensin-converting enzyme; CHF, congestive heart failure; CVD, cardiovascular disease; M, myocardial infarction; NS, not significant.

Search date May 2002

Margaret Thorogood, Melvyn Hillsdon, and Carolyn Summerbell

INTERVENTIONS

*In terms of producing the
    intended behavioural change

See glossary, p 92

Key Messages

- **Acupuncture for smoking cessation** One systematic review has found no significant difference in rates of smoking cessation at 1 year with acupuncture versus control.

- **Advice from nurses to quit smoking** One systematic review has found that advice to quit smoking versus no advice significantly increased the rate of quitting at 1 year.

- **Advice from physicians and trained counsellors to quit smoking** Systematic reviews have found that simple, one off advice from a physician during a routine consultation is associated with 2% of smokers quitting smoking and not relapsing for 1 year. Advice from trained counsellors (who are neither doctors nor nurses) increases quit rates compared with minimal intervention.

- **Advice on cholesterol lowering diet** Systematic reviews have found that advice on cholesterol lowering diet (i.e. advice to lower total fat intake or increase the ratio of polyunsaturated to saturated fatty acid) leads to a small reduction in blood cholesterol concentrations in the long term (≥ 6 months).

- **Advice on diet and exercise supported by behavioural therapy for the encouragement of weight loss** Systematic reviews and subsequent RCTs have found that a combination of advice on diet and exercise supported by behavioural therapy is probably more effective than either diet or exercise advice alone in the treatment of obesity, and might lead to sustained weight loss.

- **Advice on reducing sodium intake to reduce blood pressure** Systematic reviews have found that salt restriction significantly reduces blood pressure in people with hypertension, and have found limited evidence that salt restriction is effective in preventing hypertension. One RCT found limited evidence that advice on restricting salt intake was less effective than advice on weight reduction in preventing hypertension.

- **Anxiolytics for smoking cessation** One systematic review found no significant difference in quit rates with anxiolytics versus control.

- **Bupropion as part of a smoking cessation programme** One systematic review of antidepressants used as part of a smoking cessation programme has found that bupropion increases quit rates at 1 year.

- **Counselling people at high risk of disease to quit smoking** Systematic reviews and subsequent RCTs have found that antismoking advice improves smoking cessation in people at higher risk of smoking related disease.

- **Counselling pregnant women to quit smoking** Two systematic reviews have found that antismoking interventions in pregnant women increase abstinence rates during pregnancy and reduce the risk of low birthweight babies. Interventions without nicotine replacement were as effective as nicotine replacement in healthy non-pregnant women.

- **Counselling sedentary people to increase physical activity** We found weak evidence from systematic reviews and subsequent RCTs that counselling sedentary people increases physical activity compared with no intervention. Limited evidence from RCTs suggests that consultation with an exercise specialist rather than a physician may increase physical activity at 1 year.

Cardiovascular disorders

Changing behaviour

- **Exercise advice to women over 80 years** One RCT found that exercise advice delivered in the home by physiotherapists increased physical activity and reduced the risk of falling in women over 80 years.

- **Nicotine replacement in smokers who smoke at least 10 cigarettes daily** One systematic review and one subsequent RCT have found that nicotine replacement is an effective additional component of cessation strategies in smokers who smoke at least 10 cigarettes daily. We found no clear evidence that any method of delivery of nicotine is more effective than others. We found limited evidence from three RCTs with follow up of 2–6 years that the additional benefit of nicotine replacement treatment on quit rates reduced with time.

- **Physical exercise to aid smoking cessation** One systematic review found very limited evidence that exercise might increase smoking cessation.

- **Self help materials for people who want to stop smoking** One systematic review found that self help materials slightly improve smoking cessation compared with no intervention. It found that individually tailored materials were more effective than standard or stage based materials and that telephone counselling increased the effectiveness of postal self help materials.

- **Training health professionals to give advice on smoking cessation** One systematic review has found that training professionals increases the frequency of antismoking interventions being offered, but found no good evidence that antismoking interventions are more effective if the health professionals delivering the interventions received training. One RCT found that a structured intervention delivered by trained community pharmacists increased smoking cessation rates compared to usual care delivered by untrained community pharmacists.

DEFINITION	Cigarette smoking, diet, and level of physical activity are important in the aetiology of many chronic diseases. Individual change in behaviour has the potential to decrease the burden of chronic disease, particularly cardiovascular disease. This topic focuses on the evidence that specific interventions lead to changed behaviour.
INCIDENCE/ PREVALENCE	In the developed world, the decline in smoking has slowed and the prevalence of regular smoking is increasing in young people. A sedentary lifestyle is becoming increasingly common and the prevalence of obesity is increasing rapidly.
AIMS	To encourage individuals to reduce or abandon unhealthy behaviours and to take up healthy behaviours; to support the maintenance of these changes in the long term.
OUTCOMES	Ideal outcomes are clinical, and relate to the underlying conditions (longevity, quality of life, and rate of stroke or myocardial infarction). However, the focus of this topic and the outcomes reported by most studies are proxy outcomes, such as the proportion of people changing behaviour (e.g. stopping smoking) in a specified period.
METHODS	*Clinical Evidence* update search and appraisal May 2002.

| QUESTION | Which interventions reduce cigarette smoking? |

| OPTION | ADVICE TO QUIT SMOKING |

Systematic reviews have found that simple, one off advice from a physician during a routine consultation is associated with at least 2% of smokers quitting smoking and not relapsing for 1 year. Additional encouragement or support may increase the effectiveness of the advice (by a further 3%). Individual advice from a psychologist achieves a similar quit rate (3%), and advice from trained nurse counsellors, or from trained counsellors who are neither doctors nor nurses, increases quit rates compared with minimal intervention. We found limited evidence from one systematic review that telephone counselling may improve quit rates compared to interventions with no personal contact. One systematic review found that self help materials slightly improve smoking cessation compared with no intervention. It found that individually tailored materials were more effective than standard or stage based materials and that telephone counselling increased the effectiveness of postal self help materials.

Benefits: We found four systematic reviews[1-4] and one later RCT.[5] **Physicians:** The first review (search date 2000, 34 RCTs, 28 000 smokers) considered advice given by physicians, most often in the primary care setting, but also in hospitals and other clinics.[1] It found that brief advice improved quit rates compared to no advice (16 trials, 12 with follow up for at least 1 year; 451/7705 [5.9%] with brief advice v 241/5870 [4.1%] with no advice; meta-analysis OR 1.69, 95% CI 1.45 to 1.98; ARI 2.5%; NNT 40). Intensive advice slightly improved quit rates compared with minimal advice among smokers not at high risk of disease (10 trials, 7 with follow up for at least 1 year; OR with intensive v minimal advice 1.23, 95% CI 1.02 to 1.49). One subsequent RCT tested a brief (10 min) intervention given by general practitioners who had received a 2 hour training.[5] The intervention increased the abstinence rate at 12 months (7.3% with control v 13.4% with intervention; NNT 16; P < 0.05). **Counsellors:** The second systematic review (search date 1998, 11 RCTs) of interventions by counsellors (other than doctors and nurses) trained in smoking cessation used a broad definition of counselling, which included all contacts with a smoker that lasted at least 10 minutes. Follow up was at least 1 year for six of the RCTs, and was at least 6 months for the rest. The review found that counselling increased the rate of quitting (263/1381 [14%] quit with counselling v 194/1899 [10%] with control; OR of quitting 1.55, 95% CI 1.27 to 1.90).[2] **Nurses:** The third review (search date 2001, 22 RCTs, 5 with follow up for < 1 year) considered the effectiveness of smoking interventions delivered by a nurse. It found that advice from a nurse increased the rate of quitting by the end of follow up (meta-analysis of 18 studies: 646/4836 [13.4%] quit with advice v 405/3356 [12.1%] with control; OR 1.50, 95% CI 1.29 to 1.73).[3] **Telephone advice:** The final systematic review (search date 2000, 23 RCTs) considered counselling delivered by telephone.[4] Ten of the included trials (9 with follow up for at least 12 months) compared proactive telephone counselling versus minimum intervention (involving no person to person contact). Pooled analysis was not possible because of statistical heterogeneity among trials. However, three trials found that telephone counselling was significantly more effective than minimum intervention; four trials found a non-significant benefit, and none of the trials found significant harms of telephone counselling. **Self help materials:** We found one systematic review (search date 1999, 45 RCTs)[6] and one subsequent RCT[7] that examined effects of providing materials giving advice and information to smokers attempting to give up on their own. It found that self help materials without face to face contact slightly improved smoking cessation compared with no intervention (9 trials, 8 of them with at least 12 months' follow up; OR 1.23, 95% CI 1.02 to 1.49; NNT 100). Individually tailored materials were more effective than standard or stage based materials (8 trials, OR for cessation 1.41, 95% CI 1.14 to 1.75).[6] One subsequent RCT compared postal self help materials alone versus postal self help plus telephone counselling.[7] It found that adding telephone counselling improved quit rates at 12 months compared with self help materials alone (OR 2.2, 95% CI 1.1 to 4.6).[7]

Harms: We found no evidence of harm.

Comment: The effects of advice may appear small, but a year on year reduction of 2% in the number of smokers would represent a significant public health gain (see smoking cessation under primary prevention, p 155). In the systematic review of advice provided by nurses,[3] there was significant heterogeneity of the study results and many studies may not have been adequately randomised (7/18 studies [39%] did not specify the randomisation method and 3 [19%] used an inadequate form of randomisation).

OPTION   **NICOTINE REPLACEMENT**

One systematic review and one subsequent RCT have found that nicotine replacement is an effective component of cessation strategies in smokers who smoke at least 10 cigarettes daily. Fifteen such smokers would have to be treated with nicotine replacement to produce one extra non-smoker at 12 months, but this overestimates effectiveness because relapse will continue after 12 months. Higher dose chewing gum (4 mg) is more effective than lower dose chewing gum (2 mg) in very dependent smokers. We found no clear evidence that any one method of delivery of nicotine is more effective, or evidence of further benefit after 8 weeks' treatment with patches. Long term relapse may occur in people who quit, but the review found that the rate of relapse was not greater in those who quit with the aid of nicotine replacement. Abstinence after 1 week is a strong predictor of 12 month abstinence.

Benefits: **Abstinence at 12 months:** We found one systematic review (search date 2001) that identified 51 trials of nicotine chewing gum, 33 trials of nicotine transdermal patches, four of nicotine intranasal spray, four of inhaled nicotine, and two of sublingual tablets.[8] All forms of nicotine replacement were more effective than placebo. When the abstinence rates for all trials were pooled according to the longest duration of follow up available, nicotine replacement compared with placebo increased the odds of abstinence (1508/7674 [19.7%] with nicotine replacement v 1110/9613 [11.5%] with placebo; OR 1.66, 95% CI 1.52 to 1.81). The review found no significant difference in abstinence with different forms of nicotine replacement in indirect comparisons (OR 1.66 for nicotine chewing gum v 2.27 for nicotine nasal spray) or direct comparisons (1 RCT, inhaler v patch; OR 0.57, 95% CI 0.20 to 1.62). In trials that directly compared 4 mg with 2 mg nicotine chewing gum, the higher dose improved abstinence in highly dependent smokers (OR 2.18, 95% CI 1.49 to 3.17). High dose versus standard dose patches slightly increased abstinence (6 RCTs; OR 1.21, 95% CI 1.03 to 1.42). The review found no evidence of a difference in effectiveness for 16 hour patches versus 24 hour patches, and no difference in effect in trials where the dose was tapered compared with those where the patches were withdrawn abruptly. Use of the patch for 8 weeks was as effective as longer use, and there was very weak evidence in favour of nicotine replacement in relapsed smokers. One included RCT (3585 people) found that abstinence at 1 week was a strong predictor of 12 month abstinence (25% of those abstinent at 1 wk were abstinent at 12 months v 2.7% of those not abstinent at 1 wk).[9] One meta-analysis of relapse rates in nicotine replacement trials found that nicotine replacement increased abstinence at 12 months, but that continued nicotine replacement did not significantly affect relapse rates between 6 weeks and 12 months.[10] **Longer term abstinence:** We found three RCTs[11-13] that found nicotine replacement does not affect long term abstinence. In one RCT that compared nicotine spray versus placebo, 47 people abstinent at 1 year were followed for up to a further 2 years and 6 months, after which there was still a significant, although smaller, difference in abstinence (in the longer term 15.4% abstinent with nicotine spray v 9.3% with placebo; NNT for 1 extra person to abstain 7 at 1 year v 11 at 3.5 years).[11] The second RCT compared 5 months of nicotine patches plus nicotine spray versus the same patches plus a placebo spray. It found no significant difference between treatments after 6 years (16.2% abstinent with nicotine spray v 8.5% with placebo spray; P = 0.08).[12] The third trial compared patches delivering different nicotine doses versus placebo patches. The trial followed everyone that quit at 6 weeks for a further 4–5 years and found no significant difference in relapse between the groups. Overall, 73% of people who quit at 6 weeks relapsed.[13]

Harms: Nicotine chewing gum has been associated with hiccups, gastrointestinal disturbances, jaw pain, and orodental problems. Nicotine transdermal patches have been associated with skin sensitivity and irritation. Nicotine inhalers and nasal spray have been associated with local irritation at the site of administration. Nicotine sublingual tablets have been reported to cause hiccups, burning, smarting sensations in the mouth, sore throat, coughing, dry lips, and mouth ulcers.[14]

Changing behaviour

Comment: Nicotine replacement may not represent an "easy cure" for nicotine addiction, but it does improve the cessation rate. The evidence suggests that the majority of smokers attempting cessation fail at any one attempt or relapse over the next 5 years. Multiple attempts may be needed.

OPTION   ACUPUNCTURE

One systematic review has found no evidence that acupuncture increases rates of smoking cessation at 12 months.

Benefits: We found one systematic review (search date 2002, 22 RCTs, 4158 adults, 330 young people aged 12–18 years) comparing acupuncture with sham acupuncture, other treatment, or no treatment.[15] Seven RCTs (2701 people) reported abstinence after at least 12 months. The review found no significant difference in smoking cessation with acupuncture versus control at 12 months (OR 1.08, 95% CI 0.77 to 1.52).

Harms: None were documented.

Comment: None.

OPTION   PHYSICAL EXERCISE

One systematic review found limited evidence that exercise might increase smoking cessation.

Benefits: We found one systematic review (search date 1999, 8 RCTs) of exercise versus control interventions.[16] Four small RCTs in the review reported point prevalence of non-smoking at 12 months and found no significant benefit from exercise, but these studies were insufficiently powered to exclude a clinically important effect. One RCT (281 women) found that three exercise sessions a week for 12 weeks plus a cognitive behavioural programme (see glossary, p 92) improved continuous abstinence from smoking at 12 months compared with the behavioural programme alone (16/134 [12%] with exercise v 8/147 [5%] with control; ARR +6.5%, 95% CI −19 to +0.0; RR 2.2, 95% CI 0.98 to 4.5).[17]

Harms: None were documented.

Comment: None.

OPTION   ANTIDEPRESSANT AND ANXIOLYTIC TREATMENT

Systematic reviews have found that quit rates are significantly increased by bupropion, but not by moclobemide or anxiolytics.

Benefits: **Antidepressants:** We found one systematic review of antidepressants (search date 2001, 18 RCTs).[18] Eight of the RCTs (2649 people) reported 12 month cessation rates. It found that bupropion increased quit rates compared with placebo at 6–12 months (calculated by combining results of 4 RCTs with 12 month follow up and 3 RCTs with 6 month follow up; OR of quitting with bupropion v placebo 2.54, 95% CI 1.90 to 3.41; NNT 10). The review found no evidence of statistical heterogeneity between the two follow up times.[18] One RCT included in the review compared combined bupropion plus a nicotine patch versus patch alone. It found that combined treatment improved cessation compared with patch alone (OR 2.65, 95% CI 1.58 to 4.45), but was not more effective than bupropion alone. Another included RCT compared different doses of bupropion (100–300 mg/day) and found that cessation rate was linearly related to dose. Three other included RCTs (2 with 6 months' and 1 with 12 months' follow up) found that nortriptyline improved long term (6–12 month) abstinence rates compared with placebo (OR 2.77, 95% CI 1.73 to 4.44). One RCT of moclobemide found no significant difference in abstinence at 12 months. **Anxiolytics:** We found one systematic review of anxiolytics (search date 2000, 6 RCTs).[19] Four of the RCTs (626 people) reporting 12 month cessation rates found no significant increase in abstinence with anxiolytics versus control treatment.[19]

Harms: Headache, insomnia, and dry mouth were reported in people using bupropion.[19] Nortriptyline can cause sedation and urinary retention, and can be dangerous in overdose. One large RCT found that discontinuation rates caused by adverse events were 3.8% with placebo, 6.6% for nicotine replacement treatment, 11.9% for bupropion, and 11.4% for bupropion plus nicotine replacement treatment.[20] Anxiolytics may cause dependence and withdrawal problems, tolerance, paradoxical effects, and impair driving ability. Allergic reactions to bupropion have been reported in about 1 in 1000 people.

Comment: None.

QUESTION   **Are smoking cessation interventions more effective in people at high risk of smoking related disease?**

OPTION   **IN PREGNANT WOMEN**

Two systematic reviews have found that antismoking interventions in pregnant women increase abstinence rates and decrease the risk of giving birth to low birthweight babies. The increase in abstinence with non-nicotine replacement interventions was similar to the increase found in trials of nicotine replacement in men and non-pregnant women. One RCT found no evidence that nicotine patches increased quit rates in pregnant women compared with placebo, although birthweight was greater in babies born to mothers given active patches. One RCT found no evidence that a brief intervention delivered by midwives at the booking visit improved quit rates compared with no intervention.

Benefits: We found two systematic reviews[21,22] and three additional RCTs.[23–25] The most recent review (search date 1998, 44 RCTs) assessed smoking cessation interventions in pregnancy. It found that smoking cessation programmes improved abstinence (OR of continued smoking in late pregnancy with antismoking programmes v no programmes 0.53, 95% CI 0.47 to 0.60; NNT 16).[22] The findings were similar if the analysis was restricted to trials in which abstinence was confirmed by means other than self reporting. The review also found that antismoking programmes reduced the risk of low birthweight babies, but found no evidence of an effect on the rates of very low birthweight babies or perinatal mortality, although the power to detect such effects was low (OR for low birthweight babies 0.80, 95% CI 0.69 to 0.99). The review calculated that of 100 smokers attending a first antenatal visit, 10 stopped spontaneously and a further six to seven stopped as the result of a smoking cessation programme. Five included trials examined the effects of interventions to prevent relapse in 800 women who had quit smoking. Collectively, these trials found no evidence that the interventions reduced relapse rate.[22] One earlier systematic review (search date not stated, 10 RCTs, 4815 pregnant women)[21] of antismoking interventions included one trial of physician advice, one trial of advice by a health educator, one trial of group sessions, and seven trials of behavioural therapy based on self help manuals. Cessation rates among trials ranged from 1.9–16.7% in the control groups and from 7.1–36.1% in the intervention groups. The review found that antismoking interventions significantly increased the rate of quitting (ARI with intervention v no intervention 7.6%, 95% CI 4.3% to 10.8%).[21] One additional RCT found that nicotine patches did not significantly alter quit rates in pregnant women compared with placebo. But active patches were associated with greater birthweight in babies born to treated mothers (mean difference in birthweight with nicotine v placebo 186 g, 95% CI 35 g to 336 g).[23] The second RCT (1120 pregnant women) compared a brief (10–15 min) smoking intervention delivered by trained midwives at booking interviews versus usual care.[24] It found no significant difference in smoking behaviour between women receiving intervention versus usual care (abstinence in final 12 wks of pregnancy until birth 17% in each group; abstinence for 6 months after birth 7% with intervention v 8% with control). The intervention was difficult to implement (see comment below). The third RCT compared motivational interviewing (see glossary, p 93) with usual care in 269 women in their 28th week of pregnancy who had smoked in the past month.[25] It found no significant differences in cessation rate between intervention and control group at 34th week or at 6 months post partum.

Harms: None documented.

Comment: The recent review found that some women quit smoking before their first antenatal visit, and the majority of these will remain abstinent.[22] Recruitment to the RCT comparing midwife delivered intervention versus usual care was slow. Midwives reported that the intervention was difficult to implement because of a lack of time to deliver the intervention at the booking appointment.[24]

OPTION   **IN PEOPLE AT HIGH RISK OF DISEASE**

Systematic reviews and two subsequent RCTs have found that antismoking advice improves smoking cessation in people at high risk of smoking related disease. One RCT found no added benefit from a single session intervention that included a carbon monoxide reading.

Benefits: We found no trials in which the same intervention was used in high and low risk people. We found one systematic review (search date not stated, 4 RCTs, 13 208 healthy men at high risk of heart disease),[21] one systematic review among people admitted to hospital (search date 2000, 15 RCTs),[26] and two subsequent RCTs.[27,28] The first review found that antismoking advice improved smoking cessation rates compared with control interventions among healthy men at high risk of heart disease (ARI of smoking cessation 21%, 95% CI 10 to 31; NNT 5, 95% CI 4 to 10).[21] One early trial (223 men) that was included in the review used non-random allocation after myocardial infarction. The intervention group was given intensive advice by the therapeutic team while in the coronary care unit. The trial found that the self reported cessation rate at 1 year or more was higher in the intervention group than the control group (63% quit in the intervention group v 28% in the control group; ARI of quitting 36%, 95% CI 23 to 48).[29] The second review included seven trials (6 of them with at least 12 months' duration) of high intensity behavioural interventions (defined as contact in hospital plus active follow up for at least 1 month) among smokers admitted to hospital. The review found that active intervention increased quit rates compared to usual care (OR 1.82, 95% CI 1.49 to 2.22; NNT about 10). We found two RCTs not included in the reviews. The first compared postal advice on smoking cessation versus no intervention in men aged 30–45 years with either a history of asbestos exposure, or forced expiratory volume in 1 second in the lowest quartile for their age. Postal advice increased the self reported sustained cessation rate at 1 year compared with no intervention (5.6% with postal advice v 3.5%; P < 0.05; NNT 48).[27] The second RCT compared brief advice (consultation lasting 20–30 min plus a carbon monoxide reading) versus usual care in 540 smokers following myocardial infarction or cardiac bypass surgery.[29] At 12 months the trial found no significant difference between groups for abstinence rates (41% abstinent with usual care v 37% with intervention).[28]

Harms: None were documented.

Comment: There was heterogeneity in the four trials included in the review among healthy men at high risk of heart disease, partly because of a less intense intervention in one trial and the recording of a change from cigarettes to other forms of tobacco as success in another. One of the included trials was weakened by use of self reported smoking cessation as an outcome and non-random allocation to the intervention.[29]

QUESTION   **Does training of professionals increase the effectiveness of smoking cessation interventions?**

One systematic review has found that training professionals increases the frequency of antismoking interventions being offered, but found no good evidence that antismoking interventions are more effective if the health professionals delivering the interventions received training. One RCT found that a structured intervention delivered by trained community pharmacists increased smoking cessation rates compared to usual care delivered by untrained community pharmacists.

Benefits: We found one systematic review[30] and one subsequent RCT.[31] The review (search date 2000, 9 RCTs)[30] included eight RCTs of training medical practitioners and one RCT of training dental practitioners to give antismoking advice. All the trials took place in the USA. The training was provided on a group basis, and variously included lectures, videotapes, role plays, and discussion. The importance of setting quit dates and offering follow up was emphasised in most of the training programmes. The review found no good evidence that training professionals leads to higher quit rates in people receiving antismoking interventions from those professionals, although training increased the frequency with which such interventions were offered. Three of the trials used prompts and reminders to practitioners to deploy smoking cessation techniques, and found that prompts increased the frequency of health professional interventions.[30] The later RCT compared a structured smoking cessation intervention delivered by community pharmacists, who had received 3 hours of training versus no specific training or antismoking intervention.[31] Intervention delivered by trained pharmacists improved abstinence compared to usual care (AR of abstinence at 12 months 14.3% with intervention v 2.7% with usual care; RR 5.3; NNT 9; CIs not reported; P < 0.001).

Harms: None were documented.

Comment: The results of the systematic review should be interpreted with caution because there were variations in the way the analysis allowed for the unit of randomisation.

QUESTION Which interventions increase physical activity in sedentary people?

OPTION COUNSELLING

We found weak evidence from systematic reviews and subsequent RCTs that sedentary people can be encouraged to increase their physical activity. Interventions that encourage moderate rather than vigorous exercise, and do not require attendance at a special facility, may be more successful. Increases in walking in previously sedentary women can be sustained over at least 10 years. Brief advice from a physician may lead to short term changes in physical activity, but is probably not effective in increasing physical activity beyond 3 months. We found limited evidence from RCTs that primary care consultation with an exercise specialist may increase physical activity at 1 year compared with no advice. We found limited evidence that in primary care more intensive and prolonged advice programmes are likely to be more effective than brief advice alone, at least among women.

Benefits: We found two systematic reviews[32,33] and ten subsequent RCTs.[34–43] The first review (search date 1996, 11 RCTs based in the USA, 1699 people) assessed single factor physical activity promotion.[32] Seven trials evaluated advice to undertake exercise from home (mainly walking, but including jogging and swimming), and six evaluated advice to undertake facility based exercise (including jogging and walking on sports tracks, endurance exercise, games, swimming, and exercise to music classes). An increase in activity in the intervention groups was seen in trials in which home based moderate exercise was encouraged and regular brief follow up of participants was provided. In most of the trials participants were self selected volunteers, so the effects of the interventions may have been exaggerated. The second systematic review (search date not stated, 3 RCTs, 420 people) compared "lifestyle" physical activity interventions with either standard exercise treatment or a control group.[33] Lifestyle interventions were defined as those concerned with the daily accumulation of moderate or vigorous exercise as part of everyday life. The first RCT (60 adults, 65–85 years old) found significantly more self reported physical activity in the lifestyle group than a standard exercise group. The second RCT (235 people, 35–60 years old) found no significant difference in physical activity between the groups. The third RCT (125 women, 23–54 years old) of encouraging walking found no significant difference in walking levels at 30 months' follow up between people receiving an 8 week behavioural intervention and those receiving a 5 minute telephone call and written information about the benefits of exercise, although both groups increased walking. Nine of the additional trials involved primary care delivered interventions.[34–36,38–43] The two trials in which advice was delivered by an exercise specialist rather than a physician found significant improvement in self reported physical activity at long term (> 6 months) follow up compared with controls.[38,39] Short term improvement was found in two further trials, but not maintained at 9 months or 1 year.[35,36] Two quasi-randomised trials (776 and 1142 people in a primary care setting) tested the effect of brief physician advice plus a postal booklet on physical activity.[37,42] Both found short term improvement in self reported physical activity with the intervention versus control. One of the RCTs continued follow up after 12 months and found that a significant difference was not maintained.[37] One RCT conducted in a primary care setting (874 people) compared behavioural counselling versus behavioural counselling plus telephone support versus physician advice and brief education.[41] At 24 months, interventions including behavioural counselling significantly improved cardiorespiratory fitness compared to the briefer intervention among women, but not men (mean difference in VO_2 max for behavioural counselling plus telephone support v advice 80.7 mL/min, 99.2% CI 8.1 mL/min to 153.2 mL/min). The trial found no significant effect from adding telephone support to behavioural counselling on cardiorespiratory fitness among men or women. However, self reported activity was similar among all treatment groups, for women and men, at 24 months. One RCT (229 women) of encouraging women to increase walking found significantly increased walking in the intervention group at 10 years' follow up (86% of women available for follow up, median estimated calorie expenditure from self reported amount of walking 1344 kcal/wk with encouragement v 924 kcal/wk with no encouragement; $P = 0.01$).[44] A further RCT (260 people in a primary care setting) compared the additional offer of community walks (led by lay people) versus fitness tests and advice alone.[43] It found no significant difference in physical activity at 12 months' follow up (ARR for achieving at least 120 min moderate intensity activity per wk 6%, 95% CI −5% to +16.4%).

Harms: In the trial comparing behavioural counselling versus brief advice, 60% of participants experienced a musculoskeletal event during the 2 years of the study. About half of these required a visit to the physician. About 5% of all participants were admitted to hospital for a suspected cardiovascular event. The trial lacked a non-intervention control group.[41] We found no evidence that counselling people to increase activity levels increased adverse events compared to no counselling.

Comment: Self reporting of effects by people in a trial, especially where blinding to interventions is not possible (as is the case with advice or encouragement), is a potential source of bias. Several trials are in progress, including one in the UK, in which people in primary care have been randomised to two different methods of encouragement to increase walking or to a no intervention arm.

QUESTION What are effects of exercise advice in high risk people?

OPTION IN WOMEN AGED OVER 80 YEARS

One RCT found exercise advice increased physical activity in women aged over 80 years and decreased the risk of falling.

Benefits: We found no systematic review. One RCT (233 women > 80 years old, conducted in New Zealand) compared four visits from a physiotherapist who advised a course of 30 minutes of home based exercises three times a week that was appropriate for the individual versus a similar number of social visits.[45] After 1 year, women who had received physiotherapist visits were significantly more active than women in the control group, and 42% were still completing the recommended exercise programme at least three times a week. The mean annual rate of falls in the intervention group was 0.87 compared with 1.34 in the control group, a difference of 0.47 falls a year (95% CI 0.04 to 0.90).

Harms: No additional harms in the intervention group were reported.

Comment: None.

QUESTION What are the effects on blood cholesterol of dietary advice to reduce fat, increase polyunsaturated fats, and decrease saturated fats?

OPTION COUNSELLING

Systematic reviews have found that advice on eating a cholesterol lowering diet (i.e. advice to reduce fat intake or increase the polyunsaturated to saturated fatty acid ratio in the diet) leads to a small reduction in blood cholesterol concentrations in the long term (6 months or more). We found no evidence to support the effectiveness of such advice in primary care.

Benefits: **Effects on blood cholesterol:** We found three systematic reviews[14,46,47] and two subsequent RCTs that reported biochemical rather than clinical end points.[48,49] None of the reviews included evidence after 1996. One review (search date 1993) identified five trials of cholesterol lowering dietary advice (principally advice from nutritionists or specially trained counsellors) with follow up for 9–18 months.[46] It found a reduction in blood cholesterol concentration in the intervention group of 0.22 mmol/L (95% CI 0.05 mmol/L to 0.39 mmol/L) compared with the control group. There was significant heterogeneity (P < 0.02), with two outlying studies — one showing no effect and one showing a larger effect. This review excluded trials in people at high risk of heart disease. Another systematic review (search date 1994) identified 13 trials of more than 6 months' duration and included people at high risk of heart disease.[14] It found that dietary advice reduced blood cholesterol (mean reduction in blood cholesterol concentration with advice 4.5%, 95% CI 3.9 to 5.1; given a mean baseline cholesterol of 6.3 mmol/L, mean AR about 0.3 mmol/L). The third systematic review (search date 1996, 1 trial,[50] 76 people) found no significant difference between brief versus intensive advice from a general practitioner and dietician on blood cholesterol at 1 year.[47] The first subsequent RCT (186 men and women at high risk of coronary heart disease) compared advice on healthy eating versus no intervention. At 1 year it found no significant differences between groups in total and low density lipoprotein cholesterol concentrations for either sex, even though the reported percentage of energy from fat consumed by both women and men in the advice group decreased significantly compared with that reported by the women and men in the control group.[48] These results may reflect bias caused by self reporting of dietary intake. The second RCT, in 531 men with hypercholesterolaemia (with and without other hyperlipdaemias) and fat intake of about 35%, compared dietary advice aimed at reducing fat intake to 30% versus 26% versus 22%. All interventions were similarly effective for reducing fat intake (total fat intake after intervention about 26% in all groups).[49] **Effects on clinical outcomes:** We found two systematic reviews that reported on morbidity and mortality.[14,51] The first (search date 1994) compared 13 separate and single dietary interventions.[14] It found no significant effect of dietary interventions on total mortality (OR 0.93, 95% CI 0.84 to 1.03) or coronary heart disease mortality (OR 0.93, 95% CI 0.82 to 1.06), but found a reduction in non-fatal myocardial infarction (OR 0.77, 95% CI 0.67 to 0.90). The second review (search date 1999, 27 studies including 40 intervention arms, 30 901 person years) found dietary advice to reduce or modify dietary fat versus no dietary advice had no significant effect on total mortality (HR 0.98, 95% CI 0.86 to 1.12) or cardiovascular disease mortality (HR 0.98, 95% CI 0.77 to 1.07), but significantly reduced cardiovascular disease events (HR 0.84, 95% CI 0.72 to 0.99).[51] RCTs in which people were followed for more than 2 years showed significant reductions in the rate of cardiovascular disease events. The relative protection from cardiovascular disease events was similar in both high and low risk groups, but was significant only in high risk groups.

Harms: We found no evidence about harms.

Comment: The finding of a 0.2–0.3 mmol/L reduction in blood cholesterol in the two systematic reviews accords with the findings of a meta-analysis of the plasma lipid response to changes in dietary fat and cholesterol.[52] The analysis included data from 244 published studies (trial duration 1 day to 6 years), and concluded that adherence to dietary recommendations (30% energy from fat, < 10% saturated fat, and < 300 mg cholesterol/day) compared with average US dietary intake would reduce blood cholesterol by about 5%.

QUESTION **Does dietary advice to reduce sodium intake lead to a sustained fall in blood pressure?**

Systematic reviews and RCTs have found that salt restriction reduces blood pressure in people with normal blood pressure, and in people with hypertension. The effect was more pronounced in older people. We found no evidence of effects on morbidity and mortality.

Benefits: We found three systematic reviews[46,53,54] and three additional RCTs[55–57] about the effects of advice to restrict salt. The first systematic review (search date 1993, 5 trials with follow up for 9–18 months) compared dietary advice (mainly from nutritionists or specially trained counsellors) with control treatment. It found that the advice slightly reduced systolic blood pressure (change in blood pressure, −1.9 mm Hg systolic, 95% CI −3.0 mm Hg to −0.8 mm Hg), but not diastolic blood pressure (−1.2 mm Hg, 95% CI −2.6 mm Hg to +0.2 mm Hg).[46] The second review (search date 1998, 8 RCTs in adults over 44 years with and without hypertension) found no clearly significant systolic blood pressure changes after at least 6 months' follow up with advice on salt restriction versus no dietary advice either in people with hypertension (−2.9 mm Hg, 95% CI −5.8 mm Hg to +0.0 mm Hg) or in people without hypertension (−1.3 mm Hg, 95% CI −2.7 mm Hg to +0.1 mm Hg). Small but significant changes in mean diastolic blood pressure were found in people with hypertension (−2.1 mm Hg, 95% CI −4.0 mm Hg to −0.1 mm Hg) but not in people without hypertension (−0.8 mm Hg, 95% CI −1.8 mm Hg to +0.2 mm Hg).[53] The definitions of hypertension varied between the trials. The third review (search date 1996, 30 RCTs) found that, in people aged over 44 years defined as having hypertension, a reduction in sodium intake of 100 mmol daily resulted in a decrease of 6.3 mm Hg in systolic blood pressure and 2.2 mm Hg in diastolic pressure.[54] For younger people with hypertension, the systolic fall was 2.4 mm Hg and the diastolic fall was negligible. We found three additional RCTs that found similar results.[55–57] The first RCT (975 people) found that advice to restrict salt intake was more effective compared to usual care at 30 months (HR for hypertension, prescription of an antihypertensive drug or a cardiovascular event with advice v usual care 0.69, 95% CI 0.59 to 0.81).[55] Subgroup analysis (585 people) found no evidence that advice to reduce salt intake was more effective than advice to reduce weight among people who were overweight at baseline. The second RCT (208 people, analysis performed on 181 participants) compared weight reduction advice versus salt restriction advice versus no intervention. The weight advice group excluded people who were not overweight, whereas salt restriction and control groups included people regardless of weight. Among people of all weights, salt restriction did not significantly reduce the risk of hypertension at 7 years compared to all controls (AR for hypertension at 7 years 22.4% with advice v 32.9% with control; CI not provided; P = 0.19).

But in overweight people, weight reduction advice significantly reduced hypertension at 7 years compared to overweight control participants (AR for hypertension at 7 years 18.9% with advice v 40.5% in overweight controls; CI not provided; P = 0.02).[56] The third RCT (2382 overweight non-hypertensive people) compared advice to reduce salt versus advice to reduce weight versus both versus usual care. Compared to usual care, advice reduced blood pressure (at 6 months blood pressure decreased by 3.7/2.7 mm Hg with weight loss advice v 2.9/1.6 mm Hg with salt reduction advice v 4.0/2.8 mm Hg with both; P < 0.001 for all comparisons).[57]

Harms: None reported.

Comment: None.

QUESTION   **What are the effects of lifestyle interventions to achieve sustained weight loss?**

Systematic reviews and subsequent RCTs have found that a combination of advice on diet and exercise, supported by behavioural therapy, is probably more effective in achieving weight loss than either diet or exercise advice alone. A low energy, low fat diet is the most effective lifestyle intervention for weight loss. Combined personal and computerised tailoring of weight loss programmes may improve maintenance of weight loss. RCTs have found no significant differences in weight loss between interventions to promote physical activity. Weight regain is likely, but weight loss of 2–6 kg may be sustained over at least 2 years.

Benefits: We found three systematic reviews[58–60] and 17 additional RCTs.[55,61–76] One systematic review (search date 1995) identified 99 studies, including some that tested either dietary or physical activity interventions with or without a behavioural intervention component. The combination of diet and exercise in conjunction with behavioural therapy produced greater weight loss than diet alone. However, this finding was based on the results of one RCT, in which a mean weight loss of 3.8 kg at 1 year was observed in a group receiving diet guidelines and behavioural intervention compared with a significantly different mean loss of 7.9 kg in a group receiving the same intervention plus a programme of walking.[58] The second systematic review of the detection, prevention, and treatment of obesity (search date 1999, 11 RCTs and additional prospective cohort studies) included eight RCTs comparing dietary prescriptions with exercise, counselling, or behavioural therapy for the treatment of obesity, and three RCTs comparing dietary counselling alone with no intervention. In both comparisons, initial weight loss was followed by gradual weight regain once treatment had stopped (mean difference in weight change at least 2 years after baseline, 2–6 kg for dietary prescription trials, and 2–4 kg for dietary counselling trials).[59] The third systematic review (search date 1997) of RCTs and observational studies similarly found that a combination of diet and exercise, supported by behavioural therapy, was more effective than any one or two of these individual interventions.[60] One additional RCT compared advice on an energy restricted diet to advice on a fat restricted diet.[65] Weight loss was greater on an energy restricted diet than on the fat restricted diet at 6 months (−11.2 kg v −6.1 kg; P < 0.001) and at 18 months (−7.5 kg v −1.8 kg; P < 0.001). Seven RCTs focused on physical activity.[61–63,67-69,72] The heterogeneity of interventions makes pooling of data inappropriate, but no major differences were found between the various behavioural therapies and exercise regimes. One RCT[64] found behavioural choice therapy versus standard behavioural therapy resulted in greater weight loss at 12 months (−10.1 kg v −4.3 kg; P < 0.01). One RCT (166 people) compared standard behavioural therapy plus support from friends with standard behavioural therapy without support. It found no additional weight loss at 16 months with social support from friends (−4.7 kg v −3.0 kg, P < 0.3).[66] A further RCT (62 women) found that 1 year weight loss was greater in women following a standard versus a modified cognitive behavioural programme (−3.6 kg v 2.0 kg; P = 0.02).[71] One RCT has found that adding meal replacements to a dietician led group intervention improved weight loss at 1 year (9.1% weight loss with replacements v 4.1% without),[73] although another found that adding body image treatment did not significantly improve weight loss compared to dietician led treatment alone.[74] We found two RCTs examining effects of advice to lose weight among people who were overweight and hypertensive. The first (1191 people) found that advice reduced weight and hypertension more than no weight loss advice at 3 years (weight loss at 3 years, 1.8 kg with advice v 0.2 kg with control; RR for hypertension with advice v control 0.81, 95% CI 0.70 to 0.95). Subgroup analysis of the second RCT (585 overweight elderly people with hypertension) found that weight advice reduced body weight more than no weight advice (weight loss at 30 months 4.7 kg v 0.9 kg).[55] One large RCT (588 overweight people) compared three different cognitive behavioural approaches for tailoring lifestyle modification goals: workbook alone (no tailoring of goals); adding computerised computer kiosks with touch screen monitors to help participants tailor goals; and adding both computers and staff consultation to tailor goals. After 12 months, it found that all groups achieved a statistically significant mean weight loss from baseline. It found that combined personal and computerised tailoring improved weight loss compared with workbook alone (mean weight loss 1 kg with workbook v 2.1 kg with computerised tailoring v 3.3 kg with combined personal and computerised tailoring, P = 0.02 for workbook v combined group).[76]

Harms: The systematic reviews and RCTs provided no evidence about harms resulting from diet or exercise for weight loss.

Comment: None.

QUESTION   **What are the effects of lifestyle interventions to maintain weight loss?**

One systematic review and additional RCTs have found that most types of maintenance strategy result in smaller weight gains or greater weight losses compared with no contact. Strategies that involve personal contact with a therapist, family support, walking training programmes, or multiple interventions, or are weight focused, appear most effective.

Benefits: We found one systematic review[58] and seven additional RCTs.[77–83] The systematic review (search date 1995, 21 studies) compared different types and combinations of interventions. It found that increased contact with a therapist in the long term produced smaller weight gain or greater weight loss, and that additional self help peer groups, self management techniques, or involvement of the family or spouse may increase weight loss. The largest weight loss was seen in programmes using multiple strategies. Two additional small RCTs (102 people[77] and 100 people in two trials[81]) assessed simple strategies without face to face contact with a therapist. Frequent telephone contacts, optional food provision, continued self monitoring, urge control, or relapse prevention did not reduce the rate of weight regain. One small RCT (117 people) found that telephone contacts plus house visits did reduce the rate of weight regain compared with no intervention (3.65 kg v 6.42 kg; P = 0.048).[78] One further small RCT (80 obese women) found no difference in weight change at 1 year between participants offered relapse prevention training or problem solving compared with no further contact.[83] One RCT (82 women) compared two walking programmes (4.2 MJ/wk or 8.4 MJ/wk) plus diet counselling versus diet counselling alone following a 12 week intensive weight reduction programme.[82] Both walking programmes reduced weight regain at 1 year (reduction in weight gain compared with dietary counselling alone 2.7 kg, 95% CI 0.2 kg to 5.2 kg with low intensity programme and 2.6 kg, 95% CI 0.0 kg to 5.1 kg with high intensity programme). At 2 years, weight regain was not significantly different between high intensity programme and control, but was reduced in the low intensity group (reduction in weight gain 3.5 kg, 95% CI 0.2 kg to 6.8 kg with low intensity programme and 0.2 kg, 95% CI −3.1 kg to +3.6 kg with high intensity programme). One additional small RCT (67 people) found that people on a weight focused programme maintained weight loss better than those on an exercise focused programme (0.8 kg v 4.4 kg; P < 0.01).[79] One 5 year RCT (489 menopausal women) compared behavioural intervention in two phases aimed at lifestyle changes in diet and physical activity with lifestyle assessment. People in the intervention group were encouraged to lose weight during the first 6 months (phase I), and thereafter maintain this weight loss for a further 12 months (phase II). The intervention resulted in weight loss compared to control during the first 6 months (−8.9 lb v −0.8 lb; P < 0.05), most of which was sustained over phase II (−6.7 lb v +0.6 lb; P < 0.05).[80]

Harms: We found no direct evidence that interventions designed to maintain weight loss are harmful.

Comment: Weight regain is common. The resource implication of providing long term maintenance of any weight loss may be a barrier to the routine implementation of maintenance programmes.

QUESTION **What are the effects of lifestyle advice to prevent weight gain?**

One small RCT found that low intensity education increased weight loss. A second RCT found no significant effect on weight gain from a postal newsletter with or without a linked financial incentive. One RCT found that lifestyle advice prevented weight gain in perimenopausal women compared to assessment alone.

Changing behaviour

Benefits: We found three systematic reviews (search dates 1995,[58] 1999,[59] and not stated[84]) that included the same two RCTs[85,86] and one subsequent RCT.[87] The first RCT (219 people) compared low intensity education with a financial incentive to maintain weight versus an untreated control group. It found significantly greater average weight loss in the intervention group than in the control group (−0.95 kg with intervention v −0.14 kg with control; $P = 0.03$).[85] The second RCT (228 men and 998 women) compared a monthly newsletter versus the newsletter plus a lottery incentive versus no contact. There was no significant difference in weight gain after 3 years between the groups (1.6 kg v 1.5 kg v 1.8 kg).[86] The later RCT, which was not included in the reviews, compared lifestyle advice versus assessment alone among 535 perimenopausal women. It found that advice reduced weight gain over 2 years (weight gain 0.5 kg with advice v 11.5 kg with assessment alone).[87]

Harms: None reported.

Comment: None.

QUESTION   **What are the effects of training professionals in promoting reduction of body weight?**

One systematic review of poor quality RCTs found little evidence on the sustained effect of interventions to improve health professionals' management of obesity. One subsequent small RCT found limited evidence that training for primary care doctors in nutrition counselling plus a support programme reduced body weight of the people in their care over 1 year.

Benefits: We found one systematic review (search date 2000, 18 RCTs, 8 with follow up > 1 year)[88] and one subsequent RCT.[89] The studies in the review were heterogeneous and poor quality. The subsequent RCT (45 people) compared nutrition counselling training plus a support programme for primary care doctors versus usual care.[89] The nutrition supported intervention compared with usual care increased weight loss at 1 year (additional weight loss 2.3 kg; $P < 0.001$).

Harms: None reported.

Comment: The doctors were randomly allocated to treatment but the analysis of results was based on the people in the care of those doctors. No allowance was made for cluster bias. This increases the likelihood that the additional weight loss could have occurred by chance.

GLOSSARY

Behavioural choice therapy A cognitive behavioural intervention based on a decision making model of women's food choice. This relates situation specific eating behaviour to outcomes and goals using decision theory. The outcomes and goals governing food choice extend beyond food related factors to include self esteem and social acceptance.

Cognitive behavioural programme Traditional cognitive behavioural topics (e.g. self monitoring, stimulus control, coping with cravings and high risk situations, stress management, and relaxation techniques) along with topics of particular importance to women (e.g. healthy eating, weight management, mood management, and managing work and family).

Motivational interviewing A goal directed counselling style that helps participants to understand and resolve areas of ambivalence that impede behavioural change.

Standard behavioural therapy A behavioural weight management programme that incorporates moderate calorie restriction to promote weight loss.

REFERENCES

1. Silagy C, Stead LF. Physician advice for smoking cessation. In: The Cochrane Library, Issue 2, 2002. Oxford: Update Software. Search date 2000; primary sources Cochrane Tobacco Addiction Group Trials Register and the Cochrane Controlled Trials Register.

2. Lancaster T, Stead LF. Individual behavioural counselling for smoking cessation. In: The Cochrane Library, Issue 2, 2002. Oxford: Update Software. Search date 1998; primary sources Cochrane Tobacco Addiction Group Trials Register.

3. Rice VH, Stead LF. Nursing interventions for smoking cessation. In: The Cochrane Library, Issue 2, 2002. Oxford: Update Software. Search date 2001; primary sources Cochrane Tobacco Addiction Group Trials Register and Cinahl.

4. Stead LF, Lancaster T. Telephone counselling for smoking cessation. In: The Cochrane Library Issue 2, 2002. Oxford: Update Software. Search date 2000; primary source Cochrane Tobacco Addiction Group Trials Register.

5. Pieterse ME, Seydel ER, de Vries H, et al. Effectiveness of a minimal contact smoking cessation program for Dutch general practitioners: a randomized controlled trial. *Prev Med* 2001;32:182–190.

6. Lancaster T, Stead LF. Self help interventions for smoking cessation (Cochrane review). In: The Cochrane Library Issue 2, 2002. Oxford: Update Software. Search date 1999; primary sources previous reviews and meta-analyses, the Tobacco Addiction Review Group register of controlled trials identified from Medline Express (Silverplatter) to 1999/8 and the Science Citation Index to 9/1999.

7. Miguez MC, Vasquez FL, Becona F. Effectiveness of telephone contact as an adjunct to a self-help program for smoking cessation. A randomized controlled trial in Spanish smokers. *Addict Behav* 2002;27:139–144.

8. Silagy C, Mant D, Fowler G, et al. Nicotine replacement therapy for smoking cessation. In: The Cochrane Library, Issue 2, 2002. Oxford: Update Software. Search date 2001; primary source Cochrane Tobacco Addiction Group Trials Register.

9. Tonneson P, Paoletti P, Gustavsson G, et al. Higher dose nicotine patches increase one year smoking cessation rates: results from the European CEASE trial. *Eur Respir J* 1999;13:238–246.

10. Stapleton J. Cigarette smoking prevalence, cessation and relapse. *Stat Methods Med Res* 1998;7:187–203.

11. Stapleton JA, Sutherland G, Russell MA. How much does relapse after one year erode effectiveness of smoking cessation treatments? Long term follow up of a randomised trial of nicotine nasal spray. *BMJ* 1998;316:830–831.

12. Blondal T, Gudmundsson J, Olafsdottir I, et al. Nicotine nasal spray with nicotine patch for smoking cessation: randomised trial with six years follow up. *BMJ* 1999;318:285–289.

13. Daughton DM, Fortmann SP, Glover ED, et al. The smoking cessation efficacy of varying doses of nicotine patch delivery systems 4 to 5 years post-quit day. *Prev Med* 1999;28:113–118.

14. Ebrahim S, Davey Smith G. Health promotion in older people for the prevention of coronary heart disease and stroke. *Health promotion effectiveness reviews reries*, No 1. London: Health Education Authority, 1996. Search date 1994; primary sources Medline, hand searched reference lists, and citation search on BIDS for Eastern European trials.

15. White AR, Rampes H, Ernst E. Acupuncture for smoking cessation (Cochrane review) In: The Cochrane Library Issue 2, 2002. Oxford: Update Software. Search date 2002; primary sources Cochrane Tobacco Addiction Group Register, Medline, Psychlit, Dissertation Abstracts, Health Planning and Administration, SocialSciSearch, Smoking and Health, Embase, Biological Abstracts, and Drug.

16. Ussher MH, Taylor AH, West R, et al. Does exercise aid smoking cessation? *Addiction* 2000;95:199–208. Search date 1999; primary sources Medline, Psychlit, Dissertation Abstracts, Sports Discus, hand searched reference lists, and personal contact with research colleagues.

17. Marcus BH, Albrecht AE, King TK, et al. The efficacy of exercise as an aid for smoking cessation in women. *Arch Intern Med* 1999;159:1229–1234.

18. Hughes JR, Stead LF, Lancaster T. Antidepressants for smoking cessation. In: The Cochrane Library, Issue 2, 2002. Oxford: Update Software. Search date 2001; primary source Cochrane Tobacco Addiction Group Trials Register.

19. Hughes JR, Stead LF, Lancaster T. Anxiolytics for smoking cessation. In: The Cochrane Library, Issue 2, 2002. Oxford: Update Software. Search date 2000; primary source Cochrane Tobacco Addiction Group Trials Register.

20. Jorenby DE, Leischow SJ, Nides MA, et al. A controlled trial of sustained-release bupropion, a nicotine patch, or both for smoking cessation. *N Engl J Med* 1999;340:685–691.

21. Law M, Tang JL. An analysis of the effectiveness of interventions intended to help people stop smoking. *Arch Intern Med* 1995;155:1933–1941. Search date not stated; primary sources Medline and Index Medicus.

22. Lumley J, Oliver S, Waters E. Interventions for promoting smoking cessation during pregnancy. In: The Cochrane Library, Issue 2, 2002. Oxford: Update Software. Search date 1998; primary source Cochrane Tobacco Addiction Group Trials Register.

23. Wisborg K, Henriksen TB, Jespersen LB, et al. Nicotine patches for pregnant smokers: a randomized controlled study. *Obstet Gynecol* 2000;96:967–971.

24. Hajek P, West R, Lee A, et al. Randomized trial of a midwife-delivered brief smoking cessation intervention in pregnancy. *Addiction* 2001;96:485–494.

25. Stotts A, DiClememte CC, Dolan-Mullen P. One-to-one. A motivational intervention for resistant pregnant smokers *Addict Behav* 2002;27:275–292.

26. Rigotti NA, Munafo MR, Murphy MFG, et al. Interventions for smoking cessation in hospitalised

patients. In: The Cochrane Library, Issue 2, 2002. Oxford: Update Software. Search date 2000; primary sources Cochrane Controlled Trials Register, Centre for Disease Control Smoking and Health database, Cinahl, and experts.

27. Humerfelt S, Eide GE, Kvale G, et al. Effectiveness of postal smoking cessation advice: a randomized controlled trial in young men with reduced FEV_1 and asbestos exposure. Eur Respir J 1998;11:284–290.

28. Hajek P, Taylor TZ, Mills P. Brief intervention during hospital admission to help patients to give up smoking after myocardial infarction and bypass surgery: randomized controlled trial. BMJ 2002;324:1–6.

29. Burt A, Thornley P, Illingworth D, et al. Stopping smoking after myocardial infarction. Lancet 1974;1:304–306.

30. Lancaster T, Silagy C, Fowler G. Training health professionals in smoking cessation. In: The Cochrane Library, Issue 2, 2002. Oxford: Update Software. Search date 2000; primary source Cochrane Tobacco Addiction Group Trials Register.

31. Maguire TA, McElnay JC, Drummond A. A randomized controlled trial of a smoking cessation intervention based in community pharmacies. Addiction 2001;96:325–331.

32. Hillsdon M, Thorogood M. A systematic review of physical activity promotion strategies. Br J Sports Med 1996;30:84–89. Search date 1996; primary sources Medline, Excerpta Medica, Sport SCISearch, and hand searched reference lists.

33. Dunn AL, Anderson RE, Jakicic JM. Lifestyle physical activity interventions. History, short- and long-term effects and recommendations. Am J Prev Med 1998;15:398–412. Search date not stated; primary sources Medline, Current Contents, Biological Abstracts, The Johns Hopkins Medical Institutions Catalog, Sport Discus, and Grateful Med.

34. Goldstein MG, Pinto BM, Marcus BH, et al. Physician-based physical activity counseling for middle-aged and older adults: a randomised trial. Ann Behav Med 1999;1:40–47.

35. Harland J, White M, Drinkwater C, et al. The Newcastle exercise project: a randomised controlled trial of methods to promote physical activity in primary care. BMJ 1999;319:828–832.

36. Taylor, A, Doust, J, Webborn, N. Randomised controlled trial to examine the effects of a GP exercise referral programme in Hailsham, East Sussex, on modifiable coronary heart disease risk factors. J Epidemiol Community Health 1998;52:595–601.

37. Bull F, Jamorozik K. Advice on exercise from a family physician can help sedentary patients to become active. Am J Prev Med 1998;15:85–94.

38. Stevens W, Hillsdon M, Thorogood M, et al. Cost-effectiveness of a primary care based physical activity intervention in 45–74 year old men and women; a randomised controlled trial. Br J Sports Med 1998;32:236–241.

39. Halbert JA, Silagy CA, Finucane PM, et al. Physical activity and cardiovascular risk factors: effect of advice from an exercise specialist in Australian general practice. Med J Aust 2000;173:84–87.

40. Norris SL, Grothaus LC, Buchner DM, et al. Effectiveness of physician-based assessment and counseling for exercise in a staff model HMO. Prev Med 2000;30:513–523.

41. The Writing Group for the Activity Counseling Trial Research Group. Effects of physical activity counseling in primary care: the Activity Counseling Trial: a randomised controlled trial. JAMA 2001;286:677–687.

42. Smith BJ, Bauman AE, Bull FC, et al. Promoting physical activity in general practice: a controlled trial of written advice and information maeterials. Br J Sports Med 2000;34:262–267.

43. Lamb SE, Bartlett HP, Ashley A, et al. Can lay-led walking programmes increase physical activity in middle aged adults? A randomised controlled trial. J Epidemiol Community Health 2002;56:246–252.

44. Pereira MA, Kriska AN, Day RD, et al. A randomized walking trial in postmenopausal women. Arch Intern Med 1998;158:1695–1701.

45. Campbell AJ, Robertson MC, Gardner MM, et al. Randomised controlled trial of a general practice programme of home based exercise to prevent falls in elderly women. BMJ 1997;315:1065–1069.

46. Brunner E, White I, Thorogood M, et al. Can dietary interventions change diet and cardiovascular risk factors? A meta-analysis of randomised controlled trials. Am J Public Health 1997;87:1415–1422. Search date 1993; primary sources computer and manual searched databases and journals.

47. Tang JL, Armitage JM, Lancaster T, et al. Systematic review of dietary intervention trials to lower blood total cholesterol in free living subjects. BMJ 1998;316:1213–1220. Search date 1996; primary sources Medline, Human Nutrition, Embase, Allied and Alternative Health, hand search of Am J Clin Nutr, and reference list checks.

48. Stefanick ML, Mackey S, Sheehan M, et al. Effects of diet and exercise in men and postmenopausal women with low levels of HDL cholesterol and high levels of LDL cholesterol. N Engl J Med 1998;339:12–20.

49. Knopp RH, Retzlaff B, Walden C, et al. One year effects of increasingly fat-restricted, carbohydrate-enriched diets in lipoprotein levels in free living subjects. Proc Soc Exp Biol Med 2000;225:191–199.

50. Tomson Y, Johannesson M, Aberg H. The costs and effects of two different lipid intervention programmes in primary health care. J Intern Med 1995;237:13–17.

51. Hooper L, Summerbell CD, Higgins JPT, et al. Reduced or modified dietary fat for preventing cardiovascular disease. In: The Cochrane Library, Issue 2, 2002. Oxford: Update Software. Search date 1999; primary sources Cochrane Library, Medline, Embase, CAB Abstracts, CVRCT registry, related Cochrane Groups' Trial Registers, trials known to experts in the field, and biographies.

52. Howell WH, McNamara DJ, Tosca MA, et al. Plasma lipid and lipoprotein responses to dietary fat and cholesterol: a meta-analysis. Am J Clin Nutr 1997;65:1747–1764. Search date 1994; primary sources Medline, hand search of selected review publications, and bibliographies.

53. Ebrahim S, Davey Smith G. Lowering blood pressure: a systematic review of sustained effects of non-pharmacological interventions. J Public Health 1998;2:441–448. Search date 1998; primary sources Medline and hand searches of reference lists.

54. Fodor JG, Whitmore B, Leenen F, et al. Recommendations on dietary salt. Can Med Assoc J 1999;160(Suppl 9):29–34. Search date 1996; primary sources Medline, hand searches of reference lists, personal files, and contact with experts.

55. Whelton PK, Appel LJ, Espeland MA, et al. Sodium reduction and weight loss in the treatment of hypertension in older persons. A randomized controlled Trial of Nonpharmacologic Interventions in the Elderly (TONE). JAMA 1998;279:839–846.

56. He J, Whelton PK, Appel LJ, et al. Long-term effects of weight loss and dietary sodium reduction on incidence of hypertension. Hypertension 2000;35:544–549.

57. The Trials of Hypertension Prevention, Phase II. Effects of weight loss and sodium reduction intervention on blood pressure and hypertension incidence in overweight people with high-normal blood pressure. Arch Intern Med 1997;157:657–667.

58. Glenny A-M, O'Meara S, Melville A, et al. The treatment and prevention of obesity: a systematic review of the literature. Int J Obesity 887;21;715–737. Published in full as NHS CRD report 1997, No 10. A systematic review of interventions in the treatment and prevention of obesity. http://www.york.ac.uk/inst/crd/obesity.htm (last accessed 03/00/2002). Search date 1995; primary sources Medline, Embase, DHSS data, Current Research in UK, Science citation index, Social science citation index, Conference Proceedings index, Sigle, Dissertation Abstracts, Sport, Drug Info, AMED (Allied and alternative medicine), ASSI (abstracts and Indexes), CAB, NTIS (national technical information dB), Directory of Published Proceedings (Interdoc), Purchasing Innovations database, Health promotion database, S.S.R.U., DARE (CRD, database of systematic reviews, NEED, CRD, database of health economic reviews), and all databases searched from starting date to the end of 1995.

59. Douketis JD, Feightner JW, Attia J, et al. Periodic health examination, 1999 update. Detection, prevention and treatment of obesity. Canadian Task Force on Preventive Health Care. Can Med Assoc J 1999;160:513–525. Search date 1999; primary sources Medline, Current Contents, and hand searched references.

60. The National Heart, Lung, and Blood Institute. Clinical guidelines on the identification, evaluation, and treatment of overweight and obesity in adults. Bethesda, Maryland: National Institutes of Health, 1998; http://www.nhlbi.nih.gov/guidelines/obesity/ob_home.htm (last accessed 3 Sept 2002) Search date 1997; primary sources Medline, and hand searched reference lists.

61. Wing RR, Polley RA, Venditti E, et al. Lifestyle intervention in overweight individuals with a family history of diabetes. Diabetes Care 1998;21:350–359.

62. Anderson RE, Wadden TA, Barlett SJ, et al. Effects of lifestyle activity v structured aerobic exercise in obese women. JAMA 1999;281:335–340.

63. Jakicic JM, Winters C, Lang W, et al. Effects of intermittent exercise and use of home exercise equipment on adherence, weight loss, and fitness in overweight women. JAMA 1999;282:1554–1560.

64. Sbrocco T, Nedegaard RC, Stone JM, et al. Behavioural choice treatment promotes continuing weight loss. J Consult Clin Psychol 1999;67:260–266.

65. Harvey-Berino J. Calorie restriction is more effective for obesity treatment than dietary fat restriction. Ann Behav Med 1999;21:35–39.

66. Wing RR, Jeffery RW. Benefits of recruiting participants with friends and increasing social support for weight loss and maintenance. J Consult Clin Psychol 1999;67:132–138.

67. Jeffery RW, Wing RR, Thorson C, et al. Use of personal trainers and financial incentives to increase exercise in a behavioural weight loss program. J Consult Clin Psychol 1998;66:777–783.

68. Craighead LW, Blum MD. Supervised exercise in behavioural treatment for moderate obesity. Behav Ther 1989;20:49–59.

69. Donnelly JE, Jacobsen DJ, Heelan KS, et al. The effects of 18 months of intermittent vs. continuous exercise on aerobic capacity, body weight and composition, and metabolic fitness in previously sedentary, moderately obese females. Int J Obesity 2000;24:566–572.

70. Kunz K, Kreimel K, Gurdet G, et al. Comparison of behaviour modification and conventional dietary advice in a long-term weight reduction programme for obese women [abstract]. Diabetologia 1982;23.181.

71. Rapoport L, Clark M, Wardle J. Evaluation of a modified cognitive-behavioural programme for weight management. Int J Obesity 2000;24:1726–1737.

72. Wing R, Epstein LH, Paternostro-Bayles M, et al. Exercise in a behavioural weight control program for obese patients with type 2 (non insulin dependent) diabetes. Diabetologica 1988;31:902–909.

73. Ashley LM, St leor ST, Schrage JP, et al. Weight control in the physicians office. Arch Intern Med 2001;161:1599–1604.

74. Ramirez EM, Rosen JC. A comparison of weight control and weight control plus body image therapy for obese men and women. J Consult Clin Psychol 2001;69:444–446.

75. Stevens VJ, Obarzanek E, Cook NR, et al. for the Trials of Hypertension Prevention Research Group. Long term weight loss and changes in blood pressure: Results of the Trials of Hypertension Prevention, Phase II. Ann Intern Med 2001;134:1–11.

76. Wylie-Rosett J, Swencionis C, Ginsberg M, et al. Computerized weight loss intervention optimises staff time: the clinical and cost results of a controlled clinical trail conducted in a managed care setting. J Am Dietetic Assoc 2001;101:1155–1162.

77. Bonato DP, Boland FJ. A comparison of specific strategies for long-term maintenance following a behavioural treatment program for obese women. Int J Eat Disord 1986;5:949–958.

78. Hillebrand TH, Wirth A. Evaluation of an outpatient care program for obese patients after an inpatient treatment. Präv Rehab 1996;8:83–87.

79. Leermakers EA, Perri MG, Shigaki CL, et al. Effects of exercise-focused versus weight-focused maintenance programs on the management of obesity. Addict Behav 1999;24:219–227.

80. Simkin-Silverman LR, Wing RR, Boraz MA, et al. Maintenance of cardiovascular risk factor changes among middle aged women in a lifestyle intervention trial. Women's Health: Research on Gender, Behaviour, and Policy 1998;4:255–271.

81. Wing RR, Jeffery RW, Hellerstedt WL, et al. Effect of frequent phone contacts and optional food provision on maintenance of weight loss. Ann Behav Med 1996;18:172 176.

82. Fogelholm M, Kukkonen-Harjula K, Nenonen A, et al. Effects of walking training on weight maintenance after a very-low-energy diet in premenopausal obese women: a randomized controlled trial. Arch Intern Med 2000;160:2177–2184.

83. Perri MG, Nezu AM, McKelvey WF, et al. Relapse prevention training and problem-solving therapy in the long-term management of obesity. J Consult & Clin Psychol 2001;69:722–726.

84. Hardeman W, Griffin S, Johnston M, et al. Interventions to prevent weight gain: a systematic review of psychological models and behaviour change methods. Int J Obesity 2000;4:131–143. Search date not stated; primary sources Medline, Embase, Psychlit, The Cochrane Library, Current Contents, ERIC, HealthStar, Social Science Citation Index, and hand searched reference lists.

85. Forster JL, Jeffery RW, Schmid TL, et al. Preventing weight gain in adults: a pound of prevention. *Health Psychol* 1988;7:515–525.
86. Jeffery RW, French SA. Preventing weight gain in adults: the pound of prevention study. *Am J Public Health* 1999;89:747–751.
87. Kuller LH, Simkin-Silverman LR, Wing RR, et al. Women's health lifestyle project: a randomized clinical trial. *Circulation* 2001;103:32–37.
88. Harvey EL, Glenny A, Kirk SFL, et al. Improving health professionals' management and the organisation of care for overweight and obese people. In: The Cochrane Library, Issue 2, 2002. Oxford: Update Software. Search date 2000; primary sources Specialised Registers of the Cochrane Effective Practice and Organisation of Care Group, the Cochrane Depression, Anxiety and Neurosis Group, the Cochrane Diabetes Group, the Cochrane Controlled Trials Register, Medline, Embase, Cinahl, PsycLit, Sigle, Sociofile, Dissertation Abstracts, Resource Database in Continuing Medical Education, and Conference Papers Index.
89. Ockene IS, Hebert JR, Ockene JK, et al. Effect of physician-delivered nutrition counseling training and an office-support program on saturated fat intake, weight, and serum lipid measurements in a hyperlipidemic population: Worcester area trial for counseling in hyperlipidemia (WATCH). *Arch Intern Med* 1999;159:725–731.

Margaret Thorogood
Reader in Public Health and Preventative Medicine

Melvyn Hillsdon
Lecturer in Health Promotion

London School of Hygiene and Tropical Medicine
University of London
London
UK

Carolyn Summerbell
Reader in Human Nutrition
School of Health
University of Teesside
Middlesborough
UK

Competing interests: None declared.

Search date September 2001

William Herman

INTERVENTIONS

Key Messages

Intensive control of hyperglycaemia in people aged 13–75 years

- One systematic review and large subsequent RCTs in people with type 1 or type 2 diabetes have found strong evidence that intensive versus conventional glycaemic control significantly reduces the development and progression of microvascular and neuropathic complications. A second systematic review has found that intensive versus conventional treatment is associated with a small reduction in cardiovascular risk.

- RCTs have found that intensive treatment increases the incidence of hypoglycaemia and weight gain, without adverse impact on neuropsychological function or quality of life.

- The benefit of intensive treatment is limited by the complications of advanced diabetes (such as blindness, end stage renal disease, or cardiovascular disease), major comorbidity, and reduced life expectancy.

- Large RCTs have found that diabetic complications increase with HbA1c concentrations above the non-diabetic range.

Intensive control of hyperglycaemia in people with frequent severe hypoglycaemia

- The benefits of intensive treatment of hyperglycaemia are described above.

- It is difficult to weigh the benefit of reduced complications against the harm of increased hypoglycaemia. The risk of intensive treatment is increased by a history of severe hypoglycaemia or unawareness of hypoglycaemia, advanced autonomic neuropathy or cardiovascular disease, and impaired ability to detect or treat hypoglycaemia (such as altered mental state, immobility, or lack of social support). For people likely to have limited benefit or increased risk with intensive treatment, it may be more appropriate to negotiate less intensive goals for glycaemic management that reflect the person's self determined goals of care and willingness to make lifestyle modifications.

DEFINITION Diabetes mellitus is a group of disorders characterised by hyperglycaemia (definitions vary slightly, one current US definition is fasting plasma glucose ≥ 7.0 mmol/L or ≥ 11.1 mmol/L 2 h after a 75 g oral glucose load, on 2 or more occasions). Intensive treatment is designed to achieve blood glucose values as close to the non-diabetic range as possible. The components of such treatment are education, counselling, monitoring, self management, and pharmacological treatment with insulin or oral antidiabetic agents to achieve specific glycaemic goals.

INCIDENCE/ PREVALENCE Diabetes is diagnosed in around 5% of adults aged 20 years or older in the USA.[1] A further 2.7% have undiagnosed diabetes on the basis of fasting glucose. The prevalence is similar in men and women, but diabetes is more common in some ethnic groups. The prevalence in people aged 40–74 years has increased over the past decade.

AETIOLOGY/ RISK FACTORS Diabetes results from deficient insulin secretion, decreased insulin action, or both. Many processes can be involved, from autoimmune destruction of the β cells of the pancreas to incompletely understood abnormalities that result in resistance to insulin action. Genetic factors are involved in both mechanisms. In type 1 diabetes there is an absolute deficiency of insulin. In type 2 diabetes, insulin resistance and an inability of the pancreas to compensate are involved. Hyperglycaemia without clinical symptoms but sufficient to cause tissue damage can be present for many years before diagnosis.

PROGNOSIS Severe hyperglycaemia causes numerous symptoms, including polyuria, polydipsia, weight loss, and blurred vision. Acute, life threatening consequences of diabetes are hyperglycaemia with ketoacidosis or the non-ketotic hyperosmolar syndrome. There is increased susceptibility to certain infections. Long term complications of diabetes include retinopathy (with potential loss of vision), nephropathy (leading to renal failure), peripheral neuropathy (increased risk of foot ulcers, amputation, and Charcot joints), autonomic neuropathy (cardiovascular, gastrointestinal, and genitourinary dysfunction), and greatly increased risk of atheroma affecting large vessels (macrovascular complications of stroke, myocardial infarction, or peripheral vascular disease). The physical, emotional, and social impact of diabetes and demands of intensive treatment can also create problems for people with diabetes and their families. One systematic review (search date 1998) of observational studies in people with type 2 diabetes found a positive association between increased blood glucose concentration and mortality.[2] It found no minimum threshold level.

AIMS To slow development and progression of the microvascular, neuropathic, and cardiovascular complications of diabetes, while minimising adverse effects of treatment (hypoglycaemia and weight gain) and maximising quality of life.

OUTCOMES Quality of life; short term burden of treatment; long term clinical complications; risks and benefits of treatment. Both the development of complications in people who have previously been free of them, and the progression of complications, are used as outcomes.

Scales of severity are used to detect disease progression (e.g. 19 step scales of diabetic retinopathy; normoalbuminuria, microalbuminuria, and albuminuria for nephropathy; absence or presence of clinical neuropathy).

METHODS   *Clinical Evidence* search and appraisal September 2001.

QUESTION   **What are the effects of intensive versus conventional glycaemic control?**

One systematic review and three subsequent RCTs in people with type 1 and type 2 diabetes have found that intensive treatment compared with conventional treatment reduces development and progression of microvascular and neuropathic complications. A second systematic review in people with type 1 diabetes, and two additional RCTs in people with type 2 diabetes, found no evidence that intensive treatment increased adverse cardiovascular outcomes. Intensive treatment reduces the number of macrovascular events but has no significant effect on the number of people who develop macrovascular disease. Intensive treatment is associated with hypoglycaemia and weight gain, but does not seem to affect neuropsychological function or quality of life adversely.

Benefits: **Microvascular and neuropathic complications:** We found one systematic review (search date 1991, 16 small RCTs of type 1 diabetes)[3] and three subsequent long term RCTs [4-6] that found the relative risks of retinopathy, nephropathy, and neuropathy were all significantly reduced by intensive treatment versus conventional treatment (see table 1, p 105). In one subsequent RCT (1441 people with type 1 diabetes) about half had no retinopathy and half had mild retinopathy at baseline.[4] At 6.5 years, intensive treatment significantly reduced the progression of retinopathy and neuropathy. After a further 4 years the benefit was maintained, regardless of whether people stayed in the groups to which they were initially randomised.[7] The difference in the median HbA1c concentration for people initially randomised to intensive or conventional care narrowed. The proportion of people with worsening retinopathy and nephropathy was also significantly lower for those who had received intensive treatment. However, another subsequent RCT compared a conventional dietary treatment policy with two different intensive treatment policies based on sulphonylurea and insulin (3867 people with newly diagnosed type 2 diabetes, age 25–65 years, fasting plasma glucose 6.1–15.0 mmol/L after 3 months' dietary treatment, no symptoms of hyperglycaemia, follow up 10 years).[6] HbA1c rose steadily in both groups. Intensive treatment was associated with a significant reduction in any diabetes related end point (40.9 v 46.0 events/1000 person years; RRR 12%, 95% CI 1% to 21%), but no significant effect on diabetes related deaths (10.4 v 11.5 deaths/1000 person years; RRR +10%, 95% CI –11% to +27%) or all cause mortality (17.9 v 18.9 deaths/1000 person years; RRR +6%, 95% CI –10% to +20%). Secondary analysis found that intensive treatment was associated with a significant reduction in microvascular end points (8.6 v 11.4/1000 person years; RRR 25%, 95% CI 7% to 40%) compared with conventional treatment (see table 1, p 105).[6] **Cardiovascular outcomes:**

We found one systematic review[8] and two additional RCTs.[5,6] The systematic review (search date 1996, 6 RCTs, 1731 people with type 1 diabetes followed for 2–8 years) found that intensive insulin treatment versus conventional treatment decreased the number of macrovascular events (OR 0.55, 95% CI 0.35 to 0.88), but had no significant effect on the number of people developing macrovascular disease (OR 0.72, 95% CI 0.44 to 1.17) or on macrovascular mortality (OR 0.91, 95% CI 0.31 to 2.65).[8] The additional RCTs included people with type 2 diabetes.[5,6] In the first RCT the number of major cerebrovascular, cardiovascular, and peripheral vascular events in the intensive treatment group was half that of the conventional treatment group (0.6 v 1.3 events/100 person years), but the event rate in this small trial was low and the results were not significant.[5] In the second RCT, intensive treatment versus conventional treatment was associated with a non-significant reduction in the risk of myocardial infarction (AR 387/2729 [14%] with intensive treatment v 186/1138 [16%] with conventional treatment; RRR +13%, 95% CI –2% to +27%), a non-significant increase in the risk of stroke (AR 148/2729 [5.4%] v 55/1138 [4.8%]; RRI +12%, 95% CI –17% to +51%), and a non-significant reduction in the risk of amputation or death from peripheral vascular disease (AR 29/2729 [1.1%] v 18/1138 [1.6%]; RRR +33%, 95% CI –20% to +63%).[6]

Harms:

Hypoglycaemia: We found one systematic review[9] and three additional RCTs.[5,6,10] The systematic review (search date not stated, 14 RCTs with at least 6 months' follow up and monitoring of HbA1c, 2067 people with type 1 diabetes followed for 0.5–7.5 years) found that the median incidence of severe hypoglycaemia was 7.9 episodes/100 person years among intensively treated people and 4.6 episodes/100 person years among conventionally treated people (OR 3.0, 95% CI 2.5 to 3.6). The risk of severe hypoglycaemia was associated with the degree of HbA1c lowering in the intensive treatment groups (P = 0.005). The three additional RCTs included people with type 2 diabetes with lower baseline rates of hypoglycaemia. In the first RCT (110 people), there was no significant difference in rates of hypoglycaemia between groups.[5] In the second RCT (3867 people), the rates of major hypoglycaemic episodes per year were 0.7% with conventional treatment, 1.0% with chlorpropamide, 1.4% with glibenclamide, and 1.8% with insulin. People in the intensive treatment group had significantly more hypoglycaemic episodes than those in the conventional group (P < 0.0001).[6] In the third RCT (1704 overweight people) major hypoglycaemic episodes occurred in 0.6% of overweight people in the metformin treated group.[10] **Weight gain:** Four RCTs found more weight increase with intensive treatment than with standard treatment.[4–6,11] One RCT found weight remained stable in people with type 1 diabetes in the conventional treatment group, but body mass index increased by 5.8% in the intensive treatment group (95% CI not presented; P < 0.01).[11] In the second RCT (1441 people with type 1 diabetes) intensive treatment was associated with increased risk of developing a body weight more than 120% above the ideal (12.7 cases/100 person years with intensive treatment v 9.3 cases/100 person years with conventional treatment; RR 1.33). At 5 years, people treated intensively gained

4.6 kg more than people treated conventionally (CI not provided for weight data).[4] In the third RCT, the increase in body mass index from baseline to 6 years was not significant in either group (intensive treatment group 20.5 to 21.2 kg/m^2, conventional treatment group 20.3–21.9 kg/m^2).[5] In the fourth RCT, weight gain at 10 years was significantly higher in people with type 2 diabetes in the intensive treatment group compared with people in the conventional treatment group (mean 2.9 kg; P < 0.001), and people assigned insulin had a greater gain in weight (4.0 kg) than those assigned chlorpropamide (2.6 kg) or glibenclamide (1.7 kg).[6] We found one systematic review (search date 1996, 10 RCTs)[12] and one subsequent RCT[10] comparing metformin and sulphonylurea. Meta-analysis in the review found that sulphonylurea was associated with an increase in weight from baseline and metformin with a decrease (difference 2.9 kg, 95% CI 1.1 kg to 4.4 kg). In the subsequent RCT, overweight participants randomly assigned to intensive blood glucose control with metformin had a similar change in body weight to the conventional treatment group, and less increase in mean body weight than people receiving intensive treatment with sulphonylureas or insulin.[10] **Neuropsychological impairment:** We found no systematic review on neuropsychological impairment, but found two RCTs.[13–16] One RCT (102 people) compared intensified with standard treatment in people with type 1 diabetes. It found no cognitive impairment associated with hypoglycaemia after 3 years.[13,14] The second RCT found that intensive treatment did not affect neuropsychological performance.[15] People who had repeated episodes of hypoglycaemia did not perform differently from people who did not have repeated episodes.[16] **Quality of life:** We found three RCTs that reported quality of life in people undergoing intensive versus conventional treatment.[17–19] Together, they suggested that quality of life is lowered by complications, but is not lowered directly by intensive versus conventional treatment. The first RCT (1441 people) found that intensive treatment did not reduce quality of life in people with type 1 diabetes.[17] Severe hypoglycaemia was not consistently associated with a subsequent increase in distress caused by symptoms or decline in the quality of life. However, in the primary prevention intensive treatment group, repeated severe hypoglycaemia (3 or more events resulting in coma or seizure) tended to increase the risk of distress caused by symptoms. The second RCT (77 adolescents with type 1 diabetes) found after 1 year that behavioural intervention plus intensive diabetes management versus intensive diabetes management alone significantly improved quality of life, diabetes and medical self efficacy, and HbA1c (7.5% v 8.5%; P = 0.001).[18] The behavioural intervention included six small group sessions and monthly follow up aimed at social problem solving, cognitive behaviour modification, and conflict resolution. The third RCT of intensive versus conventional treatment of type 2 diabetes assessed quality of life in two large cross sectional samples at 8 and 11 years after randomisation (disease specific measures in 2431 people and generic measures in 3104 people), and also in a small cohort (diabetes specific quality of life measures in 374 people 6 months after randomisation and annually thereafter for 6 years).[19] The cross-sectional studies found no significant effect of intensive versus conventional treatment on scores for mood, cognitive mistakes, symptoms, work satisfaction, or general health. The longitudinal study also found no significant difference in quality of life scores other than a small increase in the number of symptoms in people allocated to conventional than to intensive treatment. In the cross sectional studies, people who had macrovascular or microvascular complications in the past year had lower quality of life than people without complications. People treated with insulin who had two or more hypoglycaemic episodes during the previous year reported more tension, more overall mood disturbance, and less work satisfaction than those with no hypoglycaemic attacks (after adjusting for age, time from randomisation, systolic blood pressure, HbA1c, and sex). It was unclear whether frequent hypoglycaemic episodes affected quality of life, or whether people with certain personality traits or symptoms simply reported increased numbers of hypoglycaemic attacks.

Comment: We found one follow up study in people with type 1 diabetes 11.4 years after randomisation.[20] In people originally randomised to intensive treatment, it found that the fall in systolic blood pressure with upright posture (one measure of cardiovascular sympathetic dysfunction) and cardiovascular parasympathetic autonomic dysfunction (regardless of how it was measured) developed at a significantly slower pace.[20]

QUESTION   What is the optimum target blood glucose?

Large RCTs in people with type 1 and type 2 diabetes have found that risk of development or progression of complications increases progressively as HbA1c increases above the non-diabetic range.

Benefits: We found no systematic review but found two large RCTs.[4,6] The first RCT (1441 people with type 1 diabetes) found that lower HbA1c was associated with a lower risk of complications.[4,21] The second RCT (3867 people with type 2 diabetes) found that, as concentrations of HbA1c were reduced, the risk of complications fell but the risk of hypoglycaemia increased.[6,19] A further analysis of the second RCT (3642 people who had HbA1c measured 3 months after the diagnosis of diabetes and who had complete data whether or not they were randomised in the trial) found that each 1% reduction in mean HbA1c was associated with reduced risk of any diabetes related microvascular or macrovascular event (RR 0.79, 95% CI 0.76 to 0.83), diabetes related death (RR 0.79, 95% CI 0.73 to 0.85), all cause mortality (RR 0.86, 95% CI 0.81 to 0.91), microvascular complications (RR 0.63, 95% CI 0.59 to 0.67), and myocardial infarction (RR 0.86, 95% CI 0.79 to 0.92).[22] These prospective observational data suggested that there is no lower glycaemic threshold for the risk of complications; the better the glycaemic control, the lower the risk of complications. They also suggested that the rate of increase of risk for microvascular disease with hyperglycaemia is greater than that for macrovascular disease.

Harms: Both RCTs found that hypoglycaemia was increased by intensive treatment.[19,21]

Comment: It is difficult to weigh the benefit of reduced complications against the harm of increased hypoglycaemia. The balance between benefits and harms of intensive treatment in type 1 diabetes may be less favourable in children under 13 years or in older adults, and in people with repeated severe hypoglycaemia or unawareness of hypoglycaemia. Similarly, the balance between benefits and harms of intensive treatment in type 2 diabetes may be less favourable in people over 65 years or in those with longstanding diabetes. The benefit of intensive treatment is limited by the complications of advanced diabetes (such as blindness, end stage renal disease, or cardiovascular disease), major comorbidity, and reduced life expectancy. The risk of intensive treatment is increased by a history of severe hypoglycaemia or unawareness of hypoglycaemia, advanced autonomic neuropathy or cardiovascular disease, and impaired ability to detect or treat hypoglycaemia (such as altered mental state, immobility, or lack of social support). For people likely to have limited benefit or increased risk with intensive treatment, it may be more appropriate to negotiate less intensive goals for glycaemic management that reflect the person's self determined goals of care and willingness to make lifestyle modifications.

REFERENCES

1. Harris MI, Flegal KM, Cowie CC, et al. Prevalence of diabetes, impaired fasting glucose, and impaired glucose tolerance in US adults: the third national health and nutrition examination survey, 1988–1994. *Diabetes Care* 1998;2:518–524.

2. Groeneveld Y, Petri H, Hermans J, et al. Relationship between blood glucose level and mortality in type 2 diabetes mellitus: a systematic review. *Diabet Med* 1999;16:2–13. Search date 1998; primary source Medline.

3. Wang PH, Lau J, Chalmers TC. Meta-analysis of effects of intensive blood glucose control on late complications of type 1 diabetes. *Lancet* 1993;341:1306–1309. Search date 1991; primary source Medline.

4. The Diabetes Control and Complications Trial Research Group. The effect of intensive treatment of diabetes on the development and progression of long-term complications in insulin-dependent diabetes mellitus. *N Engl J Med* 1993;329:977–986.

5. Ohkubo Y, Kishikawa H, Arake E, et al. Intensive insulin therapy prevents the progression of diabetic microvascular complications in Japanese patients with non-insulin-dependent diabetes mellitus: a randomized prospective 6-year study. *Diabetes Res Clin Pract* 1995;28:103–117.

6. UK Prospective Diabetes Study Group. Intensive blood-glucose control with sulphonylureas or insulin compared with conventional treatment and risk of complications in patients with type 2 diabetes. *Lancet* 1998;352:837–853.

7. The DCCT/Epidemiology of Diabetes Interventions and Complications Research Group. Retinopathy and nephropathy in patients with type 1 diabetes four years after a trial of intensive therapy. *N Engl J Med* 2000;342:381–389.

8. Lawson ML, Gerstein HC, Tsui E, et al. Effect of intensive therapy on early macrovascular disease in young individuals with type 1 diabetes. *Diabetes Care* 1999;22:B35–B39. Search date 1996; primary sources Medline, Citation Index, reference lists, and personal files.

9. Egger M, Smith GD, Stettler C, et al. Risk of adverse effects of intensified treatment in insulin-dependent diabetes mellitus: a meta-analysis. *Diabet Med* 1997;14:919–928. Search date not stated; primary sources Medline, reference lists, and specialist journals.

10. UK Prospective Diabetes Study Group. Effect of intensive blood-glucose control with metformin on complications in overweight patients with type 2 diabetes. *Lancet* 1998;352:854–865.

11. Reichard P, Berglund B, Britz A, et al. Intensified conventional insulin treatment retards the microvascular complications of insulin-dependent diabetes mellitus (IDDM): the Stockholm diabetes intervention study (SDIS) after 5 years. *J Intern Med* 1991;30:101–108.

12. Johansen K. Efficacy of metformin in the treatment of NIDDM. *Diabetes Care* 1999;22:33–37. Search date 1996; primary sources current list of medical literature, Index Medicus, Medline, Embase, and hand searched references.

13. Reichard P, Nilsson BY, Rosenqvist U. The effect of long-term intensified insulin treatment on the development of microvascular complications of diabetes mellitus. *N Engl J Med* 1993;29:304–309.

14. Reichard P, Berglund A, Britz A, et al. Hypoglycaemic episodes during intensified insulin treatment: increased frequency but no effect on cognitive function. *J Intern Med* 1991;229:9–16.

15. The Diabetes Control and Complications Trial Research Group. Effects of intensive diabetes therapy on neuropsychological function in adults in the diabetes control and complications trial. *Ann Intern Med* 1996;124:379–388.

16. Austin EJ, Deary IJ. Effects of repeated hypoglycaemia on cognitive function. A psychometrically validated reanalysis of the diabetes control and complications trial data. *Diabetes Care* 1999;22:1273–1277.

17. The Diabetes Control and Complications Trial Research Group. Influence of intensive diabetes treatment on quality-of-life outcomes in the diabetes control and complications trial. *Diabetes Care* 1996;19:195–203.

18. Grey M, Boland EA, Davidson M, Li J, Tamborlane W. Coping skills training for youth with diabetes

Cardiovascular disorders

mellitus has long-lasting effects on metabolic control and quality of life. *J Pediatr* 2000;137:107–113.

19. UK Prospective Diabetes Study Group. Quality of life in type 2 diabetic patients is affected by complications but not by intensive policies to improve blood glucose or blood pressure control (UKPDS 37). *Diabetes Care* 1999;22:1125–1136.

20. Reichard P, Jensen-Urstad K, Ericsson M, Jensen-Urstad M, Lindblad LE. Automonic neuropathy – a complication less pronounced in patients with type 1 diabetes mellitus who have lower blood glucose levels. *Diabet Med* 2000;17:860–866.

21. The Diabetes Control and Complications Trial Research Group. The absence of a glycaemic threshold for the development of long-term complications: the perspective of the diabetes control and complications trial. *Diabetes* 1996;45:1289–1298.

22. Stratton IM, Adler AI, Neil HAW, et al, on behalf of the UK Prospective Diabetes Study Group. Association of glycaemia with macrovascular and microvascular complications of type 2 diabetes (UKPDS 35): prospective observational study. *BMJ* 2000;321:405–412

William Herman
Professor of Internal Medicine and Epidemiology
University of Michigan Medical Center
Ann Arbor Michigan
USA

Competing interests: None declared.

TABLE 1 Risk (odds ratio) for development or progression of microvascular, nephropathic, and neuropathic complications with intensive versus conventional treatment. Odds ratio, number needed to treat, and confidence intervals were all calculated from data in papers (see text, p 99).

Studies	Systematic Review[3]	DCCT[4]	Kumamoto[5]	UKPDS[6]
Number of participants	16 RCTs	RCT	RCT	RCT
Type of diabetes	ND	1441	110	3857
Follow up	Type 1	Type 1	Type 2	Type 2*
Change in HbA1c	8–60 months	6.5 years	6 years	10 years
	1.4%	2.0%	2.0%	0.9%
Progression of retinopathy				
OR (95% CI)	0.49 (0.28 to 0.85)	0.39 (0.28 to 0.55)	0.25 (0.09 to 0.65)	0.66 (0.48 to 0.92)
NNT (95% CI) over duration of study	ND	5 (4 to 7)	4 (3 to 11)	10 (6 to 50)
Development of retinopathy				
OR (95% CI)	ND	0.22 (0.14 to 0.36)	ND	ND
NNT (95% CI) over duration of study	ND	6 (5 to 7)	ND	ND
Development or progression of nephropathy				
OR (95% CI)	0.34 (0.20 to 0.58)	0.50 (0.39 to 0.63)	0.26 (0.09 to 0.75)	0.54 (0.25 to 1.18)
NNT (95% CI) over duration of study	ND	7 (6 to 11)	5 (4 to 19)	ND
Development or progression of neuropathy				
OR (95% CI)	ND	0.36 (0.24 to 0.54)	ND	0.42 (0.23 to 0.78)
NNT (95% CI) over duration of study	ND	13 (11 to 18)	ND	5 (3 to 16)

*All participants had fasting plasma glucose > 6.0 mmol/L on two occasions: 93% had fasting plasma glucose ≥ 7.0 mmol/L (American Diabetes Association criterion) and 86% had fasting plasma glucose ≥ 7.8 mmol/L (World Health Organization criterion). CI, confidence interval; ND, no data.

Cardiovascular disorders

Search date February 2002

Robert McKelvie

Key Messages

Non-drug treatments

■ **Exercise** Systematic reviews have found that prescribed exercise training improves functional capacity and quality of life. One subsequent RCT has found that exercise training versus no exercise training significantly reduces fatal or non-fatal cardiac events (NNT 2, 95% CI 2 to 5), hospital readmission for heart failure (NNT 5, 95% CI 4 to 30), and mortality at 12 months (NNT 4, 95% CI 3 to 19).

■ **Multidisciplinary interventions** One systematic review has found that multidisciplinary approaches to nutrition, patient counselling, and education versus usual care significantly reduce admissions to hospital, but do not significantly reduce mortality. Analysis by each intervention found that only follow up by a multidisciplinary team reduced admissions to hospital, whereas telephone contact plus improved coordination of primary care had no significant effect.

Drug and invasive treatments

- **Amiodarone** Systematic reviews have found weak evidence suggesting that amiodarone versus placebo may reduce mortality.

- **Angiotensin converting enzyme inhibitors** Systematic reviews and RCTs have found that angiotensin converting enzyme inhibitors versus placebo significantly reduce mortality, hospital admission for heart failure, and ischaemic events. Relative benefits are similar in different groups of people, but absolute benefits are greater in people with severe heart failure. RCTs in people with asymptomatic left ventricular systolic dysfunction have found that angiotensin converting enzyme inhibitors versus placebo significantly delay the onset of symptomatic heart failure and reduce cardiovascular events over 40 months.

- **Angiotensin II receptor blockers** One systematic review has found that angiotensin receptor blockers versus placebo reduced all cause mortality and hospital admission in people with New York Heart Association class II–IV heart failure, although the difference was not significant. This may be explained by the small numbers of deaths and admissions reported. It found no significant difference in all cause mortality or hospital admission with angiotensin receptor blockers versus angiotensin converting enzyme inhibitors. It found that angiotensin receptor blockers plus angiotensin converting enzyme inhibitors versus angiotensin converting enzyme inhibitors alone reduced admission for heart failure but did not significantly reduce all cause mortality.

- **Anticoagulation** We found no RCTs of anticoagulation in people with heart failure. We found conflicting evidence from two large retrospective cohort studies.

- **Antiplatelet agents** We found no RCTs of antiplatelet agents in people with heart failure. Retrospective analyses have included too few events to establish or exclude a clinically important effect of antiplatelet agents.

- **β Blockers** Systematic reviews have found strong evidence that adding a β blocker to an angiotensin converting enzyme inhibitor significantly decreases mortality and hospital admission. Limited evidence from a subgroup analysis of one RCT found no significant effect on mortality in black people.

- **Calcium channel blockers** One systematic review has found no significant difference in mortality with second generation dihydropyridine calcium channel blockers versus placebo. RCTs comparing other calcium channel blockers versus placebo found no evidence of benefit.

- **Digoxin (improves morbidity in people already receiving diuretics and angiotensin converting enzyme inhibitors)** One large RCT in people already receiving diuretics and angiotensin converting enzyme inhibitors found that digoxin versus placebo significantly reduces the number of people admitted to hospital for worsening heart failure at 37 months (NNT 13, 95% CI 10 to 17), but did not significantly reduce mortality.

- **Implantable cardiac defibrillators (In people with heart failure and cardiac arrest)** One RCT has found good evidence that an implantable cardiac defibrillator reduces mortality in people with heart failure who have experienced a cardiac arrest.

- **Non-amiodarone antiarrhythmic drugs** Evidence extrapolated from one systematic review in people treated after a myocardial infarction suggests that other antiarrhythmic drugs (apart from β blockers) may increase mortality.

- **Positive inotropes (ibopamine, milrinone, and vesnarinone)** RCTs found that positive inotropic drugs (other than digoxin) versus placebo significantly increased mortality over 6–11 months.

Heart failure

- **Prophylactic use of implantable cardiac defibrillators in people at high risk of arrhythmia** Two RCTs have found that implantable cardiac defibrillators versus medical treatment reduce mortality in people with heart failure and at high risk of arrythmia, whereas one RCT found no significant difference in mortality.

- **Spironolactone in severe heart failure** One RCT in people with severe heart failure taking diuretics, angiotensin converting enzyme inhibitors, and digoxin has found that adding spironolactone versus placebo significantly reduces mortality after 2 years (NNT 9, 95% CI 6 to 15).

- **Treatments for diastolic heart failure** We found no RCTs in people with diastolic heart failure.

DEFINITION Heart failure occurs when abnormality of cardiac function causes failure of the heart to pump blood at a rate sufficient for metabolic requirements, or maintains cardiac output only with a raised filling pressure. It is characterised clinically by breathlessness, effort intolerance, fluid retention, and poor survival. It can be caused by systolic or diastolic dysfunction and is associated with neurohormonal changes.[1] Left ventricular systolic dysfunction (LVSD) is defined as a left ventricular ejection fraction below 0.40. It can be symptomatic or asymptomatic. Defining and diagnosing diastolic heart failure can be difficult. Recently proposed criteria include: (1) clinical evidence of heart failure; (2) normal or mildly abnormal left ventricular systolic function; and (3) evidence of abnormal left ventricular relaxation, filling, diastolic distensibility, or diastolic stiffness.[2] The clinical utility of these criteria is limited by difficulty in standardising assessment of the last criterion.

INCIDENCE/ PREVALENCE Both the incidence and prevalence of heart failure increase with age. Studies of heart failure in the USA and Europe found that under 65 years of age the incidence is 1/1000 men a year and 0.4/1000 women a year. Over 65 years, incidence is 11/1000 men a year and 5/1000 women a year. Under 65 years the prevalence of heart failure is 1/1000 men and 1/1000 women; over 65 years the prevalence is 40/1000 men and 30/1000 women.[3] The prevalence of asymptomatic LVSD is 3% in the general population.[4–6] The mean age of people with asymptomatic LVSD is lower than that for symptomatic individuals. Both heart failure and asymptomatic LVSD are more common in men.[4–6] The prevalence of diastolic heart failure in the community is unknown. The prevalence of heart failure with preserved systolic function in people in hospital with clinical heart failure varies from 13–74%.[7,8] Less than 15% of people with heart failure under 65 years have normal systolic function, whereas the prevalence is about 40% in people over 65 years.[7]

AETIOLOGY/ RISK FACTORS Coronary artery disease is the most common cause of heart failure.[3] Other common causes include hypertension and idiopathic dilated congestive cardiomyopathy. After adjustment for hypertension, the presence of left ventricular hypertrophy remains a risk factor for the development of heart failure. Other risk factors include cigarette smoking, hyperlipidaemia, and diabetes mellitus.[4] The common causes of left ventricular diastolic dysfunction are coronary artery disease and systemic hypertension. Other causes are hypertrophic cardiomyopathy, restrictive or infiltrative cardiomyopathies, and valvular heart disease.[8]

PROGNOSIS The prognosis of heart failure is poor, with 5 year mortality ranging from 26–75%.[3] Up to 16% of people are readmitted with heart failure within 6 months of first admission. In the USA it is the leading cause of hospital admission among people over 65 years old.[3] In people with heart failure, a new myocardial infarction increases the risk of death (RR 7.8, 95% CI 6.9 to 8.8); 34% of all deaths in people with heart failure are preceded by a major ischaemic event.[9] Sudden death, mainly caused by ventricular arrhythmia, is responsible for 25–50% of all deaths, and is the most common cause of death in people with heart failure.[10] The presence of asymptomatic LVSD increases an individual's risk of having a cardiovascular event. One large prevention trial found that for a 5% reduction in ejection fraction the risk ratio for mortality was 1.20 (95% CI 1.13 to 1.29), for hospital admission for heart failure it was 1.28 (95% CI 1.18 to 1.38), and for development of heart failure it was 1.20 (95% CI 1.13 to 1.26).[4] The annual mortality for patients with diastolic heart failure varies in observational studies (1.3–17.5%).[7] Reasons for this variation include age, the presence of coronary artery disease, and variation in the partition value used to define abnormal ventricular systolic function. The annual mortality for left ventricular diastolic dysfunction is lower than that found in patients with systolic dysfunction.[11]

AIMS To relieve symptoms; to improve quality of life; to reduce morbidity and mortality, with minimum adverse effects.

OUTCOMES Functional capacity (assessed by the New York Heart Association [see glossary, p 125] functional classification or more objectively by using standardised exercise testing or the 6 min walk test);[12] quality of life (assessed with questionnaires),[13] mortality; adverse effects of treatment. Proxy measures of clinical outcome (e.g. left ventricular ejection fraction and hospital readmission rates) are used only when clinical outcomes are unavailable.

METHODS Clinical Evidence update search and appraisal February 2002. Generally, RCTs with less than 500 people have been excluded because of the number of large RCTs available. If for any comparison very large RCTs exist then much smaller RCTs have been excluded, even if they have more than 500 people.

QUESTION **What are the effects of non-drug treatments?**

OPTION **MULTIDISCIPLINARY**

One systematic review has found that multidisciplinary programmes significantly reduce admissions to hospital but did not significantly reduce mortality; analysis by intervention has found that only follow up by a multidisciplinary team reduces admissions to hospital, whereas telephone contact plus improved coordination of primary care has no significant effect.

Benefits: We found one systematic review (search date 1999, 11 RCTs, 2067 people with heart failure) that compared a multidisciplinary programme versus conventional care alone.[14] Multidisciplinary programmes included non-drug treatments such as nutrition advice, counselling, patient education, and exercise training. The review found that multidisciplinary interventions significantly reduced hospital admission (406/1001 [40.6%] with multidisciplinary programme v with conventional care 474/1011 [46.9%]; RR 0.87, 95% CI 0.79 to 0.96; 11 RCTs), but did not significantly reduce mortality (104/534 [19.5%] with multidisciplinary programme v 121/572 [21.2%] with conventional care; RR 0.94, 95% CI 0.75 to 1.19; 7 RCTs). However, the hospital admission results were heterogeneous by intervention. Specialised follow up by a multidisciplinary team substantially reduced admissions to hospital (RR 0.77, 95% CI 0.68 to 0.86; 1366 people with heart failure; 9 RCTs), but there was no benefit from telephone contact plus improved coordination of primary care services (RR 1.15, 95% CI 0.96 to 1.37; 646 people with heart failure; 2 RCTs).

Harms: The review suggested that disease management programmes may fragment care such that peoples other conditions are overlooked.[14] However, it did not provide evidence to support this.

Comment: Studies were small, involved highly selected patient populations, and were usually performed in academic centres, so results may not generalise to smaller community centres. Studies lasted less than 6 months and it is not known how well people adhere to treatment over the longer term. Larger studies are needed to define the effects on morbidity and mortality of longer term multidisciplinary interventions.

OPTION   EXERCISE

Systematic reviews found that prescribed exercise training improved functional capacity and quality of life. One recent RCT also found that exercise significantly reduced adverse cardiac events.

Benefits: We found two systematic reviews (search dates 1993 and not stated),[15,16] two subsequent non-systematic reviews,[17,18] and one subsequent RCT[19] of exercise training in people with heart failure. The reviews identified 20 small RCTs that reported only proxy outcomes (maximum exercise time [see glossary, p 125] oxygen uptake, various biochemical measures, and unvalidated symptom scores) in a small number of people over a few weeks. The subsequent RCT (99 people with heart failure, 88 men) compared 12 months of exercise training versus a group with no exercise training.[19] After 12 months, exercise compared with control improved quality of life (P < 0.001), reduced fatal or non-fatal cardiac events (17/50 [34%] with training v 37/49 [76%] without exercise; ARR 42%, 95% CI 20% to 58%; RR 0.45, 95% CI 0.23 to 0.73; NNT 2, 95% CI 2 to 5), mortality (9/50 [18%] with training v 20/49 [41%] without exercise; RR 0.44, 95% CI 0.20 to 0.87; NNT 4, 95% CI 3 to 19), and reduced hospital readmission for heart failure (5/50 [10%] with training v 14/49 [29%] without exercise; ARR 19%, 95% CI 3% to 25%; RR 0.35, 95% CI 0.12 to 0.88; NNT 5, 95% CI 4 to 30).[19]

Harms: The reviews and trial reported no important adverse effects associated with prescribed exercise training.[15,17–19]

Comment: The studies were small, involved highly selected patient populations, and were performed in well resourced academic centres. The results may not generalise to smaller community centres The specific form of exercise training varied among studies and the relative merits of each strategy are unknown. The studies generally lasted less than 1 year and long term effects are unknown. Larger studies over a longer period are needed.

QUESTION **What are the effects of drug treatments in heart failure?**

OPTION **ANGIOTENSIN CONVERTING ENZYME INHIBITORS**

Two systematic reviews and recent RCTs have found that angiotensin converting enzyme inhibitors reduce mortality, hospital admission for heart failure, and ischaemic events in people with heart failure. Relative benefits are similar in different groups of people, but absolute benefits are greater in people with severe heart failure.

Benefits: We found two systematic reviews (search dates 1994 and not stated) of angiotensin converting enzyme (ACE) inhibitors versus placebo in heart failure.[20,21] The first systematic review (search date 1994, 32 RCTs, duration 3–42 months, 7105 people, New York Heart Association [see glossary, p 125] class III or IV) found that ACE inhibitors versus placebo reduced mortality (611/3870 [16%] with ACE inhibitors v 709/3235 [22%] with placebo; ARR 6%, 95% CI 4% to 8%; OR 0.77, 95% CI 0.67 to 0.88; NNT 16).[20] Relative reductions in mortality were similar in different subgroups (stratified by age, sex, cause of heart failure, and New York Heart Association class). The second systematic review (search date not stated, 5 RCTs, 12 763 people with left ventricular dysfunction or heart failure of mean duration 35 months) analysed results from individuals in long term and large RCTs that compared ACE inhibitors versus placebo.[21] Three RCTs were in people for 1 year after myocardial infarction. In these three postinfarction trials (5966 people) ACE inhibitor versus placebo significantly reduced mortality (702/2995 [23.4%] with ACE inhibitor v 866/2971 [29.1%] with placebo; OR 0.74, 95% CI 0.66 to 0.83), readmission for heart failure (355/2995 [11.9%] with ACE inhibitor v 460/2971 [15.5%] with placebo; OR 0.73, 95% CI 0.63 to 0.85), and reinfarction (324/2995 [10.8%] with ACE inhibitor v 391/2971 [13.2%] with placebo; OR 0.80, 95% CI 0.69 to 0.94). For all five trials, ACE inhibitors versus placebo reduced mortality (1467/6391 [23.0%] with ACE inhibitor v 1710/6372 [26.8%] with placebo; OR 0.80, 95% CI 0.74 to 0.87), reinfarction (571/6391 [8.9%] with ACE inhibitor v 703/6372 [11.0%] with placebo; OR 0.79, 95% CI 0.70 to 0.80), and readmission for heart failure (876/6391 [13.7%] with ACE inhibitor v 1202/6372 [18.9%] with placebo; OR 0.67, 95% CI 0.61 to 0.74). The relative benefits began soon after the start of treatment, persisted long term, and were independent of age, sex, and baseline use of diuretics, aspirin, and β blockers. Although there was a trend towards greater relative reduction in mortality or readmission for heart failure in people with lower ejection fractions, benefit was apparent over the range examined. **Other ischaemic**

events: Individual RCTs that studied high risk groups found that ACE inhibitors significantly reduced some ischaemic event rates. One RCT in people with left ventricular dysfunction found that ACE inhibitors reduced myocardial infarction (combined fatal or non-fatal myocardial infarction: 9.9% with ACE inhibitor v 12.3% with placebo; RR 0.77, 95% CI 0.61 to 0.98), hospital admission for angina (15% with ACE inhibitor v 19% with placebo; RR 0.73, 95% CI 0.60 to 0.88), and the combined end point of cardiac death, non-fatal myocardial infarction, or hospital admission for angina (43% with ACE inhibitor v 51% with placebo; RR 0.77, 95% CI 0.68 to 0.86).[9] Effects on hospital readmissions were observed shortly after starting ACE inhibitor treatment, although effects on ischaemic events were not apparent for at least 6 months and peaked at 36 months. **Dosage:** We found one large RCT (3164 people with New York Heart Association class II–IV heart failure) that compared low dose lisinopril (2.5 or 5.0 mg/day) versus high dose lisinopril (32.5 or 35 mg/day).[22] It found no significant difference in mortality (717/1596 [44.9%] with low dose v 666/1568 [42.5%] with high dose; ARR 2.4%, CI not provided; HR 0.92, 95% CI 0.80 to 1.03; P = 0.128), but found that high dose lisinopril reduced the combined outcome of death or hospital admission for any reason (1338/1596 [83.8%] events with low dose v 1250/1568 [79.7%] events with high dose; ARR 4.1%, CI not provided; HR 0.88, 95% CI 0.82 to 0.96; P = 0.002), and reduced admissions for heart failure (1576/1596 [98.7%] admissions with low dose v 1199/1568 [76.5%] admissions with high dose; ARR 22.2%; CI not provided; P = 0.002). **Comparison of different angiotensin converting enzyme inhibitors:** The first systematic review found similar benefits with different ACE inhibitors.[20]

Harms: We found no systematic review. The main adverse effects documented in large trials were cough, hypotension, hyperkalaemia, and renal dysfunction. Compared with placebo, ACE inhibitors increased the incidence of cough (37% with ACE inhibitor v 31% with placebo; ARI 7%, 95% CI 3% to 11%; RR 1.23, 95% CI 1.11 to 1.35; NNH 14), dizziness or fainting (57% with ACE inhibitor v 50% with placebo; ARI 7%, 95% CI 3% to 11%; RR 1.14, 95% CI 1.06 to 1.21; NNH 14), increased creatinine concentrations above 177 µmol/L (10.7% with ACE inhibitor v 7.7% placebo; ARI 3.0%, 95% CI 0.6% to 6.0%; RR 1.38, 95% CI 1.09 to 1.67; NNH 34), and increased potassium concentrations above 5.5 mmol/L (AR 6.4% with ACE inhibitor v 2.5% with placebo; ARI 4%, 95% CI 2% to 7%; RR 2.56, 95% CI 1.92 to 3.20; NNH 26).[23] Angioedema was not found to be more common with ACE inhibitors than placebo (3.8% taking enalapril v 4.1% taking placebo; ARI +0.3%, 95% CI −1.4% to +1.5%).[23] The trial comparing low and high doses of lisinopril found that most adverse effects were more common with high dose (no P value provided; dizziness: 12% with low dose v 19% with high dose; hypotension: 7% with low dose v 11% with high dose; worsening renal function: 7% with low dose v 10% with high dose; significant change in serum potassium concentration: 7% with low dose v 7% with high dose), although there was no difference in withdrawal rates between groups (17% discontinued with high dose v 18% with low dose). The trial found that cough was less commonly experienced with high dose compared with low dose lisinopril (cough: 13% with low dose v 11% with high dose).

Comment: The relative beneficial effects of ACE inhibitors were similar in different subgroups of people with heart failure. Most RCTs evaluated left ventricular function by assessing left ventricular ejection fraction, but some studies defined heart failure clinically, without measurement of left ventricular function in people at high risk of developing heart failure (soon after myocardial infarction) It is unclear whether there are additional benefits from adding ACE inhibitor treatment in people with heart failure who are already taking antiplatelet treatment, and of adding antiplatelet treatment in people with heart failure who are already taking an ACE inhibitor (see antiplatelet agents, p 122).

OPTION   ANGIOTENSIN II RECEPTOR BLOCKERS

One systematic review has found that angiotensin receptor blockers versus placebo reduced all cause mortality and hospital admission in people with New York Heart Association class II–IV heart failure, although the difference was not significant. This may be explained by the small numbers of deaths and admissions reported. It found no significant difference in all cause mortality or hospital admission with angiotensin receptor blockers versus angiotensin converting enzyme inhibitors. It found that angiotensin receptor blockers plus angiotensin converting enzyme inhibitors versus angiotensin converting enzyme inhibitors alone reduced admission for heart failure but did not significantly reduce all cause mortality.

Benefits: **Versus placebo:** We found one systematic review (search date 2001, 11 RCTs, 2259 people with New York Heart Association [see glossary, p 125] class II–IV, follow up 4 wks to 2 years).[24] It found that angiotensin receptor blockers versus placebo reduced all cause mortality and admission for heart failure, although the differences were not significant (all cause mortality: 7 RCTs; AR 2% with angiotensin receptor blockers v 3% with placebo; OR 0.68, 95% CI 0.38 to 1.22; admission for heart failure: 1 RCT; 8% with angiotensin receptor blockers v 12% with placebo; OR 0.67, 95% CI 0.29 to 1.51). The numbers of deaths and admissions were small, which may explain why the difference did not reach significance. **Versus angiotensin converting enzyme inhibitors:** The systematic review identified six RCTs (4682 people with New York Heart Association class II–IV, follow up 4 wks to 1.5 years) comparing angiotensin receptor blockers versus angiotensin converting enzyme (ACE) inhibitors.[24] It found no significant difference between treatments for all cause mortality or rate of admission for heart failure (all cause mortality: 6 RCTs; OR 1.09, 95% CI 0.92 to 1.29; admission for heart failure: 3 RCTs; OR 0.95, 95% CI 0.8 to 1.13). **Plus angiotensin converting enzyme inhibitors versus angiotensin converting enzyme inhibitors alone:** The systematic review identified six RCTs (5712 people with New York Heart Association class II–IV heart failure) comparing angiotensin receptor blockers plus ACE inhibitors versus ACE inhibitors alone.[24] It found that combined treatment significantly reduced hospital admission for heart failure (3 RCTs; OR 0.74, 95% CI 0.64 to 0.86). However, it found no significant difference between treatments for all cause mortality (6 RCTs; OR 1.04, 95% CI 0.91 to 1.20).

Harms: The systematic review did not report on harms.[24]

Comment: In people who are truly intolerant of ACE inhibitors the evidence supports the use of angiotensin II receptor blockers, with the expectation of at least symptomatic improvement of the heart failure.

| OPTION | POSITIVE INOTROPIC AGENTS |

One well designed RCT found that digoxin decreased the rate of hospital admissions for worsening heart failure in people already receiving diuretics and angiotensin converting enzyme inhibitors, although it found no evidence of an effect on mortality. RCTs found evidence that positive inotropic drugs other than digoxin increased mortality in people with heart failure; evidence on morbidity was less clear.

Benefits: **Digoxin:** We found one systematic review (search date 1992, 13 RCTs, duration 3–24 wks, 1138 people with heart failure and sinus rhythm)[25] and one subsequent large RCT.[26] The systematic review found that six of the 13 RCTs enrolled people without assessment of ventricular function and may have included some people with mild or no heart failure. Other limitations of the older trials included crossover designs and small sample sizes. In people who were in sinus rhythm with heart failure, the systematic review found fewer people with clinical worsening of heart failure (52/628 [8.3%] with digoxin v 131/631 [20.8%] with placebo; ARR 12.5%, 95% CI 9.5% to 14.7%; RR 0.40, 95% CI 0.29 to 0.54) but did not find a definite effect on mortality (16/628 [2.5%] with digoxin v 15/631 [2.4%] with placebo; ARR −0.2%, 95% CI −2.6% to +1.1%; RR 1.07, 95% CI 0.53 to 2.23). The subsequent large RCT (6800 people, 88% male, mean age 64 years, New York Heart Association class I–III [see glossary, p 125], 94% already taking angiotensin converting enzyme inhibitors, 82% taking diuretics) compared blinded additional treatment with either digoxin or placebo for a mean of 37 months.[26] Digoxin did not reduce all cause mortality compared with placebo (1181/3397 [34.8%] with digoxin v 1194/3403 [35.1%] with placebo; ARR +0.3%, 95% CI −2.0% to +2.6%; RR 0.99, 95% CI 0.93 to 1.06). The number of people admitted to hospital for worsening heart failure was substantially less with digoxin over 37 months (910/3397 [27%] with digoxin v 1180/3403 [35%] with placebo; ARR 8%, 95% CI 6% to 10%; RR 0.77, 95% CI 0.72 to 0.83; NNT 13, 95% CI 10 to 17), as was the combined outcome of death or hospital admission caused by worsening heart failure (1041/3397 [31%] with digoxin v 1291/3403 [38%] for placebo; ARR 7.3%, 95% CI 5.1% to 9.4%; RR 0.81, 95% CI 0.75 to 0.87; NNT 14). **Other inotropic agents:** One non-systematic review (6 RCTs, 8006 people) of RCTs found that non-digitalis positive inotropic agents increased mortality compared with placebo.[10] The largest RCT in the review (3833 people with heart failure) found increased mortality with vesnarinone 60 mg daily versus placebo over 9 months (292/1275 [23%] with vesnarinone v 242/1280 [19%] with placebo; ARI 4%, 95% CI 1% to 8%; RR 1.21, 95% CI 1.04 to 1.40; NNH 25).[10,27] Another large RCT (1088 people with heart failure) found milrinone versus placebo increased mortality over 6 months (168/561 [30%] with milrinone v 127/527 [24%] with placebo; ARI 6.0%, 95% CI 0.5% to 12.0%; RR 1.24, 95% CI 1.02 to 1.49; NNH 17).[28] A third large RCT (1906 people with heart failure) compared ibopamine versus placebo over 11 months.[29] It found that ibopamine increased mortality (232/953 [25%] with ibopamine v 193/953 [20%] with placebo; RR 1.26, 95% CI 1.04 to 1.53). The review found that some studies reported improved functional capacity and quality of life, but this was not consistent across all studies.

Harms: We found no systematic review. **Digoxin:** The RCT (6800 people) found that more people had suspected digoxin toxicity in the digoxin group versus placebo (11.9% with digoxin v 7.9% with placebo; ARI 4.0%, 95% CI 2.4% to 5.8%; RR 1.5, 95% CI 1.30 to 1.73; NNH 25).[26] The RCT found no evidence that digoxin increased the risk of ventricular fibrillation or tachycardia compared with placebo (37/3397 [1.1%] with digoxin v 27/3403 [0.8%] with placebo; ARI +0.3%, 95% CI –0.1% to +1.0%; RR 1.37, 95% CI 0.84 to 2.24). Digoxin compared with placebo increased rates of supraventricular arrhythmia (2.5% with digoxin v 1.2% with placebo; ARI 1.3%, 95% CI 0.5% to 2.4%; RR 2.08, 95% CI 1.44 to 2.99; NNH 77) and second or third degree atrioventricular block (1.2% with digoxin v 0.4% with placebo; ARI 0.8%, 95% CI 0.2% to 1.8%; RR 2.93, 95% CI 1.61 to 5.34; NNH 126). **Other inotropic agents:** Most RCTs found that inotropic agents other than digoxin increased risk of death (see benefits above).

Comment: None.

OPTION β BLOCKERS

We found strong evidence from systematic reviews that adding β blockers to standard treatment with angiotensin converting enzymes inhibitors in people with moderate and severe heart failure reduces the rate of hospital admission or death. Subgroup analysis in black people found no significant effect on mortality.

Benefits: We found two systematic reviews (search dates 2000 and not stated)[30,31] and two subsequent RCTs of the effects of β blockers in heart failure.[32,33] **In people with any severity of heart failure:** The first systematic review (search date 2000, 22 RCTs, 10 315 people with heart failure) found that β blockers versus placebo significantly reduced the risk of death (444/5273 [8.4%] with β blockers v 624/4862 [12.8%] with placebo; OR 0.65, 95% CI 0.53 to 0.80) and hospital admissions (540/5244 [10.3%] with β blockers v 754/4832 [15.6%] with placebo; OR 0.64, 95% CI 0.53 to 0.79).[30] This is equivalent to three fewer deaths and four fewer hospital admissions per 100 people treated for 1 year. The results were consistent for selective and non-selective β blockers. Sensitivity analysis and funnel plots found that the results were robust to any reasonable publication bias. **In people with severe**

heart failure: The second systematic review (search date not stated, 4 RCTs, 635 people with class IV heart failure) found that β blockers versus placebo significantly reduced the risk of death (56/313 [17.9%] with β blockers v 81/322 [25.1%] with placebo; RR 0.71, 95% CI 0.52 to 0.96). Two subsequent RCTs compared β blockers versus placebo in people with class III or IV heart failure.[32,33] The first RCT (2289 people with class IV heart failure, who were euvolemic [defined as the absence of rales and ascites and the presence of no more than minimal peripheral oedema] and who had an ejection fraction of less than 25%, but were not receiving intensive care, intravenous vasodilators, or positive inotropic drugs) compared carvedilol versus placebo over 10.4 months. It was stopped early because of a significant beneficial effect on survival that exceeded the pre-specified interim monitoring boundaries.[32] It found that β blockers significantly reduced mortality (130/1156 [11.2%] with β blockers v 190/1133 [16.8%] with placebo; RR 0.65, 95% CI 0.52 to 0.81) and the combined outcome of death or hospital admission (425/1156 [36.8%] with β blockers v 507/1133 [44.7%] with placebo; RR 0.76, 95% CI 0.67 to 0.87). The second RCT compared bucindolol versus placebo in people with severe heart failure (2708 people class III or IV heart failure and ejection fraction ≤ 35%; about 70% of the people were white and 24% were black).[33] The RCT was stopped early because of accumulated evidence from other studies of β blockers. It found that more people died with placebo but the difference did not reach significance (411/1354 [30.4%] with bucindolol v 449/1354 [33.1%] with placebo; HR 0.90, 95% CI 0.78 to 1.02). The RCT found a significant interaction of treatment effect with race (black v non-black). There was no evidence of benefit in black people (HR 1.17, 95% CI 0.89 to 1.53), although there was a significant effect for non-black people (HR 0.82, 95% CI 0.70 to 0.96).

Harms: Fears that β blockers may cause excessive problems with worsening heart failure, bradyarrhythmia, or hypotension have not been confirmed. One subsequent RCT found that fewer people with carvedilol versus placebo required permanent discontinuation of treatment because of adverse events other than death (P = 0.02).[32] Cumulative withdrawals at 1 year were 14.8% with carvedilol versus 18.5% with placebo. For the subgroup of people with recent or recurrent cardiac decompensation or severely depressed cardiac function the difference in withdrawal rates was greater (17.5% with carvedilol v 24.2% with placebo). The subsequent RCT comparing bucindolol versus placebo found that 23% in the bucindolol group and 25% of people in the placebo group permanently discontinued the medication.[33]

Comment: Good evidence was found for the use of β blockers in people with moderate symptoms (New York Heart Association class II or III [see glossary, p 125]) receiving standard treatment, including angiotensin converting enzyme inhibitors. The value of β blockers needs clarification in heart failure with preserved ejection fraction and in asymptomatic left ventricular systolic dysfunction. One recent RCT has shown that carvedilol reduced all cause mortality compared with placebo (AR for death: 12% with carvedilol v 15% with placebo; HR 0.77, 95% CI 0.60 to 0.98; P = 0.03) in 1959 people with acute myocardial infarction and left ventricular ejection fraction less than or equal to 40%.[34] The RCTs of β blockers have consistently found a mortality benefit, but it is not clear whether or not the benefit is a class effect. One recent small RCT (150 people) of metoprolol versus carvedilol found some differences in surrogate outcomes, but both drugs produced similar improvements in symptoms, submaximal exercise tolerance, and quality of life.[35] The results for non-black people were consistent between bucindolol and carvedilol. The lack of observed benefit for black people in one RCT[33] raises the possibility that there may be race specific responses to pharmacological treatment for cardiovascular disease.

OPTION	CALCIUM CHANNEL BLOCKERS

One systematic review of second generation dihydropyridine calcium channel blockers found no evidence of benefit. RCTs of other calcium channel blockers found no evidence of benefit.

Benefits: **After myocardial infarction:** See calcium channel blockers under acute myocardial infarction, p 11. **Other heart failure:** We found one systematic review (search date not stated) of second generation dihydropyridine calcium channel blockers,[36] one non-systematic review of all calcium channel blockers (3 RCTs, 1790 people with heart failure),[10] and one subsequent RCT.[37] The systematic review (18 RCTs) found two RCTs large enough to assess mortality.[36] Meta-analysis found no significant difference in mortality (1603 people; OR 0.94, 95% CI 0.79 to 1.12).[36] The largest RCT in the non-systematic review (1153 people, [New York Heart Association class III or IV — see glossary, p 125], left ventricular ejection fraction < 0.30, using diuretics, digoxin, and angiotensin converting enzyme inhibitors) found that amlodipine versus placebo had no significant effect on the primary combined end point of all cause mortality and hospital admission for cardiovascular events over 14 months (222/571 [39%] with amlodipine v 246/582 [42%] with placebo; ARR +3.4%, 95% CI –2.3% to +8.8%; RR 0.92, 95% CI 0.79 to 1.06).[10,38] Subgroup analysis of people with primary cardiomyopathy found a reduction in mortality (45/209 [22%] with amlodipine v 74/212 [35%] with placebo; ARR 13%, 95% CI 5% to 20%; RR 0.62, 95% CI 0.43 to 0.85; NNT 7). There was no significant difference in the group with heart failure caused by coronary artery disease. The second RCT (186 people, idiopathic dilated cardiomyopathy, NYHA class I–III) compared diltiazem versus placebo.[10] It found no evidence of a difference in survival with diltiazem versus placebo in those who did not have a heart transplant, although people on diltiazem had improved cardiac function, exercise capacity, and subjective quality of life. The third RCT (451 people with mild heart failure, NYHA class II or III) compared felodipine versus placebo.[10] No significant beneficial or adverse effect was found. The subsequent RCT (2590 NYHA people with class II–IV heart failure, mean follow up of 1.6 years with placebo and 1.5 with mibefradil) found that more people died with mibefradil but the difference was not significant (350/1295 [27.0%] with mibefradil v 319/1295 [24.6%] with placebo; RR 1.10, 95% CI 0.96 to 1.25).[37]

Heart failure

Harms: Calcium channel blockers have been found to exacerbate symptoms of heart failure or increase mortality in people with pulmonary congestion after myocardial infarction or ejection fraction less than 0.40 (see calcium channel blockers under acute myocardial infarction, p 11).[10] The mibefradil RCT found that in people taking digoxin, class I or II antiarrhythmics, amiodarone, or drugs associated with torsade de pointes, mibefradil increased risk of death versus placebo.[37] The review found that second generation dihydropyridine calcium channel blockers did not cause significant adverse effects.[36]

Comment: Many of the RCTs were underpowered and had wide confidence intervals. An RCT of amlodipine in people with primary dilated cardiomyopathy is in progress.

OPTION ALDOSTERONE RECEPTOR ANTAGONISTS

One large RCT of people with severe heart failure (on usual treatment including angiotensin converting enzyme inhibitors) has found that adding an aldosterone receptor antagonist (spironolactone) further reduces mortality.

Benefits: We found no systematic review. We found one RCT of spironolactone (25 mg/day) versus placebo (1663 people with heart failure, New York Heart Association class III or IV [see glossary, p 125], left ventricular ejection fraction < 0.35, all taking angiotensin converting enzyme inhibitors and loop diuretics, and most taking digoxin).[39] The trial was stopped early because of a significant reduction in the primary end point of all cause mortality with spironolactone after 2 years (mortality: 284/822 [35%] with spironolactone v 386/841 [46%] with placebo; ARR 11%, 95% CI 7% to 16%; RR 0.75, 95% CI 0.66 to 0.85; NNT 9, 95% CI 6 to 15).[39]

Harms: The RCT found no evidence that spironolactone in combination with an angiotensin converting enzyme inhibitor may result in an increased incidence of clinically significant hyperkalaemia. Gynaecomastia or breast pain were reported in 10% of men given spironolactone and 1% of men given placebo.[39]

Comment: The RCT was large and well designed. As only people with New York Heart Association functional class III or IV were included, these results cannot necessarily be generalised to people with milder heart failure.

OPTION ANTIARRHYTHMIC DRUG TREATMENT

Systematic reviews found weak evidence that amiodarone reduced total mortality in people with heart failure. Extrapolation from one systematic review in people treated after a myocardial infarction suggests that other antiarrhythmic agents may increase mortality in people with heart failure.

Benefits: **Amiodarone:** We found two systematic reviews of the effects of amiodarone versus placebo in heart failure.[40,41] The most recent review (search date 1997, 10 RCTs, 4766 people) included people with a wide range of conditions (symptomatic and asymptomatic heart failure, ventricular arrhythmia, recent myocardial infarction, and recent cardiac arrest).[40] Eight of these RCTs reported the number of deaths. The review found that treatment with amiodarone over 3–24 months reduced the risk of death from any cause compared with placebo or conventional treatment (436/2262 [19%] with amiodarone v 507/2263 [22%] with control; ARR 3%, 95% CI 0.8% to 5.3%; RR 0.86, 95% CI 0.76 to 0.96; NNT 32). This review did not perform any subgroup analyses on people with heart failure. The earlier systematic review (search date not stated) found eight RCTs (5101 people after myocardial infarction) of prophylactic amiodarone versus placebo or usual care and five RCTs (1452 people with heart failure).[41] Mean follow up was 16 months. Analysis of results from all 13 RCTs found a lower total mortality with amiodarone than control (annual mortality: 10.9% with amiodarone v 12.3% with control). The effect was significant with some methods of calculation (fixed effects model: OR 0.87, 95% CI 0.78 to 0.99) but not with others (random effects model: OR 0.85, 95% CI 0.71 to 1.02). The effect of amiodarone was significantly greater in RCTs that compared amiodarone versus usual care than in placebo controlled RCTs. Deaths classified as arrhythmic death or sudden death were significantly reduced by amiodarone compared with placebo (OR 0.71, 95% CI 0.59 to 0.85). Subgroup analysis found a significant effect of amiodarone in the five heart failure RCTs (annual mortality: 19.9% with amiodarone v 24.3% with placebo; OR 0.83, 95% CI 0.70 to 0.99). **Other antiarrhythmics:** Apart from β blockers, other antiarrhythmic drugs seem to increase mortality in people at high risk (see class I antiarrhythmic agents under secondary prevention of ischaemic cardiac events, p 189).

Harms: **Amiodarone:** Amiodarone was not found to increase the non-arrhythmic death rate (OR 1.02, 95% CI 0.87 to 1.19).[41] In placebo controlled RCTs, after 2 years 41% of people in the amiodarone group and 27% in the placebo group had permanently discontinued study medication.[41] In 10 RCTs of amiodarone versus placebo, amiodarone increased the odds of reporting adverse drug reactions compared with placebo (OR 2.22, 95% CI 1.83 to 2.68). Nausea was the most common adverse effect. Hypothyroidism was the most common serious adverse effect (7.0% with amiodarone v 1.1% with control). Hyperthyroidism (1.4% with amiodarone v 0.5% with control), peripheral neuropathy (0.5% with amiodarone v 0.2% with control), lung infiltrates (1.6% with amiodarone v 0.5% with control), bradycardia (2.4% with amiodarone v 0.8% with control), and liver dysfunction (1.0% with amiodarone v 0.4% with control) were all more common in the amiodarone group.[41] **Other antiarrhythmics:** These agents (particularly class I antiarrhythmics) may increase mortality (see class I antiarrhythmic agents under secondary prevention of ischaemic cardiac events, p 189).

Comment: **Amiodarone:** RCTs of amiodarone versus usual treatment found larger effects than placebo controlled trials.[41] These findings suggest bias; unblinded follow up may be associated with reduced usual care or improved adherence with amiodarone. Further studies are required to assess the effects of amiodarone treatment on mortality and morbidity in people with heart failure.

Heart failure

| OPTION | IMPLANTABLE CARDIAC DEFIBRILLATORS |

One RCT has found good evidence that implantable cardiac defibrillator reduces mortality in people with heart failure who have experienced a cardiac arrest. Two RCTs have found that implantable cardiac defibrillators reduce mortality compared with medical treatment in people with heart failure and at high risk of arrhythmia, whereas one RCT found no significant difference in mortality.

Benefits: We found no systematic review. We found four RCTs examining the effects of implantable cardiac defibrillators (ICDs) in people with left ventricular dysfunction.[42–45] The first RCT (1016 people resuscitated after ventricular arrhythmia plus either syncope or other serious cardiac symptom plus left ventricular ejection fraction ≤ 0.40) compared an ICD versus an antiarrhythmic drug (mainly amiodarone).[42] ICDs improved survival at 1, 2, and 3 years (1 year survival: 89.3% with ICD v 82.3% with antiarrhythmic; 2 year survival: 81.6% with ICD v 73.7% with antiarrhythmic; 3 year survival: 75.4% with ICD v 64.1% with antiarrhythmic). The second RCT included 196 people with New York Heart Association class I–III (see glossary, p 125) heart failure and previous myocardial infarction, a left ventricular ejection fraction 0.35 or less, a documented episode of asymptomatic unsustained ventricular tachycardia, and inducible non-suppressible ventricular tachyarrhythmia on electrophysiological study.[43] Ninety five people received an ICD and 101 received conventional medical treatment. The trial found that ICDs reduced mortality over a mean of 27 months (deaths: 15/95 [16%] with ICD [11 from cardiac cause] v 39/101 [39%] with conventional treatment [27 from cardiac cause]; HR 0.46, 95% CI 0.26 to 0.82). The third RCT included 1055 people aged under 80 years who were scheduled for coronary artery bypass surgery, had a left ventricular ejection fraction less than 0.36, and had electrocardiographic abnormalities. It found that ICD (446 people) at the time of bypass surgery versus no ICD (454 people) produced no significant difference in mortality over a mean of 32 months (deaths: 101/446 [23%] with ICD [71 from cardiac causes] v 95/454 [21%] with control [72 from cardiac causes]; HR 1.07, 95% CI 0.81 to 1.42).[44] The fourth RCT (1232 people with prior myocardial infarction and left ventricular ejection fraction < 0.30) compared an ICD (742 people) versus conventional medical treatment (490 people).[45] It found that ICD reduced all cause mortality after 20 months mean follow up (AR 14.2% with ICD v 19.8% with conventional treatment; HR 0.69, 95% CI 0.51 to 0.93, P = 0.016).

Harms: The RCTs found that the main adverse effects of ICDs were infection (about 5%), pneumothorax (about 2%), bleeding requiring further operation (about 1%), serious haematomas (about 3%), cardiac perforation (about 0.2%), problems with defibrillator lead (about 7%), and malfunction of defibrillator generator (about 3%).[42–45]

Comment: The RCTs were in people with reduced left ventricular function and included people with and without previous cardiac arrest or inducible arrhythmia. It is uncertain whether asymptomatic ventricular arrhythmia is in itself a predictor of sudden death in people with moderate or severe heart failure.[46] Several RCTs of prophylactic ICD treatment in people with heart failure and in survivors of acute myocardial infarction are ongoing.[47]

OPTION   ANTICOAGULATION

We found no RCTs of anticoagulation in people with heart failure. We found conflicting evidence from two large retrospective cohort studies.

Benefits: We found no systematic review and no RCTs of anticoagulation in people with heart failure. We found conflicting evidence from two large retrospective cohort studies (see comment below).[48,49]

Harms: Neither cohort study reported harms of anticoagulation.

Comment: The first retrospective analysis assessed the effect of anticoagulants used at the discretion of individual investigators in RCTs on the incidence of stroke, peripheral arterial embolism, and pulmonary embolism.[48] The first cohort was from one RCT (642 men with chronic heart failure) comparing hydralazine plus isosorbide dinitrate versus prazosin versus placebo. The second cohort was from another RCT (804 men with chronic heart failure) comparing enalapril versus hydralazine plus isosorbide dinitrate. All people were given digoxin and diuretics. The retrospective analysis found that without treatment the incidence of all thromboembolic events was low (2.7/100 people years in the first RCT; 2.1/100 people years in the second RCT) and that anticoagulation did not reduce the incidence of thromboembolic events (2.9/100 people years in the first RCT; 4.8/100 people years in the second RCT). In this group of people, atrial fibrillation was not found to be associated with a higher risk of thromboembolic events. The second retrospective analysis was from two large RCTs (2569 people with symptomatic and asymptomatic left ventricular dysfunction) that compared enalapril versus placebo.[49] The analysis found that people treated with warfarin at baseline had significantly lower risk of death during follow up (HR adjusted for baseline differences 0.76, 95% CI 0.65 to 0.89). Warfarin use was associated with a reduction in the combined outcome of death plus hospital admission for heart failure (adjusted HR 0.82, 95% CI 0.72 to 0.93). The benefit with warfarin use was not significantly influenced by the presence of symptoms, randomisation to enalapril or placebo, sex, presence of atrial fibrillation, age, ejection fraction, New York Heart Association classification (see glossary, p 125), or cause of heart failure. Warfarin reduced cardiac mortality, specifically deaths that were sudden, or associated with either heart failure or myocardial infarction. Neither of the retrospective studies was designed to determine the incidence of thromboembolic events in heart failure or the effects of treatment. Neither study included information about the intensity of anticoagulation or warfarin use. We found several additional cohort studies that showed a reduction in thromboembolic events with anticoagulation, but they all reported results for too few people to provide useful results. An RCT is needed to compare anticoagulation versus no anticoagulation in people with heart failure.

OPTION	ANTIPLATELET AGENTS

We found no RCTs. Retrospective analyses have included too few events to establish or exclude a clinically important effect of antiplatelet agents in people with heart failure. In people not taking angiotensin converting enzyme inhibitors, we found limited evidence from one retrospective cohort analysis that the incidence of thromboembolic events in people with heart failure was low and not significantly improved with antiplatelet treatment. It is unclear from two retrospective cohort analyses, whether there are additional reductions in the incidence of thromboembolic events from adding angiotensin converting enzyme inhibitor treatment to antiplatelet treatment in people with heart failure. It is unclear from one retrospective cohort analysis, whether adding antiplatelet treatment to angiotensin converting enzyme inhibitor treatment in people with heart failure is beneficial.

Benefits: We found no systematic review and no RCTs examining effects of antiplatelet agents in people with heart failure. We found two cohort studies (see comment below).[48,50]

Harms: Neither study reported harms of treatment.

Comment: **In people not taking angiotensin converting enzyme inhibitors:** We found no systematic review and no RCTs. We found one retrospective cohort analysis within one RCT in 642 men with heart failure.[48] The RCT compared hydralazine plus isosorbide dinitrate versus prazosin versus placebo in men receiving digoxin and diuretics. Aspirin, dipyridamole, or both were used at the discretion of the investigators. The number of thromboembolic events was low in both groups (only 1 stroke and no pulmonary or peripheral emboli in 184 people years of treatment with antiplatelet drugs v 21 strokes, 4 peripheral, and 4 pulmonary emboli in 1068 people years of treatment without antiplatelet drugs; 0.5 events/ 100 people years with antiplatelet agents v 2.0 events/100 people years without antiplatelet agents; P = 0.07). **In people taking angiotensin converting enzyme inhibitors:** We found no RCTs. We found two large retrospective cohort studies.[48,50] The first retrospective analysis assessed the effect of antiplatelet agents used at the discretion of individual investigators on the incidence of stroke, peripheral arterial embolism, and pulmonary embolism within one RCT.[48] The RCT (804 men with chronic heart failure) compared enalapril versus hydralazine plus isosorbide dinitrate. It found that the incidence of all thromboembolic events was low without antiplatelet treatment and, although antiplatelet agents reduced the thromboembolic rate, the difference was not significant (1.6 events/100 people years with antiplatelet agents v 2.1 events/ 100 people years with no antiplatelet agent; P = 0.48). The second cohort analysis was from two large RCTs that compared enalapril versus placebo (2569 people with symptomatic and asymptomatic left ventricular dysfunction). It found that people treated with antiplatelet agents at baseline had a significantly lower risk of death (HR adjusted for baseline differences 0.82, 95% CI 0.73 to 0.92).[50] Subgroup analysis suggested that an effect of antiplatelet agents might be present in people who were randomised to placebo (mortality HR for antiplatelet treatment at baseline v no antiplatelet treatment at baseline 0.68, 95% CI 0.58 to 0.80), but not in people randomised to enalapril (mortality HR for antiplatelet treatment v no antiplatelet treatment 1.00, 95% CI 0.85 to 1.17). Both retrospective studies have limitations common to studies with a retrospective cohort design. One study did not report on the proportions of people taking aspirin and other antiplatelet agents.[48] The other study noted that more than 95% of people took aspirin, but the dosage and consistency of antiplatelet use was not recorded.[50] One retrospective non-systematic review (4 RCTs, 96 712 people) provided additional evidence about the effect of aspirin on the benefits of early angiotensin converting enzyme inhibitors in heart failure.[51] It found a similar reduction in 30 day mortality with angiotensin converting enzyme inhibitor versus control for those people not taking aspirin compared to those taking aspirin (aspirin: OR 0.94, 95% CI 0.89 to 0.99; no aspirin: OR 0.90, 95% CI 0.81 to 1.01). However, the analysis may not be valid because the people who did not receive aspirin were older and had a worse baseline prognosis than those taking aspirin. The effects of antiplatelet treatment in combination with ACE inhibitors in people with heart failure requires further research.

QUESTION **What are the effects of angiotensin converting enzyme inhibitors in people at high risk of heart failure?**

RCTs have found good evidence that angiotensin converting enzyme inhibitors can delay development of symptomatic heart failure and reduce the frequency of cardiovascular events in people with asymptomatic left ventricular systolic dysfunction, and in people with other cardiovascular risk factors for heart failure.

Benefits: **In people with asymptomatic left ventricular systolic dysfunction:** We found no systematic review but found two RCTs. One large RCT examined an angiotensin converting enzyme (ACE) inhibitor (enalapril) versus placebo over 40 months in people with asymptomatic left ventricular systolic dysfunction (LVEF; < 0.35).[52] It found no evidence that enalapril significantly decreased total mortality and cardiovascular mortality compared with placebo (all cause mortality: 313/2111 [14.8%] with ACE inhibitor v 334/2117 [15.8%] with placebo; ARR +0.9%, 95% CI −1.3% to +2.9%; RR 0.94, 95% CI 0.81 to 1.08; cardiovascular mortality: 265/2111 [12.6%] with ACE inhibitor v 298/2117 [14.1%] with placebo; ARR +1.5%, 95% CI −0.6% to +3.3%; RR 0.89, 95% CI 0.76 to 1.04). During the study more people assigned to the placebo received digoxin, diuretics, or ACE inhibitors that were not part of the study protocol, which may have contributed to the lack of significant difference in mortality between the two groups. Compared with placebo, enalapril reduced symptomatic heart failure, hospital admission for heart failure, and fatal or non-fatal myocardial infarction (symptomatic heart failure: 438/2111 [21%] with ACE inhibitor

Heart failure

v 640/2117 [30%] with placebo; ARR 9.5%, 95% CI 7% to 12%; RR 0.69, 95% CI 0.61 to 0.77; NNT 11; admission for heart failure: 306/2111 [15%] with ACE inhibitor *v* 454/2117 [21%] with placebo; ARR 7%, 95% CI 5% to 9%; RR 0.68, 95% CI 0.59 to 0.77; NNT 14; fatal or non-fatal myocardial infarction: 7.6% with ACE inhibitor *v* 9.6% with placebo; ARR 2%, 95% CI 0.4% to 3.4%; RR 0.79, 95% CI 0.65 to 0.96).[9,52] A second RCT in asymptomatic people after myocardial infarction with documented LVSD found that an ACE inhibitor (captopril) reduced mortality and reduced the risk of ischaemic events compared with placebo.[53] **In people with other risk factors:** We found one large RCT comparing ramipril 10 mg daily versus placebo, for a mean of 5 years, in 9297 high risk people (people with vascular disease or diabetes plus one other cardiovascular risk factor) who were not known to have LVSD or heart failure.[54] It found that ramipril reduced the risk of heart failure (9.0% with ramipril *v* 11.5% with placebo; RR 0.77, 95% CI 0.67 to 0.87; P < 0.001). Ramipril also reduced the combined risk of myocardial infarction or stroke or cardiovascular death, the risk of these outcomes separately, and all cause mortality (see angiotensin converting enzyme inhibitors under secondary prevention of ischaemic cardiac events, p 189). During the trial, 496 people underwent echocardiography; 2.6% of these people were found to have ejection fraction less than 0.4. Retrospective review of charts found that left ventricular function had been documented in 5193 people; 8.1% had a reduced ejection fraction.

Harms:
We found no systematic review. The first RCT over 40 months found that a high proportion of people in both groups reported adverse effects (76% with enalapril *v* 72% with placebo).[52] Dizziness or fainting (46% with enalapril *v* 33% with placebo) and cough (34% with enalapril *v* 27% with placebo) were reported more often in the enalapril group (P value not stated). The incidence of angioedema was the same in both groups (1.4%). Study medication was permanently discontinued by 8% of the people in the enalapril group versus 5% in the placebo group (P value not stated).

Comment:
Asymptomatic LVSD is prognostically important, but we found no prospective studies that have assessed the usefulness of screening to detect its presence.

QUESTION **What are the effects of treatments for diastolic heart failure?**

We found no RCTs in people with diastolic heart failure.

Benefits:
We found no systematic review or RCTs in people with diastolic heart failure.

Harms:
We found no evidence on the harms of treatments for diastolic heart failure.

Comment:
The causes of diastolic dysfunction vary among people with diastolic heart failure. Current treatment is empirical, based on the results of small clinical studies and consists of treating the underlying cause and coexistent conditions with interventions optimised for individuals.[6,55,56] RCTs with clinically relevant outcome measures are needed to determine the benefits and harms of treatment in diastolic heart failure.

GLOSSARY

Exercise time This is the total time in seconds that a person is able to pedal in a standardised symptom limited bicycle ergonometry exercise test.

New York Heart Association classification Classification of severity by symptoms. Class I: no limitation of physical activity; ordinary physical activity does not cause undue fatigue or dyspnoea. Class II: slight limitation of physical activity; comfortable at rest, but ordinary physical activity results in fatigue or dyspnoea. Class III: limitation of physical activity; comfortable at rest, but less than ordinary activity causes fatigue or dyspnoea. Class IV: unable to carry on any physical activity without symptoms; symptoms are present even at rest; if any physical activity is undertaken, symptoms are increased.

REFERENCES

1. Poole-Wilson PA. History, definition, and classification of heart failure. In: Poole-Wilson PA, Colucci WS, Massie BM, et al, eds. Heart failure. Scientific principles and clinical practice. London: Churchill Livingstone, 1997.269–277.
2. Working Group Report. How to diagnose diastolic heart failure: European Study Group on Diastolic Heart Failure. Eur Heart J 1998;19:990–1003.
3. Cowie MR, Mosterd A, Wood DA, et al. The epidemiology of heart failure. Eur Heart J 1997;18:208–225.
4. McKelvie RS, Benedict CR, Yusuf S. Prevention of congestive heart failure and management of asymptomatic left ventricular dysfunction. BMJ 1999;318:1400–1402.
5. Bröckel U, Hense HW, Muscholl M. Prevalence of left ventricular dysfunction in the general population [abstract]. J Am Coll Cardiol 1996;27(suppl A):25.
6. Mosterd A, deBruijne MC, Hoes A. Usefulness of echocardiography in detecting left ventricular dysfunction in population-based studies (the Rotterdam study). Am J Cardiol 1997;79;103–104.
7. Vasan RS, Benjamin EJ, Levy D. Congestive heart failure with normal left ventricular systolic function. Arch Intern Med 1996;156:146–157.
8. Davie AP, Francis CM, Caruana L, et al. The prevalence of left ventricular diastolic filling abnormalities in patients with suspected heart failure. Eur Heart J 1997;18:981–984.
9. Yusuf S, Pepine CJ, Garces C, et al. Effect of enalapril on myocardial infarction and unstable angina in patients with low ejection fractions. Lancet 1992,340:1173–1178.
10. Gheorghiade M, Benatar D, Konstam MA, et al. Pharmacotherapy for systolic dysfunction: a review of randomized clinical trials. Am J Cardiol 1997;80(8B):14H–27H.
11. Gaasch WH. Diagnosis and treatment of heart failure based on LV systolic or diastolic dysfunction. JAMA 1994;271:1276–1280.
12. Bittner V, Weiner DH, Yusuf S, et al, for the SOLVD Investigators. Prediction of mortality and morbidity with a 6-minute walk test in patients with left ventricular dysfunction. JAMA 1993;270:1702–1707.
13. Rogers WJ, Johnstone DE, Yusuf S, et al, for the SOLVD Investigators. Quality of life among 5 025 patients with left ventricular dysfunction randomized between placebo and enalapril. The studies of left ventricular dysfunction. J Am Coll Cardiol 1994;23:393–400.
14. McAlister FA, Lawson FME, Teo KK, et al. A systematic review of randomized trials of disease management programs in heart failure. Am J Med 2001;110:378–384. Search date 1999; primary sources Medline, Embase, Cinahl, Sigle, Cochrane Controlled Trials Register, the Cochrane Effective Practice and Organization of Care Study Register, hand searches of bibliographies of identified studies, and personal contact with content experts.
15. Dracup K, Baker DW, Dunbar SB, et al. Management of heart failure. II. Counseling, education and lifestyle modifications. JAMA 1994;272:1442–1446. Search date 1993; primary sources Medline and Embase.
16. Piepoli MF, Flater M, Coats AJS. Overview of studies of exercise training in chronic heart failure: the need for a prospective randomized multi-centre European trial. Eur Heart J 1998;19:830–841. Search date and primary sources not stated; computer aided search performed.
17. Miller TD, Balady GJ, Fletcher GF. Exercise and its role in the prevention and rehabilitation of cardiovascular disease. Ann Behav Med 1997;19:220–229.
18. European Heart Failure Training Group. Experience from controlled trials of physical training in chronic heart failure. Protocol and patient factors in effectiveness in the improvement in exercise tolerance. Eur Heart J 1998;19:466–475.
19. Belardinelli R, Georgiou D, Cianci G, et al. Randomized, controlled trial of long-term moderate exercise training in chronic heart failure. Effects on functional capacity, quality of life, and clinical outcomes. Circulation 1999;99;1173–1182.
20. Garg R, Yusuf S, for the Collaborative Group on ACE Inhibitor Trials. Overview of randomized trials of angiotensin-converting enzyme inhibitors on mortality and morbidity in patients with heart failure. JAMA 1995;273:1450–1456. Search date 1994; primary sources Medline and correspondence with investigators and pharmaceutical companies.
21. Flather M, Yusuf S, Kober L, et al, for the ACE-Inhibitor Myocardial Infarction Collaborative Group. Long-term ACE-inhibitor therapy in patients with heart failure or left-ventricular dysfunction: a systematic overview of data from individual patients. Lancet 2000;355:1575–1581. Search date not stated; primary sources Medline, Ovid, hand searches of reference lists, and personal contact with researchers, colleagues, and principal investigators of the trials identified.
22. Packer M, Poole-Wilson PA, Armstrong PW, et al, on behalf of the ATLAS Study Group. Comparative effects of low and high doses of the angiotensin converting enzyme inhibitor, lisinopril, on morbidity and mortality in chronic heart failure. Circulation 1999;100:2312–2318.

23. SOLVD Investigators. Effect of enalapril on survival in patients with reduced left ventricular ejection fractions and congestive heart failure. *N Engl J Med* 1991;325:293–302.

24. Jong P, Demers C, McKelvie RS, et al. Angiotensin receptor blockers in heart failure: meta-analysis of randomized controlled trials. *J Am Coll Cardiol* 2002;39:463–470. Search date 2001; primary sources Medline, Embase, Biological Abstracts, International Pharmaceutical Abstracts, Cochrane Controlled Trials Database, McMaster Cardiovascular Randomized Clinical Trial Registry, and Science Citation Index.

25. Kraus F, Rudolph C, Rudolph W. Wirksamkeit von Digitalis bei Patienten mit chronischer Herzinsuffizienz und Sinusrhythmus. *Herz* 1993;18:95–117. Search date 1992; primary source Medline.

26. Digitalis Investigation Group. The effect of digoxin on mortality and morbidity in patients with heart failure. *N Engl J Med* 1997;336:525–533.

27. Cohn J, Goldstein S, Greenberg B, et al. A dose-dependent increase in mortality among patients with severe heart failure. *N Engl J Med* 1998;339:1810–1816.

28. Packer M, Carver JR, Rodeheffer RJ, et al, for the PROMISE Study Research Group. Effect of oral milrinone on mortality in severe chronic heart failure. *N Engl J Med* 1991;325:1468–1475.

29. Hampton JR, van Veldhuisen DJ, Kleber FX, et al. Randomised study of effect of ibopamine on survival in patients with advanced severe heart failure. *Lancet* 1997;349:971–977.

30. Brophy JM, Joseph L, Rouleau JL. β-blockers in congestive heart failure: a Bayesian meta-analysis. *Ann Intern Med* 2001;134:550–560. Search date 2000; primary sources Medline, Cochrane Library, Web of Science, and hand searches of reference lists from relevant articles.

31. Whorlow SL, Krum H. Meta-analysis of effect of β-blocker therapy on mortality in patients with New York Heart Association class IV chronic congestive heart failure. *Am J Cardiol* 2000;86:886–889. Search date not stated; primary sources Medline and hand searches of reference lists from relevant reviews.

32. Packer M, Coats A, Fowler MB. Effect of carvedilol on survival in severe chronic heart failure. *Engl J Med* 2001;344:1651–1658.

33. The Beta-Blocker Evaluation of Survival Trial Investigators. A trial of the β-blocker bucindolol in patients with advanced chronic heart failure. *N Engl J Med* 2001;344:1659–1667.

34. The CAPRICORN Investigators. Effect of carvedilol on outcome after myocardial infarction in patients with left ventricular dysfunction: the CAPRICORN randomized trial. *Lancet* 2001;357:1385–1390.

35. Metra M, Giubbini R, Nodari S, et al. Differential effects of β-blockers in patients with heart failure: a prospective, randomized, double-blind comparison of the long-term effects of metoprolol versus carvedilol. *Circulation* 2000;102:546–551.

36. Cleophas T, van Marum R. Meta-analysis of efficacy and safety of second-generation dihydropyridine calcium channel blockers in heart failure. *Am J Card* 2001;87:487–490. Search date not stated; primary source Medline.

37. Levine TB, Bernink P, Caspi A, et al. Effect of mibefradil, a T-type calcium channel blocker, on morbidity and mortality in moderate to severe congestive heart failure. The MACH-1 study. *Circulation* 2000;101:758–764.

38. Packer M, O'Connor CM, Ghali JK, et al, for the Prospective Randomized Amlodipine Survival Evaluation Study Group. Effect of amlodipine on morbidity and mortality in severe chronic heart failure. *N Engl J Med* 1996;335:1107–1114.

39. Pitt B, Zannad F, Remme WJ, et al, for the Randomized Aldactone Evaluation Study Investigators. The effects of spironolactone on morbidity and mortality in patients with severe heart failure. *N Engl J Med* 1999;341:709–717.

40. Piepoli M, Villani GQ, Ponikowski P, et al. Overview and meta-analysis of randomised trials of amiodarone in chronic heart failure. *Int J Cardiol* 1998;66:1–10. Search date 1997; primary source unspecified computerised literature database.

41. Amiodarone Trials Meta-Analysis Investigators. Effect of prophylactic amiodarone on mortality after acute myocardial infarction and in congestive heart failure: meta-analysis of individual data from 6500 patients in randomised trials. *Lancet* 1997;350:1417–1424. Search date not stated; primary sources literature reviews, computerised literature reviews, and discussion with colleagues.

42. The Antiarrhythmic versus Implantable Defibrillators (AVID) Investigators. A comparison of antiarrhythmic-drug therapy with implantable defibrillators I patients resuscitated from near-fatal ventricular arrhythmias. *N Engl J Med* 1997;337:1576–1583.

43. Moss AJ, Hall WJ, Cannom DS, et al. Improved survival with an implanted defibrillator in patients with coronary disease at high risk for ventricular arrhythmia. *N Engl J Med* 1996;335:1933–1940.

44. Bigger JT for The Coronary Artery Bypass Graft (CABG) Patch Trial Investigators. Prophylactic use of implanted cardiac defibrillators in patients at high risk for ventricular arrhythmias after coronary-artery bypass graft surgery. *N Engl J Med* 1997;337:1569–1575.

45. Moss AJ, Zoreba W, Hall J, et al, for the Multicenter Automatic Defibrillator Implantation Trial II Investigators. Prophylactic implantation of a defibrillator in patients with myocardial infarction and reduced ejection fraction. *N Engl J Med* 2002;346:877–883.

46. Teerlink JR, Jalaluddin M, Anderson S, et al. Ambulatory ventricular arrhythmias in patients with heart failure do not specifically predict an increased risk of sudden death. *Circulation* 2000;101:40–46.

47. Connolly SJ. Prophylactic antiarrhythmic therapy for the prevention of sudden death in high-risk patients: drugs and devices. *Eur Heart J* 1999;(suppl C):31–35.

48. Dunkman WB, Johnson GR, Carson PE, et al, for the V-HeFT Cooperative Studies Group. Incidence of thromboembolic events in congestive heart failure. *Circulation* 1993;87:94–101.

49. Al-Khadra AS, Salem DN, Rand WM, et al. Warfarin anticoagulation and survival: a cohort analysis from the studies of left ventricular dysfunction. *J Am Coll Cardiol* 1998;31:749–753.

50. Al-Khadra AS, Salem DN, Rand WM, et al. Antiplatelet agents and survival: a cohort analysis from the Studies of Left Ventricular Dysfunction (SOLVD) Trial. *J Am Coll Cardiol* 1998;31:419–425.

51. Latini R, Tognoni G, Maggioni AP, et al, on behalf of the Angiotensin-converting Enzyme Inhibitor Myocardial Infarction Collaborative Group. Clinical effects of early angiotensin-converting enzyme inhibitor treatment for acute myocardial infarction are similar in the presence and absence of aspirin. Systematic overview of individual data from 96 712 randomized patients. *J Am Coll Cardiol* 2000;35:1801–1807.

52. SOLVD Investigators. Effect of enalapril on mortality and the development of heart failure in asymptomatic patients with reduced left ventricular ejection fractions. *N Engl J Med* 1992;327:685–691.

Cardiovascular disorders

53. Rutherford JD, Pfeffer MA, Moyé LA, et al. Effects of captopril on ischaemic events after myocardial infarction. *Circulation* 1994;90:1731–1738.

54. The Heart Outcome Prevention Evaluation Study Investigators. Effects of an angiotensin-converting-enzyme inhibitor, ramipril, on cardiovascular events in high-risk patients. *N Engl J Med* 2000;342:145–153.

55. The Task Force of the Working Group on Heart Failure of the European Society of Cardiology. The treatment of heart failure. *Eur Heart J* 1997;18:736–753.

56. Tendera M. Ageing and heart failure: the place of ACE inhibitors in heart failure with preserved systolic function. *Eur Heart J* 2000;2(suppl I):I8–I14.

Robert McKelvie
Associate Professor of Medicine
McMaster University
Hamilton, ON
Canada

Competing interests: RM has been paid by AstraZeneca and Bristol-Myers Squibb to serve on steering committees and has been paid by AstraZeneca and Merck Frosst to give presentations

Cardiovascular disorders

Obesity

Search date May 2002

David Arterburn

Key Messages

- **Dexfenfluramine** One systematic review found that dexfenfluramine versus placebo promotes weight loss in healthy obese adults. Dexfenfluramine has been associated with valvular heart disease and pulmonary hypertension and is no longer marketed for use in obesity.

- **Diethylpropion** One systematic review found that diethylpropion versus placebo promotes modest weight loss in healthy obese adults. We found two case reports describing pulmonary hypertension and psychosis with diethylpropion. We found insufficient evidence on weight regain and long term safety. Diethylpropion is no longer marketed in Europe for use in obesity because of a possible link between diethylpropion and heart and lung problems that could not be totally excluded.

- **Fenfluramine** One systematic review found that fenfluramine versus placebo promotes modest weight loss in healthy obese adults. Fenfluramine has been associated with valvular heart disease and pulmonary hypertension and is no longer marketed for use in obesity.

- **Fenfluramine plus phentermine** One RCT found that fenfluramine plus phentermine versus placebo promoted weight loss. The combination of fenfluramine plus phentermine has been associated with valvular heart disease and pulmonary hypertension and is no longer marketed for use in obesity.

- **Fluoxetine** One systematic review found that fluoxetine versus placebo promotes modest weight loss in healthy obese adults. We found insufficient evidence on weight regain and long term safety of fluoxetine in obesity. One systematic review of antidepressant treatment has found an association between selective serotonin reuptake inhibitors and uncommon but serious adverse events including bradycardia, bleeding, granulocytopenia, seizures, hyponatraemia, hepatotoxicity, serotonin syndrome and extrapyramidal effects.

- **Mazindol** One systematic review found that mazindol versus placebo promotes modest weight loss in healthy obese adults. We found one case report of pulmonary hypertension diagnosed 1 year after stopping treatment with mazindol. We found one clinical evaluation of mazindol in people with stable cardiac disease that found an association between mazindol and cardiac events such as atrial fibrillation. We found insufficient evidence on weight regain and long term safety.

- **Orlistat** Systematic reviews and subsequent RCTs have found that in addition to a low calorie diet, orlistat versus placebo modestly increases weight loss in adults with obesity. Adverse effects such as oily spotting from the rectum, flatulence, and faecal urgency occurred in up to 27% of people taking orlistat. We found insufficient evidence on weight regain and long term safety.

- **Phentermine** One systematic review found that phentermine versus placebo promotes modest weight loss in healthy obese adults. We found insufficient evidence on weight regain and long term safety. Phentermine is no longer marketed in Europe for use in obesity because a link between phentermine and heart and lung problems could not be totally excluded.

- **Phenylpropanolamine** One systematic review found that phenylpropanolamine versus placebo promotes modest weight loss in healthy obese adults. One case control study found that phenylpropanolamine significantly increased risk of haemorrhagic stroke in the first 3 days of use. Phenylpropanolamine is no longer marketed for use in obesity.

- **Sibutramine** A systematic review and RCTs have found that sibutramine versus placebo promotes modest weight loss in healthy, obese adults (body mass index 25–40 kg/m^2) with diabetes, hyperlipidaemia and hypertension. One RCT has found that sibutramine is more effective than placebo for weight maintenance after weight loss in healthy, obese adults but weight regain occurs when sibutramine is discontinued. Sibutramine is no longer marketed in Italy for use in obesity because of concerns about severe adverse reactions including tachycardia, hypertension, arrhythmia, and two deaths due to cardiac arrests. One RCT found that sibutramine achieved greater weight loss than either orlistat or metformin.

- **Sibutramine plus orlistat** One RCT found no significant change in mean body weight over a 16 week period with sibutramine plus orlistat versus sibutramine alone.

DEFINITION Obesity is a chronic condition characterised by an excess of body fat. It is most often defined by the body mass index (BMI) (see glossary, p 138), a mathematical formula that is highly correlated with body fat. BMI is weight in kilograms divided by height in metres squared (kg/m^2). In the USA and UK, people with BMIs between 25–30 kg/m^2 are categorised as overweight, and those with BMIs above 30 kg/m^2 are categorised as obese.[1] Nearly 5 million US adults used prescription weight loss medication in 1996–1998. A quarter of users were not overweight, suggesting that weight loss medication may be inappropriately used. This is thought to be especially the case among women, white people, and Hispanic people.[2]

INCIDENCE/ PREVALENCE   Obesity has increased steadily in many countries since 1900. In the UK in 1994, it was estimated that 13% of men and 16% of women were obese.[1,3] In the past decade alone, the prevalence of obesity in the USA has increased from 12% in 1991 to 27% in 1999.[4]

AETIOLOGY/ RISK FACTORS   The cause of obesity includes both genetic and environmental factors. Obesity may also be induced by drugs (e.g. high dose glucocorticoids), or be secondary to a variety of neuroendocrine disorders such as Cushing's syndrome and polycystic ovary syndrome.[5]

PROGNOSIS   Obesity is a risk factor for several chronic diseases, including hypertension, dyslipidaemia, diabetes, cardiovascular disease, sleep apnoea, osteoarthritis, and some cancers.[1] The relation between increasing body weight and mortality is curvilinear, with mortality rate increasing in people with low body weight. Whether this is caused by increased mortality risk at low body weights or by unintentional weight loss is not clear.[6] Results from five prospective cohort studies and 1991 national statistics suggest that the number of annual deaths attributable to obesity among US adults is about 280 000.[7]

AIMS   To achieve realistic gradual weight loss and prevent the morbidity and mortality associated with obesity, without undue adverse effects.

OUTCOMES   We found no studies that used the primary outcomes of functional morbidity or mortality. Proxy measures include mean weight loss (kg), number of people losing 5% or more of baseline body weight, and number of people maintaining weight loss.

METHODS   *Clinical Evidence* update search and appraisal May 2002.

QUESTION   What are the effects of drug treatments in adults?

OPTION   SIBUTRAMINE

A systematic review and RCTs have found that that sibutramine versus placebo promotes modest weight loss in healthy obese adults (body mass index 25–40 kg/m[2]) with diabetes, hyperlipidaemia, and hypertension. One RCT has found that sibutramine is also more effective than placebo for weight maintenance after weight loss in healthy obese adults but weight regain occurs when sibutramine is discontinued. Sibutramine is no longer marketed in Italy for use in obesity because of concerns about severe adverse reactions including tachycardia, hypertension, arrhythmia, and two deaths due to cardiac arrests. One RCT found that sibutramine achieved greater weight loss than either orlistat or metformin. Another RCT found no significant change in mean body weight over a 16 week period with sibutramine plus orlistat versus sibutramine alone.

Benefits: **Sibutramine:** We found one systematic review (search date 2000, 11 RCTs),[8] six additional RCTs,[9–14] and five subsequent RCTs[15–19] comparing sibutramine versus placebo (see table 1, p 141). The systematic review pooled data for groups of RCTs with similar follow up.[8] The review found that sibutramine (10–20 mg daily) reduced weight more than placebo after 8 weeks (3 RCTs, 106 people, WMD sibutramine v placebo –3.4 kg, 95% CI –4.22 kg to –2.58 kg).[8] The review also pooled analyses of two 6 month trials (207 people) and found that sibutramine (10–20 mg daily) achieved weight loss of 5% or greater more frequently than placebo (RR for > 5% weight loss: sibutramine v placebo 2.1, 95% CI 1.7 to 2.6).[8] One RCT (485 healthy, obese adults) comparing sibutramine (10 or 15 mg daily) versus placebo for 52 weeks found that sibutramine reduced weight more than placebo (–4.4 kg v –6.4 kg v –1.6 kg; P < 0.01 sibutramine 10 mg or 15 mg v placebo).[11] A second RCT compared intermittent sibutramine (15 mg daily for wks 1–12, 19–30, and 37–48) versus continuous sibutramine (15 mg daily) versus placebo for 48 weeks. The RCT found no significant difference between intermittent and continuous sibutramine: both regimens reduced weight more than placebo (1001 healthy obese adults, –3.3 kg v –3.8 kg v +0.2 kg; P < 0.001 intermittent or continuous sibutramine v placebo).[10] Five RCTs found that maximal weight loss with sibutramine may be achieved as early as 12 weeks and longer duration trials suggest that weight loss continues until 24 weeks.[9–11,14,17] One RCT (605 healthy, obese adults) evaluated sibutramine for weight maintenance for 2 years.[12] People received sibutramine (10 mg daily) plus diet for 6 months; 467 people with more than 5% weight loss were then randomly assigned to sibutramine (10 mg daily) or placebo for an additional 18 months. The RCT found that a greater proportion of people maintained 80% or more of their original weight loss at 24 months with sibutramine versus placebo (43% with sibutramine v 16% with placebo; P < 0.001). Weight regain occurred when sibutramine was discontinued (73% of initial weight loss regained over 18 months).[12] Another RCT followed people for 6 months after discontinuation of sibutramine and reported 43% weight regain.[19] Three RCTs in obese adults with type 2 diabetes[13,16,18] and one RCT in obese adults with hyperlipidaemia[15] have found a significant decrease in weight with sibutramine versus placebo when used in addition to dietary modification. Two other RCTs in obese adults with hypertension have found a significant decrease in weight with sibutramine versus placebo.[9,17] **Versus orlistat or metformin**: We found one RCT (150 obese women) comparing sibutramine (20 mg daily) versus orlistat (120 mg 3 times daily) versus metformin (850 mg twice daily) for 6 months.[20] All people were also instructed to follow a reduced calorie diet. The RCT found that sibutramine achieved greater weight loss than either orlistat or metformin (–13.0 kg with sibutramine v –8.0 kg with orlistat v –9.0 kg with metformin; P < 0.0001). **Sibutramine plus orlistat**: We found one RCT (42 women who had completed 1 year of sibutramine plus lifestyle modification), which compared sibutramine (10–15 mg daily) plus orlistat (120 mg 3 times daily) versus sibutramine plus placebo.[21] Mean body weight did not change significantly in either group over a 16 week period (+0.1 kg with combined treatment v +0.5 kg with sibutramine plus placebo).

Harms: **Sibutramine:** We found no evidence about safety beyond 2 years of treatment. Sibutramine was withdrawn from the market in Italy in 2002 in response to 50 reported adverse reactions, including seven severe adverse reactions (tachycardia, hypertension, and arrhythmia) and two deaths due to cardiac arrests. To date, none of the other regulatory agencies including the Medicines Control Agency, UK; the Food & Drug Administration, USA; Health, Canada; and the Therapeutics Goods Administration, Australia have taken any regulatory actions against the drug.[22] **Versus orlistat or metformin**: One RCT reported dry mouth, insomnia, constipation, and hypertension with sibutramine and abdominal discomfort with orlistat and metformin.[20] **Sibutramine plus orlistat**: One RCT reported that people who received sibutramine plus orlistat experienced more soft stools (50%), bowel movements (50%), and oily evacuation (42.9%) than those who received sibutramine alone (9.1% with sibutramine plus orlistat, 9.1% with sibutramine alone, and 0% with placebo; $P < 0.05$).[21]

Comment: None.

OPTION   PHENTERMINE

One systematic review found that phentermine versus placebo promotes modest weight loss in healthy obese adults. We found insufficient evidence on weight regain and long term safety. Phentermine is no longer marketed in Europe for use in obesity because a link between phentermine and heart and lung problems could not be totally excluded.

Benefits: We found one systematic review (search date 1999, 6 RCTs) comparing phentermine (15–30 mg daily) versus placebo in healthy, obese adults with mean follow up of 13.2 weeks (range 2–24 wks).[23] The mean numbers of people in each arm were 32 (range 15–76) for phentermine and 29.4 (range 12–74) for placebo. The review found that phentermine produced significant weight loss (effect size < 0.8 [information presented graphically]; difference in weight loss between phentermine and placebo in the 6 RCTs ranged from 0.6–6.0 kg). The review also compared phentermine versus other agents (diethylpropion, dexfenfluramine, fenfluramine, fluoxetine, mazindol, orlistat, phenylpropanolamine, and sibutramine) and found no significant difference in effect size between phentermine and the other agents (based on 95% CIs).[23]

Harms: The systematic review did not make any comment on adverse effects.[23] We found no evidence of serious adverse reactions. Phentermine given alone has not been associated with valvular heart disease.[24] A European Commission review of the risks and benefits of phentermine concluded that randomised trials do not adequately show efficacy for weight loss. Although no new safety problems were identified with phentermine, the Commission commented that a link between phentermine and "heart and lung problems could not be totally excluded". As a result of this report and subsequent regulatory actions, phentermine has been withdrawn from the market in Europe. [25]

Comment: Most of the people treated with phentermine received additional lifestyle treatment.[23] High withdrawal rates have been reported for phentermine.

| OPTION | MAZINDOL |

One systematic review found that mazindol versus placebo promotes modest weight loss in healthy obese adults. We found one case report of pulmonary hypertension diagnosed 1 year after stopping treatment with mazindol. We found one clinical evaluation of mazindol in people with stable cardiac disease that found an association between mazindol and cardiac events such as atrial fibrillation. We found insufficient evidence on weight regain and long term safety.

Benefits: We found one systematic review (search date 1999, 22 RCTs) comparing mazindol (1–3 mg daily) versus placebo in healthy obese adults with mean follow up of 11.0 weeks (range 2–20 wks).[23] The mean number of people in each arm was 24 (range 8–50) for mazindol and 18 (range 8–30) for placebo. The review found that mazindol produced weight loss that was significantly different from placebo (effect size < 0.8 [information presented graphically]; difference in weight loss between mazindol and placebo in the 22 RCTs ranged from 0.1–7.3 kg). The review also compared mazindol versus other agents (diethylpropion, dexfenfluramine, fenfluramine, fluoxetine, orlistat, phenylpropanolamine, phentermine, and sibutramine) and found no significant difference in effect size between mazindol and the other agents except sibutramine and fenfluramine (based on 95% CIs).[23]

Harms: The systematic review did not comment on adverse effects.[23] We found a single case report of pulmonary hypertension diagnosed 12 months after stopping mazindol that had been taken for 10 weeks.[26] One clinical evaluation in people with stable cardiac disease found an association between mazindol and cardiac events (3 episodes of atrial fibrillation and 2 of syncope in 15 people receiving mazindol for 12 wks).[27] The frequency of serious adverse events with this agent remains unclear.

Comment: None.

| OPTION | DIETHYLPROPION |

One systematic review found that diethylpropion versus placebo promotes modest weight loss in healthy obese adults. We found two case reports describing pulmonary hypertension and psychosis with diethylpropion. We found insufficient evidence on weight regain and long term safety. Diethylpropion is no longer marketed in Europe for use in obesity because a link between diethylpropion and heart and lung problems could not be totally excluded.

Benefits: We found one systematic review (search date 1999, 9 RCTs) comparing diethylpropion (75 mg daily) versus placebo in healthy, obese adults with mean follow up of 17.6 weeks (range 6–52 wks).[23] The mean number of people in each arm was 22 (range 5–32) for diethylpropion and 18 (range 4–29) for placebo. The review found that diethylpropion produced weight loss that was significantly different from placebo (effect size < 0.8 [information presented graphically]; difference in weight loss between diethyl-propion and placebo in the 9 RCTs ranged from 1.6–11.5 kg). The review also compared diethylpropion versus other agents (dexfen-fluramine, fenfluramine, fluoxetine, mazindol, orlistat, phenylpropa-nolamine, phentermine, and sibutramine) and found no significant difference in effect size between diethylpropion and the other agents (based on 95% CIs).[23]

Harms: The systematic review did not comment on adverse effects.[23] Case reports have described pulmonary hypertension and psychosis in users of diethylpropion.[28,29] The frequency of serious adverse events with this agent remains unclear. A European Commission review of the risks and benefits of diethylpropion concluded that randomised trials do not adequately show efficacy for weight loss. Although no new safety problems were identified with diethylpro-pion, the Commission commented that a link between diethylpro-pion and "heart and lung problems could not be totally excluded". As a result of this report and subsequent legal actions, diethylpro-pion has been withdrawn from the market in Europe.[25]

Comment: None.

OPTION   **FLUOXETINE**

One systematic review found that fluoxetine versus placebo promotes modest weight loss in healthy obese adults. We found insufficient evidence on weight regain and long term safety of fluoxetine in obesity. One systematic review of antidepressant treatment has found an association between selective serotonin reuptake inhibitors and uncommon but serious adverse events including bradycardia, bleeding, granulocytopenia, seizures, hyponatraemia, hepatotoxicity, serotonin syndrome, and extrapyramidal effects.

Benefits: We found one systematic review (search date 1999) comparing fluoxetine (32.5–60.0 mg daily) versus placebo.[23] This review included 11 RCTs in healthy, obese adults with mean follow up of 27.5 weeks (range 6–60 wks). The mean number of people in each arm was 55.2 (range 9–136) for fluoxetine and 55.7 (range 9–136) for placebo. The review found that fluoxetine produced significant weight loss (effect size < 0.8 [information presented graphically]; difference in weight loss between fluoxetine and placebo in the 11 RCTs ranged from 0.2–7.4 kg). The review also compared fluoxetine versus other agents (diethylpropion, dexfenfluramine, fenfluramine, mazindol, orlistat, phe-nylpropanolamine, phentermine, and sibutramine) and found no sig-nificant difference in effect size between fluoxetine and the other agents except sibutramine and fenfluramine (based on 95% CIs).[23]

Harms: One systematic review did not comment on adverse effects.[23] One RCT (not included in the systematic review[23]) comparing fluoxetine versus placebo for obesity reported more frequent gastrointestinal symptoms, sleep disturbance, sweating, tremor, amnesia, and thirst in the active treatment groups (frequency of events not provided).[30] One systematic review (search date 1998) of antidepressant treatment found that selective serotonin reuptake inhibitors were associated with a 10–15% incidence of anxiety, diarrhoea, dry mouth, headache, and nausea. The review also found an association between selective serotonin reuptake inhibitors and uncommon but serious adverse events including bradycardia, bleeding, granulocytopenia, seizures, hyponatraemia, hepatotoxicity, serotonin syndrome, and extrapyramidal effects (see glossary, p 138).[31]

Comment: None.

OPTION   **FENFLURAMINE OR DEXFENFLURAMINE**

One systematic review found that fenfluramine, dexfenfluramine, or fenfluramine plus phentermine versus placebo promotes modest weight loss in healthy obese adults. Dexfenfluramine, fenfluramine, and fenfluramine plus phentermine have been associated with valvular heart disease and pulmonary hypertension and are no longer marketed for use in obesity.

Benefits: **Fenfluramine:** We found one systematic review (search date 1999) comparing fenfluramine (39–120 mg daily) versus placebo.[23] This review included 14 RCTs in healthy obese adults with mean follow up of 9.7 weeks (range 4–18 wks). The mean number of people in each arm was 20 (range 5–58) for fenfluramine and 21.2 (range 6–68) for placebo. The review found that fenfluramine produced significant weight loss (effect size > 0.8 [information presented graphically]; difference in weight loss between fenfluramine and placebo in the 14 RCTs ranged from 0.1–5.0 kg). The review found no significant difference in effect size between fenfluramine and the other agents but fenfluramine produced significantly better weight loss compared with other agents except sibutramine (based on 95% CIs).
Dexfenfluramine: We found one systematic review (search date 1999) comparing dexfenfluramine (30–130 mg daily) versus placebo.[23] This review included 14 RCTs in healthy, obese adults with mean follow up of 30 weeks (range 4–56 wks). The mean number of people in each arm was 46.6 (range 5–295) for dexfenfluramine and 44.1 (range 5–268) for placebo. The review found that dexfenfluramine produced weight loss that was significantly different from placebo (effect size < 0.8 [information presented graphically]; difference in weight loss between dexfenfluramine and placebo in the 14 RCTs ranged from 0.2–10.0 kg). The review found no significant difference in effect size between dexfenfluramine and the other agents except sibutramine and fenfluramine (based on 95% CIs).
Fenfluramine plus phentermine: We found one RCT (121 people, 30–80% overweight), which found that a combination of phentermine (15 mg daily) plus fenfluramine (60 mg daily) reduced weight more than placebo after treatment for 6 months (–14.3 kg with phentermine plus fenfluramine v –4.6 kg with placebo; mean difference –9.7 kg, 95% CI –12.0 to –7.4 kg). The trial found that weight loss ceased at 18 weeks of treatment; weight regain was noted after 60 weeks of treatment.[32]

Harms: **Dexfenfluramine, fenfluramine, fenfluramine plus phentermine:** These agents have been associated with valvular heart disease and primary pulmonary hypertension,[33,34] and are no longer marketed.[35] One 25 centre retrospective cohort study in 1473 people found prevalence rates and relative risk of aortic regurgitation of 8.9% with dexfenfluramine (RR 2.18, 95% CI 1.32

to 3.59; NNH 20) and 13.7% with phentermine plus fenfluramine (RR 3.34, 95% CI 2.09 to 5.35; NNH 10) compared with 4.1% with no treatment.[36] At 1 year follow up using repeat echocardiography of 1114 people (75.6% of people recruited), more of the dexfenfluramine and fenfluramine plus phentermine group had decreased aortic regurgitation versus controls (6.4% with dexfenfluramine v 1.7% controls; P < 0.001; 4.5% with fenfluramine plus phentermine; P = 0.03).[37] One prospective study (1072 people) found no significant increase in the risk of valvular heart disease in people taking dexfenfluramine for less than 3 months compared with those taking placebo (sustained release dexfenfluramine RR 1.6, 95% CI 0.8 to 3.4; regular dexfenfluramine RR 1.4, 95% CI 0.7 to 3.0, when compared with placebo).[38] At 1 year follow up, repeat echocardiography of 914 people (83.5% of people recruited) revealed more people had a reduction in aortic regurgitation in both dexfenfluramine groups versus placebo (5.1% sustained release dexfenfluramine; P = 0.002 and 6.4% regular dexfenfluramine; P < 0.001).[39] One case control study (95 people with primary pulmonary hypertension and 355 matched controls) found a history of fenfluramine use was associated with increased risk of primary pulmonary hypertension (OR 6.3, 95% CI 3.0 to 13.2). The odds ratio was higher among people who had taken fenfluramine in the past year (OR 10.1, 95% CI 3.4 to 29.9), and among people treated for more than 3 months (OR 23.1, 95% CI 6.9 to 77.7).[40]

Comment: None.

| OPTION | PHENYLPROPANOLAMINE |

One systematic review found that phenylpropanolamine versus placebo promotes modest weight loss in healthy obese adults. One case control study found that phenylpropanolamine significantly increased risk of haemorrhagic stroke in the first 3 days of use. Phenylpropanolamine is no longer marketed for use in obesity.

Benefits: We found one systematic review (search date 1999) comparing phenylpropanolamine (57–75 mg daily) versus placebo.[23] This review included 7 RCTs in healthy obese adults with mean follow up of 7.4 weeks (range 2–14 wks). The mean number of people in each arm was 23.5 (range 8–36) for phenylpropanolamine and 22.4 (range 10–36) for placebo. The review found that phenylpropanolamine produced significant weight loss (effect size < 0.8 [information presented graphically]; difference in weight loss between phenylpropanolamine and placebo in the 7 RCTs ranged from 0.3–2.0 kg). The review also compared phenylpropanolamine versus other agents (diethylpropion, dexfenfluramine, fenfluramine, fluoxetine, mazindol, orlistat, phentermine, and sibutramine) and found no significant difference in effect size between phenylpropanolamine and the other agents except sibutramine and fenfluramine (based on 95% CIs).[23]

Harms: A case control study (men and women aged 18–49 years) found that phenylpropanolamine used as an appetite suppressant increased the risk of haemorrhagic stroke within the first 3 days of use (adjusted OR 15.9, lower confidence limit 2.04; P = 0.013).

For the association between phenylpropanolamine in appetite suppressants and risk for haemorrhagic stroke among women, the adjusted odds ratio was 16.6 (lower confidence limit 2.2; P = 0.011).[41] Phenylpropanolamine is no longer marketed for use in obesity.[42]

Comment: None.

| OPTION | ORLISTAT |

Systematic reviews and subsequent RCTs have found that in addition to a low calorie diet, orlistat versus placebo modestly increases weight loss in adults with obesity. Adverse effects such as oily spotting from the rectum, flatulence, and faecal urgency occurred in up to 27% of people taking orlistat. We found insufficient evidence on weight regain and long term safety.

Benefits: We found two systematic reviews (search dates 2000),[43,44] one licensing review[45] and three additional RCTs.[46–48] The most comprehensive of the three reviews included 14 RCTs and pooled data for groups of RCTs with similar study designs.[44] Studies were excluded if they did not analyse separately people who were not overweight or obese. The 11 published RCTs in the systematic review (5124 adults with mean body mass index [see glossary, p 138] > 30 kg/m^2) found no significant difference in weight after 12 weeks between orlistat (50–60 mg 3 times daily) plus reduced calorie diet versus placebo plus diet (2 RCTs: WMD - 1.24 kg, 95% CI −2.65 kg to +0.16 kg).[44] However, higher dose orlistat (120 mg 3 times daily) was associated with greater weight loss than placebo at 12 weeks (1 RCT: mean weight loss 4.74 kg with orlistat v 2.98 kg with placebo; CI not provided; P = 0.001).[44] The two included 6 month trials were not pooled. In the first, 119 people received orlistat (120 mg 3 times daily) or placebo. All people received a calorie restricted diet. At 6 months, orlistat reduced weight more than placebo (mean weight loss: 10.75 kg with orlistat v 7.34 kg with placebo; P < 0.05).[49] The second RCT with 6 months' follow up compared orlistat (30, 60, 120, or 240 mg 3 times daily) versus placebo among 605 people on a reduced calorie diet. All doses of orlistat significantly increased weight loss at 6 months compared with placebo (weight loss from baseline: 6.5% with placebo v 8.5% with orlistat 30 mg; P value not provided; v 8.8% with orlistat 60 mg; P ≤ 0.002; v 9.8% with orlistat 120 mg; P ≤ 0.001; v 9.3% with orlistat 240 mg; P ≤ 0.001).[50] Pooled analysis of four trials with 1 year follow up (2111 people) found that orlistat (120 mg 3 times daily) reduced weight more than placebo (WMD for weight change with orlistat v placebo −2.90 kg, 95% CI −3.61 kg to −2.19 kg).[44] Two RCTs were not included in the 1 year pooled analysis. In these trials, 901 people were placed on a reduced calorie diet and were also randomised to orlistat (120 mg 3 times daily) versus placebo. Both found that orlistat increased weight loss compared with placebo (AR for > 10% weight loss from baseline at 1 year: 35% with orlistat v 21% with placebo; P = 0.02;[51] 30% with orlistat v 16% with placebo; P < 0.001[52]). The review found similar results at 2 years. Two trials were pooled examining change in body weight at 2 years using orlistat (120 mg 3 times daily) versus placebo. People taking orlistat had significantly greater weight loss (WMD −3.19 kg, 95% CI −4.25 kg to −2.12 kg).[44] We found one RCT that compared effects of orlistat (30, 60, and 120 mg 3 times daily) versus placebo on weight regain after 6 months of diet plus exercise counselling.[44] It found that orlistat reduced weight regain compared with placebo (P < 0.001 for orlistat 120 mg v placebo). We identified three additional RCTs.[46–48] The first (46 people) compared orlistat (120 mg 3 times daily) versus placebo for 52 weeks. Orlistat reduced weight more than placebo (mean weight reduction at 6 months 8.6 kg with orlistat v 5.5 kg with placebo; P value and CI not provided). The second additional RCT (376 adults with type 2 diabetes, hypercholesterolaemia, or hypertension) found that dietary counselling plus orlistat (120 mg 3 times daily) versus placebo significantly increased the proportion of people who lost 5% or more of their initial body weight (54% with orlistat v 41% with placebo; P < 0.001), but did not significantly increase weight reduction of 10% or more (AR 19% v 14.6%).[47] The third additional RCT (294 people with hypercholesterolaemia) compared orlistat (120 mg 3 times daily) versus placebo for 24 weeks. Mean weight loss for the orlistat group was 4.66 kg versus 1.88 kg for the placebo group (P < 0.001).[48]

Harms: Common adverse events such as oily spotting from the rectum, flatulence, and faecal urgency were more common with orlistat than placebo (22–27% with orlistat v 1–7% with placebo).[53] Subsequent RCTs have identified similar rates of gastrointestinal adverse events. The review found that gastrointestinal adverse events were more common with orlistat than placebo and that orlistat was also associated with lower serum levels of fat soluble vitamins, such that vitamin supplements were sometimes deemed necessary.[44]

Comment: People in six of the seven trials in one systematic review were selected for participation after losing weight on a preliminary low calorie diet with placebo for 4–5 weeks before randomisation.[53] Because of the high rates of gastrointestinal adverse effects associated with orlistat, authors have queried whether blinded evaluation is possible. At the end of a "double blinded" 16 week trial, 22/26 people correctly identified their treatment group.[21]

GLOSSARY

Body mass index Expressed as weight in kilograms divided by height in metres squared (kg/m^2). In the USA and UK, individuals with body mass indexes of 25–30 kg/m^2 are considered overweight; those with body mass indexes above 30 kg/m^2 are considered obese.

Extrapyramidal effects Include acute dystonia, a Parkinsonism-like syndrome, and akathisia.

Serotonin syndrome Clinical features include agitation, ataxia, diaphoresis, diarrhoea, fever, hyper-reflexia, myoclonus, shivering, and changes in mental status. The occurrence and severity of syndrome does not seem to be dose related.

REFERENCES

1. National Institutes of Health. Clinical guidelines on the identification, evaluation, and treatment of overweight and obesity in adults: the Evidence Report. Bethesda, Maryland: US Department of Health and Human Services, 1998.

2. Khan LK, Serdula MK, Bowman BA, et al. Use of prescription weight loss pills among U.S. adults in 1996–1998. Ann Int Med 2001;134:282–286.

3. University of York, NHS Centre for Reviews and Dissemination. A systematic review of the

interventions for the prevention and treatment of obesity, and the maintenance of weight loss. York, England: NHS Centre for Reviews and Dissemination, 1997. Search date 1995; primary sources Medline, Embase, Bids, Dare, Psychlit, bibliographies of review articles, and contributions from peer reviewers.

4. Prevalence of overweight and obesity among adults: United States, 1999. US Department of Health and Human Services, Centers for Disease Control and Prevention, Hyattsville, MD. National Center for Health Statistics; 2000.

5. Bray GA. Obesity: etiology. UpToDate [serial on CD-ROM] 2000;8(1). UpToDate Inc, Wellesley, Massachusetts, USA.

6. Bray GA. Obesity: overview of therapy for obesity. UpToDate [serial on CD ROM] 2000;8(1). UpToDate Inc, Wellesley, Massachusetts, USA.

7. Allison DB, Fontaine KR, Manson JE, et al. Annual deaths attributable to obesity in the United States. JAMA 1999;282:1530–1538.

8. University of York, NHS Centre for Reviews and Dissemination. A systematic review of the clinical effectiveness of sibutramine and orlistat in the management of obesity. York, UK: NHS Centre for Reviews and Dissemination, 2000. Search date 2000.

9. McMahon FG, Fujioka K, Singh BN, et al. Efficacy and safety of sibutramine in obese white and African American patients with hypertension: a 1-year, double-blind, placebo-controlled multicenter trial. Arch Int Med 2000;160:2185–2191.

10. Wirth A, Krause J. Long-term weight loss with sibutramine: a randomized controlled trial. JAMA 2001;286:1331–1339.

11. Smith IG, Goudler MA. Randomized placebo-controlled trial of long-term treatment with sibutramine in mild to moderate obesity. J Fam Pract 2001;50:505–512.

12. James WP, Astrup A, Finer N, et al. Effect of sibutramine on weight maintenance after weight loss: a randomized trial. STORM Study Group. Sibutramine Trial of Obesity Reduction and Maintenance. Lancet 2000;356:2119–2125.

13. Fujioka K, Seaton TB, Rowe E, et al. Weight loss with sibutramine improves glycaemic control and other metabolic parameters in obese patients with type 2 diabetes. Diabetes Obes Metab 2000;2:175–187.

14. Apfelbaum M, Vague P, Ziegler O, et al. Long-term maintenance of weight loss after a very-low calorie diet: a randomized blinded trial of the efficacy and tolerability of sibutramine. Am J Med 1999;106:179–184.

15. Dujovne CA, Zavoral JH, Rowe E, et al. Effects of sibutramine on body weight and serum lipids: a double-blind, randomized, placebo-controlled study in 322 overweight and obese patients with dyslipidemia. Am Heart J 2001;142:489–497.

16. Gokcel A, Karakose H, Ertorer EM, et al. Effects of sibutramine in obese female subjects with type 2 diabetes and poor blood glucose control. Diabetes Care 2001;24:1957–1960.

17. McMahon FG, Weinstein SP, Rowe E, et al. Sibutramine is safe and effective for weight loss in obese patients whose hypertension is well controlled with angiotensin-converting enzyme inhibitors. J Hum Hypertens 2002;16:5–11.

18. Serrano-Rios M, Melchionda N, Moreno-Carretero E. Role of sibutramine in the treatment of obese type 2 diabetic patients receiving sulphonylurea therapy. Diabet Med 2002;19:119–124.

19. Fanghanel G, Cortinas L, Sanchez-Reyes L, et al. Second phase of a double-blind study clinical trial on sibutramine for the treatment of patients suffering from essential obesity: 6 months after treatment cross-over. Int J Obesity 2001;25:741–747.

20. Gokcel A, Gumurdulu Y, Karakose H, et al. Evaluation of the safety and efficacy of sibutramine, orlistat, and metformin in the treatment of obesity. Diabetes Obes Metab 2002;4:49–55.

21. Wadden TA, Berkowitz RI, Womble LG, et al. Effects of sibutramine plus orlistat in obese women following 1 year of treatment by sibutramine alone: a placebo-controlled trial. Obes Res 2000;8:431–437.

22. Health Sciences Authority. Centre for Pharmaceutical Administration. Drug Alerts. Updated Report on Sibutramine. Information page. http://www.hsa.gov.sg/hsa/CPA/CPA_pharma_drugalerts.htm#12 (last accessed 3 Sept 2002).

23. Haddock CK, Poston WSC, Dill PL, et al. Pharmacotherapy for obesity: a quantitative analysis of four decades of published randomized clinical trials. Int J Obes 2002;26:262–273. Search date 1999; primary sources Medline, PsychInfo, handsearching, and personal contact with individual authors.

24. Gaasch WH, Aurigemma GP. Valvular heart disease induced by anorectic drugs. UpToDate [serial on CD-ROM] 2000;8(3). UpToDate Inc, Wellesley, Massachusetts, USA.

25. Medicines Control Agency. Committee on Safety in Medicines. Important safety message: European withdrawal of anorectic agents/appetite suppressants: new legal developments, no new safety issues: licences for phentermine and amfepramone being withdrawn May 2001. Information page. http://www.mca.gov.uk/ourwork/monitorsafequalmed/safetymessages/anorectic.htm (last accessed 3 Sept 2002).

26. Hagiwara M, Tsuchida A, Hyakkoku M, et al. Delayed onset of pulmonary hypertension associated with an appetite suppressant, mazindol: a case report. Jpn Circ 2000;64:218–221.

27. Bradley MH, Blum NJ, Scheib RJ. Mazindol in obesity with known cardiac disease: a clinical evaluation. J Int Med Res 1974;2:347–349.

28. Thomas SH, Butt AY, Corris PA, et al. Appetite suppressants and primary pulmonary hypertension in the United Kingdom. Br Heart J 1995;74:660–663.

29. Little JD, Romans SE. Psychosis following readministration of diethylpropion: a possible role for kindling? Int Clin Psychopharmacol 1993;8:67–70.

30. Goldstein DJ, Rampey AH Jr, Enas GG, et al. Fluoxetine: a randomized clinical trial in the treatment of obesity. Int J Obes 1994;18:129–135.

31. Mulrow CD, Williams JW Jr, Trivedi M, et al. Treatment of depression – newer pharmacotherapies. Psychopharmacol Bull 1998;34:409–795. Search date 1998; primary sources the Cochrane Collaboration Depression, Anxiety and Neurosis (CCDAN) Review Group register of trials, and bibliographies of trial and review articles.

32. Weintraub M. Long term weight control study: the National Heart, Lung, and Blood Institute funded multimodal intervention study. Clin Pharmacol Ther 1992;51:581–646.

33. Poston WS, Foreyt JP. Scientific and legal issues in fenfluramine/dexfenfluramine litigation. J Texas Med 2000;96:48–56.

34. Connolly HM, Crary JL, McGoon MD, et al. Valvular heart disease associated with fenfluramine-phentermine. *N Engl J Med* 1997;337:581–588.

35. Scheen AJ, Lefebvre PJ. Pharmacological treatment of obesity: present status. *Int J Obes Relat Metab Disord* 1999;23(suppl 1):47–53.

36. Gardin JM, Schumacher D, Constantine G, et al. Valvular abnormalities and cardiovascular status following exposure to dexfenfluramine and phentermine/fenfluramine. *JAMA* 2000;283:1703–1709.

37. Gardin JM, Weissman NJ, Leung C, et al. Clinical and echocardiographic follow-up of patients previously treated with dexfenfluramine or phentermine/fenfluramine. *JAMA* 2001;286:2011–2014.

38. Weissman NJ, Tighe JF, Gottdiener JS, et al. An assessment of heart-valve abnormalities in obese patients taking dexfenfluramine, sustained-release dexfenfluramine, or placebo. Sustained release dexfenfluramine study group. *N Engl J Med* 1998;339:725–732.

39. Weissman NJ, Panza JA, Tighe JF, et al. Natural history of valvular regurgitation 1 year after discontinuation of dexfenfluramine therapy. *Ann Intern Med* 2001;134:267–273.

40. Abenhaim L, Moride Y, Brenot F, et al. Appetite-suppressant drugs and the risk of primary pulmonary hypertension. International primary pulmonary hypertension study group. *N Engl J Med* 1996;335:609–616.

41. Horwitz RI, Brass LM, Kernan WN, et al. Phenylpropanolamine and risk of hemorrhagic stroke: final report of the hemorrhagic stroke project. http://www.fda.gov/ohrms/dockets/ac/00/backgrd/3647b1_tab19.doc (last accessed 3 Sept 2002).

42. Food and Drug Administration. Center for Drug Evaluation and Research. Phenylpropanolamine (PPA) information page. http://www.fda.gov/cder/drug/infopage/ppa/ (last accessed 3 September 2002).

43. Lucas KH, Kaplan-Machlis B. Orlistat: a novel weight loss therapy. *Ann Pharmacother* 2001;35:314–328. Search date 2000; primary sources Medline, Roche Laboratories, organisational guidelines, National Institutes of Health and Food and Drug Administration web sites, Doctor's Guide online, and reference sections of published articles.

44. O'Meara S, Riemsma R, Shirran L, et al. A rapid and systematic review of the clinical effectiveness and cost-effectiveness of orlistat in the management of obesity. *Health Technol Assess* 2001;5:1–81. Search date 2000; primary sources Amed, Biosis, British Nursing Index, the Cochrane Library, Cinahl, Dare, DH-Data, EconLit, Embase, Health Management Information Service, HTA database, Index to Scientific and Technical Proceedings, King's Fund database, Medline, National Research Register, NEED, Health Economic Evaluations Database, Science Citation Index, Social Science Citation Index, Internet searches, reference lists of relevant reviews, and contact with the authors of conference abstracts.

45. European Agency for the Evaluation of Medicinal Products. Committee for proprietary medicinal products. European public assessment report (EPAR) – Xenical. London: European Agency for the Evaluation of Medicinal Products, 1998.

46. James WPT, Avenell A, Broom J, et al. A one-year trial to assess the value of orlistat in the management of obesity. *Int J Obes Relat Metab Disord* 1997;21(suppl 3):S24–S30.

47. Lindgarde F. The effect of orlistat on body weight and coronary heart disease risk profile in obese patients: the Swedish Multimorbidity Study. *J Int Med* 2000;248:245–254.

48. Muls E, Kolanowski J, Scheen A, et al. The effects of orlistat on weight and on serum lipids in obese patients with hypercholesterolemia: a randomized, double-blind, placebo-controlled, multicentre study. *Int J Obes* 2001;25:1713–1721.

49. Micic D, Ivkovic-Lazar T, Dragojevic R, et al. Orlistat, a gastrointestinal lipase inhibitor, in therapy of obesity with concomitant hyperlipidemia. *Med Pregl* 1999;52:323–333.

50. Van Gaul LF, Broom JI, Enzi G, et al. Efficacy and tolerability of orlistat in the treatment of obesity: a 6-month dose-ranging study. *Eur J Clin Pharmacol* 1998;54:125–132.

51. Finer N, James WPT, Kopelman PG, et al. One-year treatment of obesity: a randomized, double-blind, placebo-controlled, multicentre study of orlistat, a gastrointestinal lipase inhibitor. *Int J Obes* 2000;24:306–313.

52. Sjostrom L, Rissanen A, Anderson T, et al. Randomised placebo-controlled trial of orlistat for weight loss and prevention of weight regain in obese patients. *Lancet* 1998;352:167–173.

53. Anonymous. Orlistat: no hurry. *Can Fam Physician* 1999;45:2331–2351. Search date 1999; primary sources Medline, Embase, Reactions, the Cochrane Library, hand searches of international journals, the Prescribe Library, and clinical pharmacology reference texts, and personal contact with Produits Roche, the European Medicines Evaluation Agency, and Food and Drug Administration committees.

David Arterburn
Health Services Research Fellow
Health Services Research and Development
VA Puget Sound Health Care System
Department of Veterans Affairs
Seattle
USA

Competing interests: None declared. The views expressed in this article are those of the authors and do not necessarily represent the views of the US Department of Veterans Affairs.

TABLE 1 Unpooled RCTs comparing sibutramine versus placebo for weight loss (see text, p 130).

Trial duration	Study	Number of people	Special population	Lifestyle modification	Intervention	Mean weight change (kg)	P value
24 weeks	15	322	Obese with hyperlipidaemia	Diet	Placebo	−0.6	
					Sibutramine 20 mg daily	−4.9	P < 0.05
	13	175	Obese with type 2 diabetes	Diet	Placebo	−0.4	
					Sibutramine 20 mg daily	−3.7	P < 0.05
	16	60	Obese with type 2 diabetes	Diet	Placebo	0.91	
					Sibutramine 10 mg daily	−9.61	P < 0.0001
	18	134	Obese with type 2 diabetes	Diet	Placebo	−1.7	
					Sibutramine 15 mg daily	−4.5	P < 0.001
48 weeks	10	1001	Healthy, obese	None	Placebo	0.2	
					Continuous sibutramine 15 mg daily	−3.8	P < 0.001
					Intermittent sibutramine 15 mg daily	−3.3	P < 0.001
52 weeks	11	485	Healthy, obese	Diet	Placebo	−1.6	
					Sibutramine 10 mg daily	−4.4	P < 0.01
					Sibutramine 15 mg daily	−6.4	P < 0.001
	17	220	Obese with hypertension	Diet	Placebo	−0.4	
					Sibutramine 20 mg daily	−4.5	P < 0.05
	9	224	Obese with hypertension	Diet	Placebo	−0.5	
					Sibutramine 20 mg daily	−4.4	P < 0.05

Search date December 2001

Sonia Anand and Mark Creager

Cardiovascular disorders

Key Messages

- **Antiplatelet treatment** Systematic reviews have found that antiplatelet agents versus control treatments significantly reduce the rate of major cardiovascular events over an average of about 2 years. Systematic reviews have found that antiplatelet agents versus placebo or no treatments significantly reduce the risk of arterial occlusion and reduce the risk of revascularisation procedures. The balance of benefits and harms is in favour of treatment for most people with symptomatic peripheral arterial disease, because as a group they are at much greater risk of cardiovascular events.

- **Bypass surgery** One systematic review found that surgery versus percutaneous transluminal angioplasty significantly improved primary patency after 12–24 months, but found no significant difference after 4 years. The review found no significant difference in mortality after 12–24 months. One systematic review found that surgery versus thrombolysis significantly reduced the number of amputations and the number of people reporting ongoing ischaemic pain, but found no significant difference in mortality after 1 year. Although the consensus view is that bypass surgery is the most effective treatment for people with debilitating symptomatic peripheral arterial disease, we found inadequate evidence from RCTs reporting long term clinical outcomes to confirm this view.

- **Cilostazol** Four RCTs in people with intermittent claudication have found that cilostazol versus placebo significantly improves initial claudication distance and absolute claudication distance measured on a treadmill and significantly reduces the proportion of people with symptoms that do not improve. One RCT with a high withdrawal rate found that pentoxifylline versus cilostazol significantly increased the number of people who had no change or deterioration in the initial claudication distance and the absolute claudication distance.

- **Exercise** Systematic reviews in people with chronic stable claudication have found that regular exercise at least three times weekly versus no exercise significantly improves total walking distance and maximal exercise time after 3–12 months.

- **Pentoxifylline** Systematic reviews of small RCTs of variable quality in people with intermittent claudication have found that pentoxifylline versus placebo increases the walking distance by a small amount. One subsequent RCT with a high withdrawal rate found no significant difference in walking distance between pentoxifylline versus placebo, but found that pentoxifylline versus placebo significantly increased the number of people who had no change or deterioration in the initial claudication distance and the absolute claudication distance.

- **Percutaneous transluminal angioplasty (transient benefit only)** Two small RCTs in people with mild to moderate intermittent claudication found limited evidence that angioplasty versus no angioplasty significantly improved walking distance after 6 months but found no significant difference after 2 or 6 years. Four RCTs in people with femoral to popliteal artery stenoses have found no significant difference with angioplasty alone versus angioplasty plus stent placement in patency rates, occlusion rates or clinical improvement.

- **Smoking cessation (based on consensus of opinion)** RCTs of advice to stop smoking are unlikely to be conducted. The consensus view is that smoking cessation improves symptoms in people with intermittent claudication. One systematic review has found observational evidence that continued cigarette smoking by people with intermittent claudication is associated with progression of symptoms, poor prognosis after bypass surgery, amputation, and need for reconstructive surgery. Another systematic review found no good evidence from controlled studies about the effects of advice to stop smoking.

DEFINITION Peripheral arterial disease arises when there is significant narrowing of arteries distal to the arch of the aorta. Narrowing can arise from atheroma, arteritis, local thrombus formation, or embolisation from the heart or more central arteries. This topic includes treatment options for people with symptoms of reduced blood flow to the leg that are likely to arise from atheroma. These symptoms range from calf pain on exercise (intermittent claudication), to rest pain, skin ulceration, or ischaemic necrosis (gangrene) in people with critical ischaemia (see glossary, p 152).

INCIDENCE/ PREVALENCE Peripheral arterial disease is more common in people aged over 50 years than in younger people, and is more common in men than women. The prevalence of peripheral arterial disease of the legs (assessed by non-invasive tests) is about 3% in people under the age of 60 years, but rises to over 20% in people over 75 years.[1] The overall annual incidence of intermittent claudication is 1.5–2.6/ 1000 men a year and 1.2–3.6/1000 women a year.[2]

AETIOLOGY/ RISK FACTORS Factors associated with the development of peripheral arterial disease include age, gender, cigarette smoking, diabetes mellitus, hypertension, hyperlipidaemia, obesity, and physical inactivity. The strongest association is with smoking (RR 2.0–4.0) and diabetes (RR 2.0–3.0).[3] Acute limb ischaemia (see glossary, p 151) may result from thrombosis arising within a peripheral artery or from embolic occlusion.

PROGNOSIS The symptoms of intermittent claudication can resolve spontane-ously, remain stable over many years, or progress rapidly to critical limb ischaemia. About 15% of people with intermittent claudication eventually develop critical leg ischaemia, which endangers the viability of the limb. The incidence of critical limb ischaemia in Denmark and Italy in 1990 was 0.25–0.45/1000 people a year.[4,5] Coronary heart disease is the major cause of death in people with peripheral arterial disease of the legs. Over 5 years, about 20% of people with intermittent claudication have a non-fatal cardiovas-cular event (myocardial infarction [MI], or stroke).[6] The mortality rate of people with peripheral arterial disease is two to three times higher than that of age and sex matched controls. Overall mortality after the diagnosis of peripheral arterial disease is about 30% after 5 years and 70% after 15 years.[6]

AIMS To reduce symptoms (intermittent claudication), local complica-tions (arterial leg ulcers, critical leg ischaemia), and general com-plications (MI and stroke).

OUTCOMES **Local outcomes:** Proportion of people with adverse outcomes including a decline in claudication distance, amputation, or adverse effects of treatment, the mean improvement in claudication dis-tance measured on a treadmill or by some other specified means. **General outcomes:** Rates of MI, stroke, and other major cardio-vascular events.

METHODS *Clinical Evidence* search and appraisal December 2001.

QUESTION **What are the effects of treatments for people with chronic peripheral arterial disease?**

OPTION ANTIPLATELET AGENTS

Systematic reviews have found strong evidence that antiplatelet agents versus control treatments significantly reduce the rate of major cardiovascular events over an average of about 2 years. Systematic reviews have found that antiplatelet agents versus placebo or no treatments significantly reduce the risk of arterial occlusion and the risk of revascularisation procedures. The balance of benefits and harms is in favour of treatment for most people with symptomatic peripheral arterial disease, because as a group they are at much greater risk of cardiovascular events.

Benefits: **Peripheral arterial disease complications:** We found two system-atic reviews,[7,8] one of which has subsequently been updated.[9] The first systematic review (search date 1997, 42 RCTs; 9214 people with intermittent claudication [see glossary, p 152], bypass surgery of the leg, or peripheral artery angioplasty) found that antiplatelet treatment compared with no additional treatment significantly reduced the risk of arterial occlusion over 19 months (RRR 0.30; P < 0.00001).[9] The second systematic review (search date 1998, 54 RCTs) found that aspirin versus placebo reduced the number of arterial occlusions and that ticlopidine reduced the risk of revascularisation procedures.[8] **Cardiovascular events:** We found two systematic reviews.[9,10] The first review (search date 1997, 42 RCTs; 9214 people) found that antiplatelet treatment versus control treatment significantly reduced the combined outcome of vascular death, myocardial infarction, or stroke over an average of 2 years (280/4844 [6.0%] with antiplatelet treatment v 347/4662 [7%] with control; RR 0.78, 95% CI 0.67 to 0.90; NNT 61, 95% CI 38 to 153).[9] The second systematic review (search date 1999, 39 RCTs) found that antiplatelet treatment versus control significantly reduced the absolute event rate for the combined end point of myocardial infarction, stroke, or vascular death (6.5% with antiplatelet treatment v 8.1% with control; OR 0.78, 95% CI 0.63 to 0.96).[10]

Harms: The first review (search date 1990; 35 RCTs; 8098 people with peripheral arterial disease) found no significant difference with antiplatelet treatment versus control treatment in the risk of non-fatal major bleeds (14/2545 [0.55%] v 9/2243 [0.40%]; RR 1.37, 95% CI 0.60 to 3.16).[7] The second review (search date 1999, 36 RCTs, 8449 people with peripheral disease) found no significant difference with antiplatelet treatment versus placebo in major bleeding (47/4349 [1%] with antiplatelet treatment v 33/4100 [< 1%] with placebo; OR 1.40, 95% CI 0.90 to 2.20), and found no significant difference with aspirin versus other antiplatelet agents in major bleeding (68/3467 [2%] with aspirin v 59/3561 [2%] with other antiplatelet agents; RR 1.18, 95% CI 0.84 to 1.67).[10] The number of events was too low to exclude a clinically important increase in major bleeding.[7,10] Across a wide range of people, antiplatelet agents have been found to increase significantly the risk of major haemorrhage (see harms of antiplatelet agents under primary prevention, p 155).

Comment: We found no evidence about the effects of combined clopidogrel and aspirin versus a single antiplatelet agent in people with peripheral arterial disease. Peripheral arterial disease increases the risk of cardiovascular events, so for most people the risk of bleeding is outweighed by the benefits of regular antiplatelet use.

OPTION EXERCISE

Systematic reviews in people with chronic stable claudication have found that regular exercise at least three times weekly versus no exercise significantly improves total walking distance and maximal exercise time after 3–12 months.

Benefits: **Walking exercise versus no exercise:** We found two systematic reviews of exercise versus no exercise in people with chronic stable intermittent claudication (see glossary, p 152) (search dates 1996,[11] and not stated;[12] see comment below). The first review found that exercise programmes (at least 30 min walking as far as claudication permits, at least 3 times weekly, for 3–6 months in people also being treated with surgery, aspirin, or dipyridamole) versus no exercise significantly increased both the initial claudication distance (see glossary, p 152) (4 RCTs; 94 people; difference of means 139 m, 95% CI 31 m to 247 m) and the absolute claudication distance (see glossary, p 151) (5 RCTs; 115 people; difference of means 179 m, 95% CI 60 m to 298 m) after 3–12 months.[13] Control treatments were placebo tablets (2 RCTs) or "instructed to continue with normal lifestyle". The second review (10 RCTs, including all those in the first review) found that exercise versus no exercise increased maximal exercise time (3 RCTs; 53 people; WMD 6.5 min, 95% CI 4.4 to 8.7 min).[12] **Different types of exercise:** All the RCTs included in the systematic reviews involved walking exercise. We found one RCT (67 people with moderate to severe intermittent claudication), which compared arm versus leg exercise of similar intensity.[13] A third group of 15 people was given no exercise, but this group was not created by random allocation. The RCT found no significant difference with arm versus leg exercises in initial claudication distance (122% with arm exercise v 93% with leg exercise) and absolute claudication distance (47% with arm exercise v 50% with leg exercise) although both groups improved after 6 weeks.

Harms: Neither review gave details of any observed harms of the exercise programmes.[11,14]

Comment: The RCTs in the systematic reviews had low drop out rates.[11,12] Blinding of participants was not possible. Blinding of assessors is not clear from the reviews. Most (5/6) exercise programmes in the second review occurred under supervision.[12] We found one further systematic review of 21 observational studies or RCTs of exercise in 564 people with peripheral arterial disease.[14] This review calculated effects based on the differences in claudication difference after and before exercise treatment, but it made no allowance for any spontaneous improvement that might have occurred in the participants. It reported large increases with exercise in the initial claudication distance (126–351 m) and in the absolute claudication distance (325–723 m), but these estimates were based on observational data. An ongoing Australian RCT is examining the effect of exercise treatment in 1400 men.[12] The benefit from arm exercise remains unconfirmed, but suggests that improved walking may be caused by generally improved cardiovascular function rather than local changes of the peripheral circulation.

OPTION	SMOKING CESSATION

RCTs of advice to stop smoking are unlikely to be conducted. The consensus view is that smoking cessation improves symptoms in people with intermittent claudication. One systematic review has found observational evidence that continued cigarette smoking by people with intermittent claudication is associated with progression of symptoms, poor prognosis after bypass surgery, amputation, and need for reconstructive surgery. Another systematic review found no good evidence from controlled studies about the effects of advice to stop smoking.

Benefits: We found no RCTs.

Harms: The reviews did not report on harms (see comment below).[11,15]

Comment: RCTs of advice to stop smoking are unlikely to be conducted, although the consensus view is that smoking cessation improves symptoms in people with intermittent claudication (see glossary, p 152). We found one systematic review (search date 1996; 4 observational studies; 866 people) of advice to quit cigarette smoking versus no advice.[11] The intervention in all the studies was advice to stop smoking. One large observational study in the systematic review found no significant increase in absolute claudication distance (see glossary, p 151) after cessation of smoking.[11] Two other studies found conflicting results about the risk of deteriorating from moderate to severe claudication in people who successfully quit smoking compared with current smokers. The fourth study provided no numerical results. Overall, the review found no good evidence to confirm or refute the consensus view that advice to stop smoking improves symptoms in people with intermittent claudication. An older systematic review (search date 1989) concluded that most of the evidence on the effects of smoking cessation derives from observational studies that have found among cigarette smokers increased risk of onset of intermittent claudication, progression of symptoms, poor progress after bypass surgery, amputation, and the need for reconstructive surgery.[15]

OPTION	CILOSTAZOL

Four RCTs in people with intermittent claudication have found that cilostazol versus placebo significantly improves initial claudication distance and absolute claudication distance measured on a treadmill and significantly reduces the proportion of people with symptoms that do not improve. One RCT with a high withdrawal rate found that pentoxifylline versus cilostazol significantly increased the number of people who had no change or deterioration in the claudication distance, the initial claudication distance, and the absolute claudication distance.

Benefits: We found no systematic review. **Versus placebo:** We found four RCTs comparing cilostazol versus placebo (see comment below) (see table 1, p 154).[16-19] The RCTs found that cilostazol versus placebo significantly reduced the risk of claudication being rated as unchanged, worsened, or unsure at the end of each trial (4 RCTs; 1091 people; no heterogeneity; combined RR using fixed effects model 0.71, 95% CI 0.63 to 0.81), and significantly improved the initial claudication distance (see glossary, p 152) (by 38–80 m) and the absolute claudication distance (see glossary, p 151) (by 28–84 m). **Versus pentoxifylline:** See benefits of pentoxifylline, p 148.

Harms: The most recent RCT reported that cilostazol versus placebo significantly increased the number of people who withdrew from the trial because of adverse effects or concerns about safety (39/227 [17%] with cilostazol v 24/239 [10%] with placebo; RR 1.71, 95% CI 1.06 to 2.75; ARI 7.1%, 95% CI 0.9% to 13.3%; NNH 14, 95% CI 8 to 111).[16] Side effects of cilostazol included headache (28% v 12% with placebo), diarrhoea (19% v 8%), abnormal stools (15% v 5%), palpitations (17% v 2%), and dizziness.[16-19] Cilostazol is a phosphodiesterase inhibitor; RCTs have found that other phosphodiesterase inhibitors (milrinone, vesnarinone) are associated with increased mortality in people with heart failure. However, results aggregated from other studies have not found an excess of cardiovascular events with cilostazol.[20]

Comment: Although the overall results of cilostazol versus placebo indicate a significant effect of cilostazol on increasing walking distance, the RCTs have some weakness of their methods, which may limit the

Cardiovascular disorders

applicability of the results.[16–19] Firstly, none of the RCTs evaluated cilostazol beyond 24 weeks. In addition, the RCTs all had moderate withdrawal rates after randomisation (up to 28.9%).[17] All four RCTs found that withdrawals were more common with cilostazol than placebo (61/227 [27%] v 38/239 [16%] with placebo; RR 1.69, 95% CI 1.18 to 2.43; ARI 11%, 95% CI 4% to 18%).[16–19] To allow for these problems, the authors performed an intention to treat analysis using "last available observation carried forward". However, the analysis did not include the 35 people with no observations to carry forward, and the effects of the difference in withdrawals between the groups was not explored adequately (e.g. if people with worsening claudication were more likely to withdraw, then the observed differences may be artefactual). Although cilostazol appears promising, the exact balance of its benefits and harms remains unclear.

| OPTION | PENTOXIFYLLINE |

Systematic reviews of small RCTs of variable quality in people with intermittent claudication have found that pentoxifylline versus placebo increases the walking distance by a small amount. One subsequent RCT with a high withdrawal rate found no significant difference in walking distance between pentoxifylline versus placebo, but found that pentoxifylline versus cilostazol significantly increased the number of people who had no change or deterioration in the initial claudication distance and the absolute claudication distance.

Benefits: We found two systematic reviews,[11,21] and one subsequent RCT.[16] The first review (search date 1994, 29 RCTs of people with Fontaine's classification stage II or III intermittent claudication [see glossary, p 152] for at least 3 months) included RCTs only if they were placebo controlled and double blinded, and used pentoxifylline 600–1800 mg daily for 2–26 weeks.[21] The review found that pentoxifylline versus placebo significantly increased both the initial claudication distance (see glossary, p 152) and the absolute claudication distance (see glossary, p 151) (see table 2, p 154). The second systematic review found similar results (see table 2, p 154).[11] The subsequent RCT (438 people; see comment below) found no significant difference with pentoxifylline versus placebo in the number of people who had no change or deterioration in the claudication distance (72/212 [34%] with pentoxifylline v 68/226 [30%] with placebo; RR 1.13, 95% CI 0.86 to 1.48), the initial claudication distance (202 m with pentoxifylline v 180 m with placebo; mean difference 22 m; P for change from baseline = 0.07), or the absolute claudication distance (308 m with pentoxifylline v 300 m with placebo; mean difference 8 m; P for change from baseline = 0.82) after 24 weeks (see table 2, p 154).[16] **Versus cilostazol:** The subsequent RCT (see comment below) found that pentoxifylline versus cilostazol significantly increased the number of people who had no change or deterioration in the claudication distance (72/212 [34%] with pentoxifylline v 47/205 [23%] with cilostazol; RR 1.48, 95% CI 1.08 to 2.03; ARR 11%,

95% CI 2.4% to 20%; NNT 9, 95% CI 5 to 42), the initial claudication distance (202 m with pentoxifylline v 218 m with cilostazol; mean difference −16 m; P = 0.0001), and the absolute claudication distance (308 m with pentoxifylline v 350 m with cilostazol; mean difference −42 m; P = 0.0005) after 24 weeks.[16]

Harms: The subsequent RCT found that pentoxifylline versus placebo significantly increased the number of people who withdrew from the RCT because of adverse effects or concerns about safety (44/232 [19%] with pentoxifylline v 24/239 [10%] with placebo; RR 1.89, 95% CI 1.19 to 3.00; ARI 8.9%, 95% CI 2.6% to 15.3%; NNH 12, 95% CI 7 to 39).[16] Side effects of pentoxifylline included sore throat (14% v 7%), dyspepsia, nausea, diarrhoea (8% v 5% with placebo; P = 0.31), and vomiting.[16] No life threatening side effects of pentoxifylline have been reported, although RCTs have been too small to date to assess this reliably.

Comment: The systematic reviews contained many RCTs in common.[11,21] Results from the subsequent RCT,[16] have been published in numerous articles without stating clearly whether any contain additional results.[17–19] The subsequent RCT had a high withdrawal rate after randomisation, which could act as a potential source of bias (60/232 [26%] with pentoxifylline v 61/237 [26%] with cilostazol). In all RCTs, withdrawals were more common with pentoxifylline (60/232 [26%] v 38/239 [16%] with placebo; RR 1.63, 95% CI 1.13 to 2.34; ARI 10%, 95% CI 3% to 17%). To allow for these problems, the published analysis performed an intention to treat analysis using "last available observation carried forward". However, the analysis did not include the 33 people with no observations to carry forward, and the effects of the difference in withdrawals between the groups was not explored adequately (e.g. if people with worsening claudication were more likely to withdraw, then the observed differences may be artefactual). The available evidence is not good enough to define clearly the effects of pentoxifylline.

OPTION   PERCUTANEOUS TRANSLUMINAL ANGIOPLASTY

Two small RCTs in people with mild to moderate intermittent claudication found limited evidence that angioplasty versus no angioplasty significantly improved walking distance after 6 months but found no significant difference after 2 or 6 years. Four RCTs in people with femoral to popliteal artery stenoses have found no significant difference with angioplasty alone versus angioplasty plus stent placement in patency rates, occlusion rates, or clinical improvement.

Benefits: **Percutaneous transluminal agioplasty (PTA) versus no PTA:** We found one systematic review (search date not stated; 2 RCTs; 78 men and 20 women with mild to moderate intermittent claudication [see glossary, p 152]) of PTA of the aortoiliac or femoral-popliteal arteries versus no angioplasty.[22] The first RCT identified by the review found that PTA versus no PTA significantly increased the median claudication distance after 6 months (667 m v 172 m; P < 0.05), but found no significant difference in median claudication distance or quality of life after 2 years.[23] The second RCT found that PTA versus

Cardiovascular disorders

an exercise programme significantly increased the absolute claudication distance (see glossary, p 151) at 6 months (130 m v 50 m; WMD 80 m), but found no significant difference in absolute claudication distance after 6 years (180 m v 130 m; WMD 50 m; P > 0.05).[24,25] **PTA versus PTA plus stents:** We found no systematic review, but found five RCTs.[26–30] One RCT (279 people with intermittent claudication and iliac artery stenosis) compared PTA plus routine stent placement versus PTA plus selective stent placement.[26] It found no significant difference in short or long term patency rates. The other four RCTs included people with femoral to popliteal artery stenoses and compared PTA alone versus PTA plus stent placement.[27–30] The first of these four RCTs (51 people) found no significant differences in primary patency assessed by colour flow duplex ultrasound (62% with PTA plus stent v 74% with PTA alone; P = 0.22) or in the occlusion rate (5/24 [21%] with PTA plus stent v 7% [2/27] with PTA alone; P = 0.16).[27] The second RCT (53 people) found no significant difference in primary patency after 34 months' follow up (68.4% with PTA v 62% with PTA plus stent placement). The third RCT (32 people) found no significant difference in "clinical improvement" after 1 year (71% with PTA v 60% with PTA plus stent placement; P = 0.17).[30] The fourth RCT (141 people, 154 limbs) found no significant difference in primary patency as determined by angiography after 1 year (63% with PTA v 63% with PTA plus stent placement).[28]

Harms: Prospective cohort studies have found that PTA complications include puncture site major bleeding (3.4%), pseudoaneurysms (0.5%), limb loss (0.2%), renal failure secondary to intravenous contrast (0.2%), cardiac complications such as myocardial infarction (0.2%), and death (0.2%).[31,32]

Comment: This limited evidence suggests transient benefit from angioplasty versus no angioplasty. The longer term effects of angioplasty or stent placement on symptoms, bypass surgery, and amputation remain unclear. Angioplasty and selective stent placement appear to be an appropriate strategy for selected iliac stenoses.[21] The long term patency of femoral-popliteal angioplasties is poor, and there is no evidence that the addition of stents confers any additional benefit.[28–30]

OPTION	BYPASS SURGERY

One systematic review found that surgery versus percutaneous transluminal angioplasty significantly improved primary patency after 12–24 months, but found no significant difference after 4 years. The review found no significant difference in mortality after 12–24 months. One systematic review found that surgery versus thrombolysis significantly reduced the number of amputations and the number of people reporting ongoing ischaemic pain, but found no significant difference in mortality after 1 year. Although the consensus view is that bypass surgery is the most effective treatment for people with debilitating symptomatic peripheral arterial disease, we found inadequate evidence from RCTs reporting long term clinical outcomes to confirm this view.

Benefits:	**Surgery versus exercise:** We found no RCTs (see comment below). **Surgery versus percutaneous transluminal angioplasty (PTA):** We found one systematic review (search date not stated, 2 RCTs, 365 people with chronic progressive peripheral arterial disease), which found no significant difference with surgery versus PTA in mortality after 12–24 months (OR 1.08, 95% CI 0.61 to 1.89).[33] The review found that surgery versus PTA significantly improved primary patency after 12–24 months (OR 0.62, 95% CI 0.39 to 0.99), but found no significant difference in primary patency after 4 years (P = 0.14). The review found no significant difference in mortality or amputation rates. **Surgery versus thrombolysis:** We found one systematic review (search date not stated, 1 RCT, with acute limb ischaemia), which compared surgery versus thrombolysis using tissue plasminogen activator or urokinase.[33] The review found no significant difference in mortality after 1 year (OR 1.59, 95% CI 0.70 to 3.59). The review found that surgery versus thrombolysis significantly reduced the number of amputations (OR 0.19, 95% CI 0.06 to 0.59) and significantly reduced the number of people reporting ongoing ischaemic pain (OR 0.30, 95% CI 0.17 to 0.50) after 1 year. **Surgery versus PTA plus stent placement:** We found no RCTs of surgery versus PTA plus stent placement that reported long term outcomes.
Harms:	Surgery versus PTA increased early procedural complications. Among people having aortoiliac surgery, perioperative mortality (within 30 days of the procedure) was 3.3%, and complications having a major health impact occurred in 8.3%.[34] Among people having infrainguinal bypass surgery, perioperative mortality was about 2% and serious complications occurred in 8%.[35] Among people having PTA with or without stent placement, perioperative mortality was about 1% and serious complications occurred in about 5%.[36]
Comment:	The RCTs are small, have different follow up periods, and assessed different outcomes. Indirect comparisons from observational studies of proxy outcomes (primary patency rates) suggest that for aortoiliac stenosis or occlusion, greater patency rates 5 years after intervention are achieved with surgery (6250 [89%] people) compared with PTA (1300 [34–85%] people) or compared with combined PTA and stent placement (816 [54–74%] people).[30–32] Too few people with infrainguinal lesions were included in the RCTs to provide good evidence about surgical management. Indirect comparisons of proxy outcomes in people with infrainguinal lesions suggest worse results after PTA (after 5 years patency 38%, range 34–42%) compared with surgery (patency 80%).[37] Although the consensus view is that bypass surgery is the most effective treatment for people with debilitating symptomatic peripheral arterial disease, we found inadequate evidence from RCTs reporting long term clinical outcomes to confirm this view.

GLOSSARY

Absolute claudication distance Also known as the total walking distance; the maximum distance a person can walk before stopping.

Acute limb ischemia An ischemic process which threatens the viability of the limb, and is associated with pain, neurologic deficit, inadequate skin capillary circulation, and/or inaudible arterial flow signals by Doppler examination. This acute process often leads to hospitalisation.

Ankle–brachial index The ratio of the systolic blood pressure in the leg over the systolic blood pressure in the arm.

Critical limb ischemia results in a breakdown of the skin (ulceration or gangrene) or pain in the foot at rest. Critical limb ischemia corresponds to the Fontaine classification III and IV.

Fontaine's classification I: asymptomatic; II: intermittent claudication (see below); II-a: pain free, claudication walking > 200 metres; II-b: pain free, claudication walking < 200 metres; III: rest/nocturnal pain; IV: necrosis/gangrene.

Initial claudication distance The distance a person can walk before the onset of claudication symptoms.

Intermittent claudication Pain, stiffness, or weakness in the leg that develops on walking, intensifies with continued walking until further walking is impossible, and is relieved by rest.

REFERENCES

1. Fowkes FGR, Housely E, Cawood EH, et al. Edinburgh Artery Study: prevalence of asymptomatic and symptomatic peripheral arterial disease in the general population. *Int J Epidemiol* 1991;20:384–392.

2. Kannel WB, McGee DL. Update on some epidemiological features of intermittent claudication. *J Am Geriatr Soc* 1985;33:13–18.

3. Maurabito JM, D'Agostino RB, Sibersschatz, et al. Intermittent claudication: a risk profile from the Framingham Heart Study. *Circulation* 1997;96:44–49.

4. Catalano M. Epidemiology of critical limb ischemia: north Italian data. *Eur J Med* 1993;2:11–14.

5. Ebskov L, Schroeder T, Holstein P. Epidemiology of leg amputation: the influence of vascular surgery. *Br J Surg* 1994;81:1600–1603.

6. Leng GC, Lee AJ, Fowkes FG, et al. Incidence, natural history and cardiovascular events in symptomatic and asymptomatic peripheral arterial disease in the general population. *Int J Epidemiol* 1996;25:1172–1181.

7. Antiplatelet Trialists' Collaborative overview of randomized trials of antiplatelet therapy. I: prevention of death, myocardial infarction, and stroke by prolonged antiplatelet therapy in various categories of patients. *BMJ* 1994;308:81–106. Search date 1990; primary sources Medline, Current Contents, hand searches of reference lists of trials and review articles, journal abstracts and meeting proceedings, trial register of the International Committee on Thrombosis and Haemostasis, and personal contacts with colleagues and antiplatelet manufacturers.

8. Girolami B, Bernardi E, Prins MH, et al. Antithrombotic drugs in the primary medical management of intermittent claudication: a meta-analysis. *Thromb Haemost* 1999;81:715–722. Search date 1998; primary sources Medline and hand searches.

9. Antithrombotic, Trialists' Collaboration Collaborative meta-analysis of randomised trials of antiplatelet therapy for prevention of death, myocardial infarction, and stroke in high risk patients. BMJ 2002; 324:71–86. Search date: 1997 Primary sources: Medline, Embase, Derwent, Scisearch, Biosis, the Cochrane Stroke and Peripheral Vascular Disease Group Registers, handsearching of journals, abstracts, and proceedings of meetings, reference lists of trials and review articles and personal contact with colleagues, including representatives of pharmaceutical companies.

10. Robless P, Mikhailidis D, Stansby G. Systematic review of antiplatelet therapy for the prevention of myocaridla infarction, stroke, or vascular death in patients with peripheral vascular disease. *British Journal of Surgery* 2001;88:787–800.

11. Girolami B, Bernardi E, Prins M, et al. Treatment of intermittent claudication with physical training, smoking cessation, pentoxifylline, or nafronyl: a meta-analysis. *Arch Intern Med* 1999;159:337–345. Search date 1996; primary sources Medline and hand searches of reference lists.

12. Leng GC, Fowler B, Ernst E. Exercise for intermittent claudication In: The Cochrane Library, Issue 3, 2000. Oxford: Update Software. Search date not stated; primary sources Peripheral Vascular Diseases Group trials register, Embase, reference lists of relevant articles, and personal contact with principal investigators of trials.

13. Walker RD, Nawaz S, Wilkinson CH, et al. Influence of upper- and lower-limb exercise training on cardiovascular function and walking distances in patients with intermittent claudication. *J Vasc Surg* 2000;31:662–669.

14. Gardner A, Poehlman E. Exercise rehabilitation programs for the treatment of claudication pain. *JAMA* 1995;274:975–980. Search date 1993; primary sources Medline and hand searches of bibliographies of reviews, textbooks, and studies located through the computer search.

15. Radack K, Wyderski RJ. Conservative management in intermittent claudication. *Ann Intern Med* 1990;113:135–146. Search date 1989; primary sources Index Medicus, Medline, textbooks, and experts.

16. Dawson DL, Cutler BS, Hiatt WR, et al. A comparison of cilostazol and pentoxifylline for treating intermittent claudication. *Am J Med* 2000;109:523–530.

17. Money SR, Herd A, Isaacsohn JL, et al. Effect of cilostazol on walking distances in patients with intermittent claudication cause by peripheral vascular disease. *J Vasc Surg* 1998;27:267–275.

18. Beebe HG, Dawson D, Cutler B, et al. A new pharmacological treatment for intermittent claudication. *Arch Intern Med* 1999;159:2041–2050.

19. Dawson D, Cutler B, Meeisner M, et al. Cilostazol has beneficial effects in treatment of intermittent claudication. *Circulation* 1998;98:678–686.

20. Hiatt WR. Medical treatment of peripheral arterial disease and claudication. *N Engl J Med* 2001;344:1608–1621.

21. Hood S, Mohur D, Barber G. Management of intermittent claudication with pentoxifylline: a meta-analysis of randomized controlled trials. *Can Med Assoc J* 1996;155:1053–1059. Search date 1994; primary sources Medline and hand searches of references lists.

22. Fowkes FG, Gillespie IN. Angioplasty (versus non surgical management) for intermittent claudication. In: The Cochrane Library, Issue 3, 2000. Oxford: Update Software. Search date not stated; primary sources Cochrane Peripheral Vascular Diseases Group Trials Register, Embase, reference lists of relevant articles and conference proceedings, and personal contact with principal investigators of trials.

23. Whyman MR, Fowkes FGR, Kerracher EMG, et al. Randomized controlled trial of percutaneous transluminal angioplasty for intermittent claudication. *Eur J Vasc Endovasc Surg* 1996;12:167–172.

24. Creasy TS, McMillan PJ, Fletcher EWL, et al. Is percutaneous transluminal angioplasty better than exercise for claudication? Preliminary results of a prospective randomized trial. *Eur J Vasc Surg* 1990;4:135–140.

25. Perkins JMT, Collin J, Creasy TS, et al. Exercise training versus angioplasty for stable claudication. Long and medium term results of a prospective, randomized trial. *Eur J Vasc Endovasc Surg* 1996;11:409–413.

26. Teteroo E, van der Graef Y, Bosch J, et al. Randomized comparison of primary stent placement versus primary angioplasty followed by selective stent placement in patients with iliac artery occlusive disease. *Lancet* 1998;351:1153–1159.

27. Vroegindeweij D, Vos L, Tielbeek A, et al. Balloon angioplasty combined with primary stenting versus balloon angioplasty alone in femoropopliteal obstructions: a comparative randomized study. *Cardiovasc Intervent Radiol* 1997;20:420–425.

28. Cejna M, Thurnher S, Illiasch H, et al. PTA versus palmaz stent placement in femeropopliteal artery obstructions: a multicenter prospective randomised study. *Journal of Vascular and interventional radiology* 2001;12:23–31.

29. Grimm J, Muller-Hulsbeck S, Jahnke T, et al. Randomized study to compare PTA alone versus PTA with Palmaz stent placement for femoropopliteal lesions. *J Vasc Interv Radiol* 200;12:935–42.

30. Zdanowski Z, Albrechtsson U, Lundin A, et al. Percutaneous transluminal angioplasty with or without stenting for femoropopliteal occlusions? A randomized controlled study. *Int Angiol* 1999;18:251–5.

31. Becker GJ, Katzen BT, Dake MD. Noncoronary angioplasty. *Radiology* 1989;170:921–940.

32. Matsi PJ, Manninen HI. Complications of lower-limb percutaneous transluminal angioplasty: a prospective analysis of 410 procedures on 295 consecutive patients. *Cardiovasc Intervent Radiol* 1998;21:361–366.

33. Leng GC, Davis M, Baker D. Bypass surgery for chronic lower limb ischemia. Cochrane Library Issue 2, 2002. Oxford: Update Software. Search date 2001; primary sources: Cochrane peripheral vascular diseases group trials register, medline, EMBASE, reference lists of various articles and contact with trial investigators.

34. De Vries SO, Hunink MG. Results of aortic bifurcation grafts for aortoiliac occlusive disease: a meta-analysis. *J Vasc Surg* 1997;26:558–569. Search date 1996; primary sources Medline and hand searches of review articles, original studies, and a vascular surgery textbook.

35. Johnston KW, Rae M, Hogg-Johnston SA, et al. Five-year results of a prospective study of percutaneous transluminal angioplasty. *Ann Surg* 1987;206:403–413.

36. Bosch J, Hunink M. Meta-analysis of the results of percutaneous transluminal angioplasty and stent placement for aortoiliac occlusive disease. *Radiology* 1997;204:87–96. Search date not stated; primary sources Medline and hand searches of reference lists.

37. Johnson KW. Femoral and popliteal arteries. reanalysis of results of balloon angioplasty. *Radiology* 1992;183:767–771.

Sonia Anand
Assistant Professor of Medicine
McMaster University
Hamilton
Canada

Mark Creager
Associate Professor of Medicine
Harvard Medical School
Boston
USA

Competing interests: None declared.

TABLE 1 Cilostazol 200 mg daily versus placebo (see text pp 147, 148).

Ref	Duration (wks)	Number of people			People self rated as worsened, unchanged, or unsure	Absolute claudication distance (m)	Initial claudication distance (m)
		Randomised	Protocol violation	Withdrawn			
16	24	466	35	64	47/205 (23%) v 68/226 (30%); RR 0.76 (95% CI 0.55 to 1.05)	350 v 300 (P < 0.001)	218 v 180 (P = 0.02)
17	16	298	59	27	53/119 (45%) v 78/120 (65%); RR 0.68 (95% CI 0.54 to 0.87)	333 v 281	NA
18	24	516	23	75	80/171 (47%) v 106/169 (63%); RR 0.75 (95% CI 0.61 to 0.91)	259 v 175 (P < 0.001)	138 v 96 (P < 0.001)
19	12	81	4	15	27/54 (50%) v 22/27 (81%); RR 0.61 (95% CI 0.45 to 0.85)	113 v 85 (P = 0.007)	232 v 152 (P = 0.002)

m, metres; NA, not available; ref, reference.

TABLE 2 Systematic reviews and a subsequent RCT of pentoxifylline versus placebo (see text, p 148).

Ref	Number of RCTs (people)	Initial claudication distance (m)	Absolute claudication distance (m)
11	13 (600)	21 (95% CI 0.7 to 41)	44 (95% CI 14 to 74)
16	1 (471)	22 (95% CI NA)	8 (95% CI NA)
21	11 (612)	29 (95% CI 13 to 46)	48 (95% CI 18 to 79)

NA, not available; ref, reference.

INTERVENTIONS

Likely to be beneficial
Physical activity............159
Eating more fruit and
    vegetables..............161
Smoking cessation 164

Trade off between benefits and harms
Aspirin in low risk people 176
Anticoagulant treatment
    (warfarin) 178

Unknown effectiveness
Antioxidants (other than
    betacarotene) 162

Likely to be ineffective or harmful
Betacarotene 162

INTERVENTIONS AIMED AT LOWERING BLOOD PRESSURE
Beneficial
Antihypertensive drug treatments in
    people with hypertension . . .171
Diuretics in high risk people . . .173

Likely to be beneficial
Physical activity............166

Low fat, high fruit and vegetable
    diet..................167
Reduced alcohol consumption .167
Dietary salt restriction 168
Smoking cessation 169
Weight loss...............169
Potassium supplementation . . .170
Fish oil supplementation 170

Unknown effectiveness
Calcium supplementation 171
Magnesium supplementation . .171

INTERVENTIONS AIMED AT LOWERING CHOLESTEROL CONCENTRATIONS
Likely to be beneficial
Cholesterol reduction in high risk
    people 174
Low fat diet 174

Covered elsewhere in *Clinical Evidence*
See cardiovascular disease in
    diabetes, p 46

Primary prevention

Key Messages

Exercise

- **Physical activity** Observational studies have found that moderate to high physical activity significantly reduces coronary heart disease and stroke. They also found that sudden death soon after strenuous exercise was rare, more common in sedentary people, and did not outweigh the benefits.

Diet

- **Antioxidants (other than betacarotene)** Observational studies found insufficient evidence on the effects of vitamin C, vitamin E, copper, zinc, manganese, or flavonoids. Two RCTs found no significant difference in mortality after about 6 years with vitamin E supplements versus placebo.
- **Betacarotene** RCTs found no evidence that betacarotene supplements are effective, and have found that they may be harmful.
- **Eating more fruit and vegetables** Observational studies have found that consumption of fruit and vegetables reduces ischaemic heart disease and stroke. The size and nature of any real effect is uncertain.

Smoking

- **Smoking cessation** Observational studies have found a strong association between smoking and overall mortality and ischaemic vascular disease. Several large cohort studies have found that the increased risk associated with smoking falls after stopping smoking. The risk can take many years to approach that of non-smokers, particularly in those with a history of heavy smoking.

Antithrombotic drugs

- **Anticoagulant treatment (warfarin)** One RCT found that the benefits and harms of oral anticoagulation among individuals without symptoms of cardiovascular disease were finely balanced, and that net effects were uncertain.
- **Aspirin in low risk people** We found insufficient evidence to identify which asymptomatic individuals would benefit overall and which would be harmed by regular treatment with aspirin. Benefits are likely to outweigh risks in people at higher risk.

Interventions aimed at lowing blood pressure

- **Antihypertensive drug treatments in people with hypertension** Systematic reviews have found that initial treatment with diuretics, angiotensin converting enzyme inhibitors, or β blockers reduce morbidity and mortality, with minimal adverse effects. The biggest benefit was seen in those with the highest baseline risk. We found limited evidence from two systematic reviews that diuretics, β blockers, and angiotensin converting enzyme inhibitors reduced coronary heart disease and heart failure more than calcium channel antagonists. However, calcium channel antagonists reduced risk of stroke more than the other agents. One RCT found no significant difference in coronary heart disease outcomes with α blockers versus diuretics, but found that α blockers significantly increased cardiovascular events, particularly congestive cardiac failure at 4 years.
- **Calcium supplementation** We found no RCTs examining the effects of calcium supplementation on morbidity or mortality. We found insufficient evidence on the effects of calcium supplementation specifically in people with hypertension. One systematic review in people with and without hypertension found that calcium supplementation may reduce systolic blood pressure by small amounts.

- **Dietary salt restriction** We found no RCTs of the effects of salt restriction on morbidity or mortality. One systematic review has found that a low salt diet versus a usual diet may lead to modest reductions in blood pressure, with more benefit in people older than 45 years than in younger people (see table 1, p 185).

- **Diuretics in high risk people** Systematic reviews have found that diuretics versus placebo significantly decrease the risk of fatal and non-fatal stroke, cardiac events, and total mortality. The biggest benefit is seen in people with the highest baseline risk. Systematic reviews have found no significant difference in mortality or morbidity with diuretics versus β blockers.

- **Fish oil supplementation** We found no RCTs examining the effects of fish oil supplementation on morbidity or mortality. One systematic review has found that fish oil supplementation in large doses of 3 g daily modestly lowers blood pressure.

- **Low fat, high fruit and vegetable diet** We found no systematic review and no RCTs examining the effects of low fat, high fruit and vegetable diet on morbidity or mortality of people with raised blood pressure. One RCT found that a low fat, high fruit and vegetable diet versus control diet modestly reduced blood pressure.

- **Magnesium supplementation** We found no RCTs examining the effects of magnesium supplementation on morbidity or mortality. We found limited and conflicting evidence on the effect of magnesium supplementation on blood pressure in people with hypertension and normal magnesium concentrations.

- **Physical activity** We found no RCTs examining the effects of exercise on morbidity or mortality. One systematic review has found that aerobic exercise versus no exercise reduces blood pressure.

- **Potassium supplementation** We found no RCTs examining the effects of potassium supplementation on morbidity or mortality. One systematic review has found that a daily potassium supplementation of about 60 mmol (2 g, which is about the amount contained in 5 bananas) reduces blood pressure by small amounts.

- **Reduced alcohol consumption** We found no RCTs examining the effects of reducing alcohol consumption on morbidity or mortality. One systematic review in moderate drinkers (25–50 drinks/wk) found inconclusive evidence regarding effects of alcohol reduction on blood pressure.

- **Smoking cessation** Observational studies have found that smoking is a significant risk factor for cardiovascular disease. We found no direct evidence specifically in people with hypertension that stopping smoking decreases blood pressure.

- **Weight loss** We found no RCTs examining the effects of weight loss on morbidity and mortality. One systematic review and additional RCTs have found that modest weight reduction in obese people with hypertension may lead to modest reductions in blood pressure.

Interventions aimed at lowering cholesterol

- **Cholesterol reduction in high risk people** Systematic reviews have found that reducing cholesterol concentration in asymptomatic people lowers the rate of cardiovascular events. RCTs have found that the magnitude of the benefit is related to an individual's baseline risk of cardiovascular events, and to the degree of cholesterol lowering, rather than to the individual's cholesterol concentration.

Primary prevention

■ **Low fat diet** Systematic reviews and RCTs have found that combined use of cholesterol lowering diet and lipid lowering drugs reduces cholesterol concentration more than lifestyle interventions alone.

DEFINITION Primary prevention in this context is the long term management of people at increased risk but with no evidence of cardiovascular disease. Clinically overt ischaemic vascular disease includes acute myocardial infarction, angina, stroke, and peripheral vascular disease. Many adults have no symptoms or obvious signs of vascular disease, even though they have atheroma and are at increased risk of ischaemic vascular events because of one or more risk factors (see aetiology below).

INCIDENCE/ According to the World Health Report 1999, ischaemic heart
PREVALENCE disease was the leading single cause for death in the world, the leading single cause for death in high income countries and second to lower respiratory tract infections in low and middle income countries. In 1998 it was still the leading cause for death, with nearly 7.4 million estimated deaths a year in member states of the World Health Organization. This condition had the eighth highest burden of disease in the low and middle income countries (30.7 million disability adjusted life years).[1]

AETIOLOGY/ Identified major risk factors for ischaemic vascular disease include
RISK FACTORS increasing age, male sex, raised low density lipoprotein cholesterol, reduced high density lipoprotein cholesterol, raised blood pressure, smoking, diabetes, family history of cardiovascular disease, obesity, and sedentary lifestyle. For many of these risk factors, observational studies show a continuous gradient of increasing risk of cardiovascular disease with increasing levels of the risk factor, with no obvious threshold level. Although by definition event rates are higher in high risk people, of all ischaemic vascular events that occur in the population, most occur in people with intermediate levels of absolute risk because there are many more of them than there are people at high risk; see Appendix 1.[2]

PROGNOSIS A study carried out in Scotland found that about half of people who suffer an acute myocardial infarction die within 28 days, and two thirds of acute myocardial infarctions occur before the person reaches hospital.[3] The benefits of intervention in unselected people with no evidence of cardiovascular disease (primary prevention) are small because in such people the baseline risk is small. However, absolute risk of ischaemic vascular events varies dramatically, even among people with similar levels of blood pressure or cholesterol. Estimates of absolute risk can be based on simple risk equations or tables; see Appendix 1.[4,5]

AIMS To reduce morbidity and mortality from cardiovascular disease, with minimum adverse effects.

OUTCOMES Incidence of fatal and non-fatal cardiovascular events (including coronary, cerebrovascular, renal, and eye disease, and heart failure). Surrogate outcomes include changes in levels of individual risk factors, such as blood pressure.

METHODS *Clinical Evidence* update search and appraisal March 2002.

QUESTION Does physical activity reduce the risk of vascular events in asymptomatic people?

Charles Foster and Michael Murphy

We found strong observational evidence that moderate to high levels of physical activity reduce the risk of non-fatal and fatal coronary heart disease and stroke. People who are physically active (those who undertake moderate levels of activity daily or almost daily, e.g. walking) typically experience 30–50% reductions in relative risk of coronary heart disease compared with people who are sedentary after adjustment for other risk factors. The absolute risk of sudden death after strenuous activity is small (although greatest in people who are habitually sedentary) and does not outweigh observed benefits.

Benefits: **Effects of physical activity on coronary heart disease:** We found no RCTs. Three systematic reviews (search dates 1995[6] and not stated[7,8]) evaluated observational studies and found increased risk of coronary heart disease (CHD) in sedentary compared with active people. Since 1992, 17 large, well conducted prospective, non randomised studies, with follow up periods ranging from 18 months to 29 years, have specifically examined the association between physical activity and risk of non-fatal or fatal CHD.[9–25] The studies found that risk declined with increasing levels of physical activity (for examples of activity levels see table 1, p 185) (AR for CHD death in people with sedentary lives [rare or no physical activity] 70/10 000 person-years v 40/10 000 person-years in people with the highest level of activity [> 3500 kcal/wk]; absolute benefit of high levels of physical activity 30 lives saved/10 000 person-years). A new observational study of women found that at least 1 hour of walking a week predicted lower risk compared to no walking a week (OR 0.49, 95% CI 0.28 to 0.86).[26] **Effects of physical fitness on coronary heart disease:** We found no RCTs. One systematic review (search date not stated) identified seven large, well designed prospective, non-randomised studies of the effects of physical fitness on CHD.[27] All used reproducible measures of physical fitness. Five studies adjusted for other CHD risk factors. These found an increased risk of death from CHD in people with low levels of physical fitness compared with those with high levels (RR of death lowest quartile v highest quartile ranged from 1.2–4.0). Most studies reported only baseline measures of physical fitness; thus, not accounting for changes in fitness. One recent large follow up study found lower risk among people who increased their fitness level (RR for cardiovascular disease death compared with those whose level of fitness did not change 0.48, 95% CI 0.31 to 0.74).[28] One recent study showed that high fitness levels seem to slow down the development of atherosclerosis compared to those with lower levels of fitness.[29] A new meta-analysis examining fitness and activity as separate risk factors for CHD concluded that being unfit warrants consideration as a risk factor.[30] **Effects of physical activity on stroke:** We found no RCTs and no systematic review of observational studies. We found 12 observational studies (published between 1990 and 1999), based on 3680 strokes among North American, Japanese, and European populations.[31–44] Most of these found that moderate activity was associated with reduced risk of stroke compared with inactivity (RR of stroke, moderate activity v inactivity about 0.5). One cohort study from Japan found that "heavy" physical activity reduced the risk of stroke compared with "moderate" activity (RR of stroke, "heavy" v "moderate" activity about 0.3; P < 0.05).[42] In most studies, the benefits were greater in older people and in men. Most studies were conducted in white men in late middle age, which potentially limits their applicability to other groups of people. The results usually persisted after adjustment for other known risk factors for stroke (blood pressure, blood lipids, body mass index, and smoking) and after exclusion of people with pre-existing diseases that might limit physical activity and increase risk of stroke. The more recent studies found maximum reduction in the risk of stroke with moderate as opposed to high levels of physical exercise levels.

Harms: No direct evidence of harm was reported in the studies described. We found two studies in people who had experienced non-fatal myocardial infarction, conducted in the USA and Germany. Each involved more than 1000 events and found that 4–7% of these events occurred within 1 hour of strenuous physical activity.[45–47] Strenuous activity was estimated to have raised the relative risk of acute myocardial infarction between two- and sixfold in the hour after activity, with risks returning to baseline after that. However, the absolute risk remained low, variously estimated at six deaths per 100 000 middle aged men a year[48] or 0.3–2.7 events per 10 000 person hours of exercise.[49] Both studies found that the relative risk of acute myocardial infarction after strenuous activity was much higher in people who were habitually sedentary (RR 107, 95% CI 67 to 171) compared with the relative risk in those who engaged in heavy physical exertion on five or more occasions a week (RR 2.4, 95% CI 1.5 to 3.7).[46] Injury is likely to be the most common adverse event, but we found too few population data to measure its risk.

Comment: Findings from these observational studies should be interpreted with caution. The studies varied in definitions of levels of activity and fitness. The level of activity or fitness experienced by each person was not experimentally assigned by an investigator (as in an RCT) but resulted from self selection. Active (or fit) people are likely to differ from inactive (or unfit) people in other ways that also influence their risk of cardiovascular disease. Confounding of this type can be partially controlled by adjustment for other known risk factors (such as age, smoking status, and body mass index), but it is likely that some residual confounding will remain, which could overestimate the effect of exercise. The studies have found that the absolute risk of sudden death during or immediately after physical activity is small and does not outweigh the observed benefits.

QUESTION **What intensity and frequency of physical activity improves fitness?**

Charles Foster and Michael Murphy

Small RCTs found that at least moderate intensity exercise (equivalent to brisk walking) is necessary to improve fitness. We found insufficient evidence on the effects of short bouts of exercise several times daily compared with longer daily bouts.

Benefits: **Intensity:** We found no systematic review. Numerous small RCTs of varying quality have been conducted in different subpopulations. In general, these found that over a period of 6–12 months low intensity activity programmes produced no measurable changes in maximum oxygen consumption (Vo_2max), whereas moderate intensity activity programmes (equivalent to brisk walking) typically produced improvements of 20% in oxygen consumption in sedentary people. Table 1, p 185 gives the intensity of effort required for a range of physical activities. Two recent RCTs compared structured aerobic exercise (such as step classes and aerobics classes) with lifestyle activity programmes (such as regular walking and using stairs instead of lifts) among obese women[50] and sedentary men and women.[51] Both studies reported similar, significant changes in measures of cardiovascular fitness and blood pressure with each intervention, and these changes were sustained for at least 2 years after intervention. One prospective follow up study of women previously involved in a randomised trial of physical activity found that women who start a programme of regular walking maintain higher levels of physical activity 10 years after the intervention.[52] **Frequency:** We found no systematic review. One RCT (36 men) compared 8 weeks of a single daily session of 30 minutes of exercise versus three daily sessions of 10 minutes each.[53] It found no significant difference in fitness benefit between groups.

Harms: None reported.

Comment: None.

QUESTION	What are the effects of dietary interventions on the risk of myocardial infarction and stroke in asymptomatic people?

Andy Ness

OPTION	EATING MORE FRUIT AND VEGETABLES

Cohort studies have found that eating more fruit and vegetables reduces the risk of myocardial infarction and stroke. The size and nature of any real protective effect is uncertain.

Benefits: **Ischaemic heart disease:** We found no RCTs. We found three systematic reviews of observational studies.[54–57] With addition of recently published studies[58–66] to those reported in the first review (search date 1995),[54] a protective association was observed for ischaemic heart disease in 14/25 (56%) cohort studies. In the second review (search date not stated),[55] the authors calculated a summary measure of the protective association of 15% between those above the 90th centile and those below the 10th centile for fruit and vegetable consumption. In the third review (search date 1998),[56,57] the authors estimated that increased intake of fruit and vegetables of about 150 g daily was associated with a reduced risk of coronary heart disease of 20–40%. The validity of these estimates has been questioned. One large, high quality cohort study found that eating more vegetables was associated with decreased coronary mortality ($\geq$ 117 g vegetables/day v < 61 g vegetables/day: RR 0.66, 95% CI 0.46 to 0.96; for fruit, the association was

Cardiovascular disorders

Primary prevention

more modest and not significant ($\geq$ 159 g fruit/day v < 75 g fruit/day: RR 0.77, 95% CI 0.54 to 1.12).[67] **Stroke:** We found no RCTs but we found two systematic reviews examining the evidence from observational studies for stroke.[54,56,57] With addition of recently published studies[58–65,67] to those reported in the first review (search date 1995),[54] a protective association was observed in 10/16 (63%) cohort studies for stroke. In the second review (search date not stated),[56,57] the authors estimated that increased intake of fruit and vegetables of about 150 g daily was associated with a reduced risk of stroke of 0–25%. The basis for this estimate is not clear. One large, high quality cohort study in US health professionals found that increased fruit and vegetable intake was associated with a decreased risk of ischaemic stroke (RR per daily serving of fruit and vegetables 0.94, 95% CI 0.90 to 0.99; RR in the fifth of the population eating the most fruit and vegetables v the fifth eating the least 0.69, 95% CI 0.52 to 0.92).[68]

Harms:　　　None were identified.

Comment:　Lack of RCT evidence and deficiencies in the data available from observational studies mean that the size and nature of any real protective effect is uncertain.[69,70] The observed associations could be the result of confounding as people who eat more fruit and vegetables often come from higher socioeconomic groups and have other healthy lifestyles.[71]

OPTION　**ANTIOXIDANTS**

We found no evidence of benefit from betacarotene supplements, and RCTs suggest that they may be harmful. Other antioxidant supplements may be beneficial, but we found insufficient RCT evidence to support their use.

Benefits:　**Betacarotene:** We found one systematic review of prospective studies and RCTs (search date not stated, published in 1997), which did not pool data because of heterogeneity among studies.[72] Most prospective cohort studies of betacarotene found a modest protective association with increased intake,[72–75] although several large RCTs of betacarotene supplementation found no evidence of benefit.[75,76] **Vitamin C (ascorbic acid):** We found two systematic reviews (search dates not stated[72] and 1996[77]), which mostly included the same studies, and seven subsequent prospective studies.[62,72,78–82] Three of 14 cohort studies found a significant protective association between vitamin C and coronary heart disease, and 2/11 (18%) studies found a protective association between vitamin C and stroke. We found no large RCTs of vitamin C supplementation alone. Two large RCTs of multivitamin supplements have been carried out in Linxian, China.[72,83–85] One RCT (that was included in the reviews) was carried out in 29 584 people drawn from the general population who were randomised by using a factorial design to one of four arms: arm A — retinol (10 000 IU) and zinc (22.5 mg); arm B — riboflavin (riboflavine) (5.2 mg) and niacin (40 mg); arm C — ascorbic acid (120 mg) and molybdenum (30 µg); and arm D — betacarotene (15 mg), selenium (50 µg), and vitamin E (30 mg). After 6 years the RCT found that people allocated to arm D (betacarotene, selenium, and vitamin E) reduced all cause mortality and death because of stroke (RR for death from any cause arm D v other arms 0.91, 95% CI 0.84 to 0.99). It found no reduction in stroke or all cause mortality among the other arms.[72] The other RCT (subsequent to the reviews) included 3318 people with oesophageal dysplasia who were randomised to placebo or a multivitamin supplement that contained 14 vitamins and 12 minerals, including vitamin C (180 mg), vitamin E (60 IU [1 IU = 0.67 mg]), betacarotene (15 mg), and selenium (50 μg). After 6 years it found that the supplement did not significantly reduce stroke or death from all causes (RR for all cause mortality 0.93, 95% CI 0.75 to 1.16; RR for stroke 0.67, 95% CI 0.37 to 1.07).[83,84] **Vitamin E:** We found one systematic review and additional prospective studies.[71] Eight large cohort studies (5 of which were included in the review) have examined the association between vitamin E intake and ischaemic heart disease. Six found a significant protective association,[72,80,86] whereas two found no significant association.[62,87] In three studies the protective association was with dietary vitamin E.[72,84] In the others it was either wholly or mainly with vitamin E supplements.[72,87] In the review, the largest RCT of vitamin E alone versus placebo (in 29 133 Finnish smokers) found that vitamin E did not significantly reduce mortality compared with placebo (RR for death 0.98, 95% CI 0.91 to 1.05) after 5–8 years. (See vitamin C above for the results of the Linxian RCTs.)[72,83–85] Since the review was published the Primary Prevention project (4495 people at high risk of cardiovascular disease in a factorial design to vitamin E [300 mg/day] and aspirin) followed them up for 3.6 years. The trial was stopped early because of the results in the aspirin arm. There was no significant reduction in the risk of cardiovascular events or all cause mortality with vitamin E (RR for all cardiovascular events with vitamin E 0.94, 95% CI 0.77 to 1.16; RR for death from all causes 0.93, 95% CI 0.51 to 1.23).[88] Four cohort studies found no association between vitamin E intake and stroke.[79,81,82,89] In the α-tocopherol and betacarotene supplement RCT (28 519 male Finnish smokers) no significant reduction in overall stroke incidence or stroke mortality was found in those receiving vitamin E (RR of stroke incidence 0.93, 95% CI 0.83 to 1.05; RR of stroke death 1.29, 95% CI 0.94 to 1.76) after 6 years. There was a reduction in incidence from cerebral infarction, but no significant reduction in mortality due to cerebral infarction (RR for cerebral infarction 0.86, 95% CI 0.75 to 0.99; RR for death due to cerebral infarction 0.81, 95% CI 0.49 to 1.32) and an increase in mortality from subarachnoid haemorrhage (RR for subarachnoid haemorrhage 1.50, 95% CI 0.97 to 2.32; RR death 2.81, 95% CI 1.37 to 5.79) and non significant increase in mortality from haemorrhagic stroke (RR 1.64, 95% CI 0.93 to 2.90).[90] **Antioxidant minerals:** We found little epidemiological evidence about the cardioprotective effect of copper, zinc, or manganese on the heart.[91] Cohort studies reported an increased risk of ischaemic heart disease in people with low blood selenium concentrations.[92] Most of these were carried out in Finland, a country with low intakes of antioxidants.[93] (See vitamin C above for the results of the Linxian RCTs.)[72,83–85] **Flavonoids:** We found no

Cardiovascular disorders

Primary prevention

systematic review. We found five cohort studies,[93–97] three of which reported a reduced risk of ischaemic heart disease with increased flavonoid intake.[93–95] One of four observational studies reported a reduced risk of stroke with increased flavonoid intake.[57,79,89,94]

Harms: Several large RCTs found that betacarotene supplements may increase cardiovascular mortality (pooled data from 4 RCTs, RR for cardiovascular death 1.12, 95% CI 1.04 to 1.22).[75] Explanations for these results include use of the wrong isomer, the wrong dose, or a detrimental effect on other carotenoid levels.[98,99]

Comment: RCTs of antioxidants such as betacarotene and vitamin E have not produced any evidence of benefit. Routine use of antioxidant supplements is not justified by the currently available evidence. More RCTs of antioxidant supplementation are underway.[100]

QUESTION **By how much does smoking cessation, or avoiding starting smoking, reduce risk?**

Julian J Nicholas

Observational studies have found that cigarette smoking is strongly related to overall mortality. We found evidence from both observational and randomised studies that cigarette smoking increases the risk of coronary heart disease and stroke. The evidence is strongest for stroke.

Benefits: Several large cohort studies examining the effects of smoking have been reviewed extensively by the US Surgeon General[101] and the UK Royal College of Physicians.[102] The reviews concluded that cigarette smoking was causally related to disease and that smoking cessation substantially reduced the risk of cancer, respiratory disease, coronary heart disease (CHD), and stroke. **Death from all causes:** The longest prospective cohort study, in 34 439 male British doctors whose smoking habits were periodically assessed over 40 years (1951–1991), found a strong association between smoking and increased mortality. It found that smokers were about three times more likely to die in middle age (45–64 years) and twice as likely to die in older age (65–84 years) compared with lifelong non-smokers (CI not provided).[103] The prospective nurses' health study followed 117 001 middle aged female nurses for 12 years. It found that the total mortality in current smokers was nearly twice that in lifelong non-smokers (RR of death 1.87, 95% CI 1.65 to 2.13).[104] **Coronary heart disease:** One review (published in 1990) identified 10 cohort studies, involving 20 million person-years of observation.[101] All studies found a higher incidence of CHD among smokers (pooled RR of death from CHD compared with non-smokers 1.7, CI not provided).[101] People smoking more than 20 cigarettes daily were more likely to have a coronary event (RR 2.5, CI not provided).[102] Middle aged smokers were more likely to experience a first non-fatal acute myocardial infarction compared with people who had never smoked (RR in men 2.9, 95% CI 2.4 to 3.4; RR in women 3.6, 95% CI 3.0 to 4.4).[105,106] One RCT of advice encouraging smoking cessation in 1445 men aged 40–59 years found that more men given advice to stop smoking gave up cigarettes (mean absolute reduction in men continuing to smoke after advice v control 53%). The RCT found no evidence that men given advice to stop smoking had a significantly lower mortality from CHD (RR 0.82, 95% CI 0.57 to 1.18).[107] The wide confidence intervals mean that there could have been anything from a 43% decrease to an 18% increase in rates of CHD death in men given advice to quit, regardless of whether they actually gave up smoking. **Stroke:** One systematic review (search date 1998) found 32 studies (17 cohort studies with concurrent or historical controls, 14 case control studies, and one hypertension intervention RCT).[108] It found good evidence that smoking was associated with an increased risk of stroke (RR of stroke in cigarette smokers v non-smokers 1.5, 95% CI 1.4 to 1.6).[108] Smoking was associated with an increased risk of cerebral infarction (RR 1.92, 95% CI 1.71 to 2.16) and subarachnoid haemorrhage (RR 2.93, 95% CI 2.48 to 3.46), and a reduced risk of intracerebral haemorrhage (RR 0.74, 95% CI 0.56 to 0.98). The relative risk of stroke in smokers versus non-smokers was highest in those aged under 55 years (RR 2.90, 95% CI 2.40 to 3.59) and lowest in those aged over 74 years (RR 1.11, 95% CI 0.96 to 1.28).

Harms: We found no evidence that stopping smoking increases mortality in any subgroup of smokers.

Comment: We found no evidence of publication or other overt bias that may explain the observed association between smoking and stroke. There was a dose related effect the number of cigarettes smoked and the relative risk for stroke, consistent with a causal relation. The absolute risk reduction from stopping smoking will be highest for those with the highest absolute risk of vascular events.

| QUESTION | How quickly do risks diminish when smokers stop smoking? |

Julian J Nicholas

Observational studies have found that the risk of death and cardiovascular events falls when people stop smoking. The risk can take many years to approach that of non-smokers, particularly in those with a history of heavy smoking.

Benefits: **Death from all causes:** In people who stopped smoking, observational studies found that death rates fell gradually to lie between those of lifelong smokers and people who had never smoked. Estimates for the time required for former smokers to bring their risk of death in line with people who had never smoked varied among studies but may be longer than 15 years.[109] Actuarial projections from one study among British doctors predicted that life expectancy would improve even among people who stopped smoking in later life (≥ 65 years).[103] **Coronary heart disease:** Observational studies found that, in both male and female ex-smokers, the risk of coronary events rapidly declined to a level comparable with that of people who had never smoked after 2–3 years and was independent of the number of cigarettes smoked before quitting.[101] **Stroke:** The US Surgeon General's review of observational studies found that the risk of stroke decreased in ex-smokers compared with smokers (RR of stroke, smokers v ex-smokers 1.2, CI not provided) but remained raised for 5–10 years after cessation compared with those who had never smoked (RR of stroke ex-smokers v never smokers 1.5, CI not provided).[101] One recent study in 7735 middle aged British men found that 5 years after smoking cessation the risk of stroke in previously light smokers (< 20 cigarettes/day) was identical to that of lifelong non-smokers, but the risk in previously heavy smokers (> 21 cigarettes/day) was still raised compared with lifelong non-smokers (RR of stroke, previously heavy smokers v never smokers 2.2, 95% CI 1.1 to 4.3).[110] One observational study in 117 001 middle aged female nurses also found a fall in risk on stopping smoking and found no difference between previously light and previously heavy smokers (RR in all former smokers 2–4 years after stopping smoking 1.17, 95% CI 0.49 to 2.23).[104]

Harms: We found no evidence that stopping smoking increases mortality in any subgroup of smokers.

Comment: For a review of the evidence on methods of changing smoking behaviour, see secondary prevention of ischaemic cardiac events, p 189.

QUESTION   What are the effects of lifestyle changes in asymptomatic people with primary hypertension?

Cindy Mulrow and Mike Pignone

OPTION   PHYSICAL ACTIVITY

One systematic review has found that aerobic exercise reduces blood pressure.

Benefits: We found no RCTs examining the effects of exercise on morbidity, mortality, or quality of life. One systematic review (search date 2001, 54 RCTs, 2419 sedentary adults aged > 18 years) examined the effects on blood pressure of at least 2 weeks of regular exercise versus no exercise.[111] Compared with non-exercising control groups, groups randomised to aerobic exercise reduced their systolic blood pressure by 3.8 mm Hg (95% CI 2.7 mm Hg to 5.0 mm Hg) and diastolic blood pressure by 2.6 mm Hg (95% CI 1.8 mm Hg to 3.4 mm Hg). Reductions in blood pressure were seen in hypertensive and non-hypertensive people, and in overweight and normal weight people. RCTs with interventions lasting longer than 6 months in adults aged 45 years or over with hypertension found non-significant mean reductions in blood pressure, with wide confidence intervals (systolic reduction 0.8 mm Hg, 95% CI 5.9 mm Hg reduction to 4.2 mm Hg increase).[112]

Harms: Musculoskeletal injuries can occur, but their frequency was not documented.

Comment: Many adults find aerobic exercise programmes difficult to sustain. The clinical significance of the observed reductions in blood pressure is uncertain. The type and amount of exercise most likely to result in benefits are unclear, with some recent studies showing some benefits with simple increases in lifestyle activity. One cohort study (173 men with hypertension) found that "regular heavy activity several times weekly" compared with no or limited spare time physical activity reduced all cause and cardiovascular mortality (all cause mortality RR 0.43, 95% CI 0.22 to 0.82; cardiovascular mortality RR 0.33, 95% CI 0.11 to 0.94).[113]

OPTION **LOW FAT, HIGH FRUIT AND VEGETABLE DIET**

We found no systematic review and no RCTs examining the effects of low fat, high fruit and vegetable diet on morbidity or mortality in people with primary hypertension. One RCT found that a low fat, high fruit and vegetable diet modestly reduced blood pressure.

Benefits: We found no systematic review and no RCTs examining the effects of low fat, high fruit and vegetable diet on morbidity or mortality in people with primary hypertension. For evidence from cohort studies in asymptomatic people in general see question on effects of dietary interventions, p 161. One RCT (459 adults with systolic blood pressures of < 160 mm Hg and diastolic blood pressures of 80–90 mm Hg) compared effects on blood pressure of three diets (control diet low in both magnesium and potassium v fruit and vegetable diet high in both potassium and magnesium v combination of the fruit and vegetable diet with a low fat diet high in both calcium and protein).[114] After 8 weeks the fruit and vegetable diet reduced systolic and diastolic blood pressure compared with the control diet (mean change in systolic blood pressure 2.8 mm Hg, 97.5% CI −4.7 mm Hg to −0.9 mm Hg; mean change in diastolic blood pressure −1.1 mm Hg, 97.5% CI −2.4 mm Hg to +0.3 mm Hg). The combination diet also reduced systolic and diastolic blood pressure compared with the control diet (mean change in systolic blood pressure −5.5 mm Hg, 97.5% CI −7.4 mm Hg to −3.7 mm Hg; mean change in diastolic blood pressure −3.0 mm Hg, 97.5% CI −4.3 to −1.6 mm Hg).

Harms: We found no direct evidence that a low fat, high fruit and vegetable diet is harmful.

Comment: The RCT was of short duration and people were supplied with food during the intervention period.[114] Other studies have found that long term maintenance of particular diets is difficult for many people, although low fat, high fruit and vegetable diets may have multiple benefits (see changing behaviour, p 74).

OPTION **REDUCED ALCOHOL CONSUMPTION**

One systematic review found inconclusive evidence regarding effects of alcohol reduction on blood pressure.

Benefits: We found no RCTs examining the effects of reducing alcohol consumption on morbidity or mortality. Over 60 population studies have reported associations between alcohol consumption and blood pressure; the relation was found to be generally linear, although several studies reported a threshold effect at about two to three standard drinks daily.[115] Any adverse effect of up to two drinks daily on blood pressure was found to be either small or non-existent. One systematic review (search date 1999, 7 RCTs, 751 people with hypertension; mainly men) found that data were inconclusive on the benefits of reducing alcohol among moderate to heavy drinkers (25–50 drinks/wk).[116]

Harms: We found no direct evidence that reducing alcohol intake to as few as two drinks daily was harmful.

Comment: Most data were from observational studies. RCTs were small and lacked reliable information about adherence. Substantial reductions in alcohol use in both control and intervention groups were observed, with limited ability to detect differences between groups.

OPTION	SALT RESTRICTION

One systematic review has found that salt restriction may lead to modest reductions in blood pressure, with more benefit in people older than 45 years than in younger people.

Benefits: We found no RCT examining the effects of salt restriction on morbidity or mortality. We found one systematic review (search date 1997, 58 RCTs, 2161 people with hypertension, age 23–73 years)[117] and two subsequent RCTs,[118,119] which examined the effects of salt restriction on blood pressure. Interventions were low salt diets with or without weight reduction. People in the control groups took their usual diet. Changes in salt intake varied among RCTs in the systematic review; a mean reduction in sodium intake of 118 mmol (6.7 g) daily for 28 days led to reductions of 3.9 mm Hg (95% CI 3.0 mm Hg to 4.8 mm Hg) in systolic blood pressure and 1.9 mm Hg (95% CI 1.3 mm Hg to 2.5 mm Hg) in diastolic blood pressure.[117] One RCT (875 people with hypertension, age 60–80 years, duration 30 months) found that a mean decrease in salt intake of about 40 mmol (2.4 g) daily reduced systolic blood pressure by 2.6 mm Hg (95% CI 0.4 mm Hg to 4.8 mm Hg) and diastolic blood pressure by 1.1 mm Hg (95% CI 0.3 mm Hg rise in diastolic to 2.5 mm Hg fall).[118] Another RCT (412 people with systolic/diastolic blood pressure > 120/80 mm Hg, mean age 48 years, duration 30 days) that tested three different target levels of sodium intake (150, 100, and 50 mmol/day) found significantly lower systolic blood pressure levels with lower sodium intakes.[119] An earlier systematic review (search date 1994) identified 28 RCTs in 1131 people with hypertension. It found that lesser reductions of 60 mmol/day led to smaller reductions in systolic/diastolic blood pressure of 2.2/ 0.5 mm Hg and found greater effects in RCTs in which mean age was over 45 years (6.3/2.2 mm Hg).[120]

Harms: We found no direct evidence that low salt diets may increase morbidity or mortality.

Comment: Small RCTs tended to report larger reductions in systolic and diastolic blood pressure than larger RCTs. This may be explained by publication bias or less rigorous methodology in small RCTs.[120]

OPTION SMOKING CESSATION

Epidemiological data clearly identify that smoking is a significant risk factor for cardiovascular disease. We found no direct evidence that stopping smoking decreases blood pressure in people with hypertension.

Benefits: We found no direct evidence that stopping smoking reduces blood pressure in people with hypertension, although we found good evidence that, in general, smoking cessation reduces risk of cardio-vascular disease (see question on how much does smoking cessa-tion, or avoiding starting smoking, reduce risk, p 164).

Harms: We found insufficient evidence in this context.

Comment: None.

OPTION WEIGHT LOSS

One systematic review and additional RCTs have found that modest weight reductions of 3–9% of body weight are achievable in motivated middle aged and older adults, and may lead to modest reductions in blood pressure in obese people with hypertension. Many adults find it difficult to maintain weight loss.

Benefits: We found no RCTs examining the effects of weight loss on morbidity and mortality. We found one systematic review (search date 1998, 18 RCTs, 2611 middle aged people, mean age 50 years, mean weight 85 kg, mean systolic/diastolic blood pressure 152/98 mm Hg, 55% men)[121] and two subsequent RCTs[122,123] that examined the effects of weight loss on blood pressure. In the systematic review, caloric intakes ranged from 450–1500 kcal daily; most diets led to weight reductions of 3–9% of body weight. Combined data from the six RCTs that did not vary antihypertensive regimens during the intervention period found that reducing weight reduced systolic and diastolic blood pressures (mean reduction in systolic pressure, weight loss v no weight loss 3.0 mm Hg, 95% CI 0.7 mm Hg to 6.8 mm Hg; mean reduction in diastolic blood pressure, weight loss v no weight loss 2.9 mm Hg, 95% CI 0.1 mm Hg to 5.7 mm Hg). RCTs that allowed adjustment of antihypertensive regimens found that lower doses and fewer antihypertensive drugs were needed in the weight reduction groups compared with control groups. The two subsequent RCTs found that sustained weight reduction of 2–4 kg significantly reduced systolic blood pressure at 1–3 years by about 1 mm Hg.[122,123]

Harms: We found no direct evidence that intentional gradual weight loss of less than 10% of body weight is harmful in obese adults with hypertension.

Comment: None.

Primary prevention

OPTION   **POTASSIUM SUPPLEMENTATION**

One systematic review has found that a daily potassium supplementation of about 60 mmol (2 g, which is about the amount contained in 5 bananas) is feasible for many adults and reduces blood pressure by small amounts.

Benefits: We found no RCTs examining the effects of potassium supplementation on morbidity or mortality. One systematic review (search date 1995, 21 RCTs, 1560 adults with hypertension, age 19–79 years) compared the effects on blood pressure of potassium supplements (60–100 mmol potassium chloride daily) versus placebo or no supplement.[124] It found that, compared with the control interventions, potassium supplements reduced systolic and diastolic blood pressures (mean decrease in systolic blood pressure with potassium supplements 4.4 mm Hg, 95% CI 2.2 mm Hg to 6.6 mm Hg; mean decrease in diastolic blood pressure 2.5 mm Hg, 95% CI 0.1 mm Hg to 4.9 mm Hg).

Harms: We found no direct evidence of harm in people without kidney failure and in people not taking drugs that increase serum potassium concentration. Gastrointestinal adverse effects such as belching, flatulence, diarrhoea, or abdominal discomfort occurred in 2–10% of people.[124]

Comment: None.

OPTION   **FISH OIL SUPPLEMENTATION**

One systematic review has found that fish oil supplementation in large doses of 3 g daily modestly lowers blood pressure.

Benefits: We found no RCTs examining the effects of fish oil supplementation on morbidity or mortality. One systematic review (search date not stated, 7 brief RCTs, 339 people with hypertension, mainly middle aged white men, mean age 50 years) compared effects on blood pressure of fish oil (usually 3 g daily as capsules) versus no supplements or "placebo".[125] The contents of placebo capsules varied among RCTs. Some used oil mixtures containing omega-3 polyunsaturated fatty acids, some without. The review found that fish oil supplements reduced blood pressure compared with control interventions (mean decrease in systolic blood pressure in treatment *v* control 4.5 mm Hg, 95% CI 1.2 mm Hg to 7.8 mm Hg, and mean decrease in diastolic blood pressure in treatment *v* control 2.5 mm Hg, 95% CI 0.6 mm Hg to 4.4 mm Hg).

Harms: Belching, bad breath, fishy taste, and abdominal pain occurred in about a third of people taking high doses of fish oil.[125]

Comment: The RCTs were of short duration and used high doses of fish oil. Such high intake may be difficult to maintain. We found no evidence of beneficial effect on blood pressure at lower intakes.

| OPTION | CALCIUM SUPPLEMENTATION |

We found insufficient evidence on the effects of calcium supplementation specifically in people with hypertension. One systematic review in people both with and without hypertension found that calcium supplementation may reduce systolic blood pressure by small amounts.

Benefits: We found no RCTs examining the effects of calcium supplementation on morbidity or mortality. One systematic review (search date 1994, 42 RCTs, 4560 middle aged people) compared the effects on blood pressure of calcium supplementation (500–2000 mg/day) versus placebo or no supplements [126] It found that calcium supplements reduced blood pressure by a small amount (mean systolic blood pressure reduction, supplement v control 1.4 mm Hg, 95% CI 0.7 mm Hg to 2.2 mm Hg; mean diastolic reduction 0.8 mm Hg, 95% CI 0.2 mm Hg to 1.4 mm Hg).

Harms: Adverse gastrointestinal effects, such as abdominal pain, were generally mild and varied among particular preparations.

Comment: Data relating specifically to people with hypertension are limited by few studies with small sample sizes and short durations.

| OPTION | MAGNESIUM SUPPLEMENTATION |

We found no RCTs examining the effects of magnesium supplementation on morbidity or mortality. We found limited and conflicting evidence on the effect of magnesium supplementation on blood pressure in people with hypertension and normal magnesium concentrations.

Benefits: We found no RCTs examining the effects of magnesium supplementation on morbidity or mortality. A few small, short term RCTs found mixed results on effects on blood pressure reduction.

Harms: We found insufficient evidence.

Comment: None.

| QUESTION | What are the effects of drug treatment in primary hypertension? |

Cindy Mulrow and Mike Pignone

| OPTION | ANTIHYPERTENSIVE DRUGS VERSUS PLACEBO |

Many systematic reviews have found that drug treatment decreases the risk of fatal and non-fatal stroke, cardiac events, and total mortality in specific populations of people. The biggest benefit is seen in people with highest baseline risk of cardiovascular disease.

Benefits: We found many systematic reviews. One review (search date 1997, 17 RCTs with morbidity and mortality outcomes, duration > 1 year, 37 000 people) found that antihypertensive drugs versus placebo produced variable reductions of systolic/diastolic blood pressure that averaged about 12–16/5–10 mm Hg.[127] It found evidence of benefit in total death rate, cardiovascular death rate, stroke, major coronary events, and congestive cardiac failure, but the absolute results depended on age and the severity of the hypertension (see target diastolic blood pressure below). The biggest benefit was seen in those with the highest baseline risk. The RCTs mainly compared placebo versus diuretics (usually thiazides with the addition of amiloride or triamterene) and versus β blockers (usually atenolol or metoprolol) in a stepped care approach. One systematic review (search date 1999, 8 RCTs, 15 693 people) found that, in people aged over 60 years with systolic hypertension, treatment of systolic pressures greater than 160 mm Hg decreased total mortality and fatal and non-fatal cardiovascular events.[128] Absolute benefits were greater in men than women, in people aged over 70 years, and in those with prior cardiovascular events or wider pulse pressure. The relative hazard rates associated with a 10 mm Hg higher initial systolic blood pressure were 1.26 (P = 0.0001) for total mortality, 1.22 (P = 0.02) for stroke, but only 1.07 (P = 0.37) for coronary events. Active treatment reduced total mortality (RR 0.87, 95% CI 0.78 to 0.98; P = 0.02).[128] **Target diastolic blood pressure:** We found one RCT (18 790 people, mean age 62 years, diastolic blood pressures 100–115 mm Hg), which aimed to evaluate the effects on cardiovascular risk of target diastolic blood pressures of 90, 85, and 80 mm Hg.[129] However, mean achieved diastolic blood pressures were 85, 83, and 81 mm Hg, which limited power to detect differences among groups. There were no significant differences in major cardiovascular events among the three groups.

Harms: **Mortality and major morbidity:** One systematic review (search date 1997) comparing diuretics and β blockers versus placebo found no increase in non-cardiovascular mortality in treated people.[127] **Quality of life and tolerability:** One systematic review (search date 1990)[130] and several recent RCTs found that quality of life was not adversely affected and may be improved in those who remain on treatment.[131]

Comment: RCTs included people who were healthier than the general population, with lower rates of cardiovascular risk factors, cardiovascular disease, and comorbidity. People with higher cardiovascular risk can expect greater short term absolute risk reduction than seen in the RCTs, whereas people with major competing risks such as terminal cancer or end stage Alzheimer's disease can expect smaller risk reduction. In the systematic review,[127] five of the RCTs were in middle aged people with mild to moderate hypertension. Seven of the RCTs were in people older than 60 years. On average, every 1000 person-years of treatment in older adults prevented five strokes (95% CI 2 to 8), three coronary events (95% CI 1 to 4), and four cardiovascular deaths (95% CI 1 to 8). Drug treatment in middle aged people prevented one stroke (95% CI 0 to 2) for every 1000 person-years of treatment and did not significantly affect coronary events or mortality. One meta-analysis (7 RCTs, 40 233 people with hypertension) found an increased risk of total and cardiovascular mortality with diastolic blood pressure levels below 85 mm Hg that was not related to antihypertensive treatment.[132]

OPTION COMPARING ANTIHYPERTENSIVE DRUG TREATMENTS

Systematic reviews have found that initial treatment with diuretics, angiotensin converting enzyme inhibitors, or β blockers reduce morbidity and mortality, with minimal adverse effects. RCTs found no significant morbidity or mortality differences among these agents. We found limited evidence from two systematic reviews that diuretics, β blockers, and angiotensin converting enzyme inhibitors reduced coronary heart disease and heart failure more than calcium channel antagonists. However, calcium channel antagonists reduced risk of stroke more than the other agents. One RCT found that a thiazide diuretic is superior to an α blocker in reducing cardiovascular events, particularly congestive heart failure.

Benefits: β **Blockers versus diuretics:** One systematic review (search date 1995, > 48 000 people) identified RCTs comparing effects of high and low dose diuretics versus β blockers.[133] A second systematic review (search date 1998) was limited to 10 RCTs in 16 164 elderly people.[134] These reviews did not summarise direct comparisons of diuretics versus β blockers but compared results of RCTs that used diuretics versus preferred treatment versus results of RCTs that used β blockers as preferred treatment. The reviews found no significant difference between diuretics and β blockers for lowering blood pressure. They found that diuretics reduced coronary events, but found no evidence that β blockers reduced coronary events. **Comparison of β blockers, diuretics, angiotensin converting enzyme inhibitors, and calcium channel antagonists:** One systematic review (search date 2000, 8 RCTs) compared different antihypertensive regimens, and found no significant differences in outcome among people initially treated with β blockers, diuretics, or angiotensin converting enzyme (ACE) inhibitors.[135] However, it found that β blockers or diuretics decreased coronary events compared with calcium channel antagonists and increased stroke rate, although there was no significant difference for all cause mortality (OR for mortality, β blockers or diuretics v calcium channel antagonists 1.01, 95% CI 0.92 to 1.11). ACE inhibitors did not significantly alter all cause mortality or stroke rate compared with calcium channel antagonists, but decreased coronary events (OR for ACE inhibitors v calcium channel antagonist 1.03, 95% CI 0.91 to 1.18 for all cause mortality; 1.02, 95% CI 0.85 to 1.21 for stroke; 0.81, 95% CI 0.68 to 0.97 for coronary events).[135] A second review of similar trials (search date 2001, 9 RCTs, 62 605 hypertensive people) found that diuretics, β blockers, ACE inhibitors, and calcium channel antagonists were all associated with similar reductions in cardiovascular risk.[136] However, calcium channel antagonists reduced risk of stroke and increased risk of myocardial infarction compared with other agents (RR for stroke 0.87, 95% CI 0.76 to 0.99; RR for myocardial infarction 1.19, 1.04 to 1.37).[136] **Comparison of α blockers and diuretics:** A double blind RCT (24 335 high risk people with hypertension), which was included in the systematic review[136], found no significant differences in coronary heart disease outcomes between doxazosin, an α blocker, compared with chlortalidone (chlorthalidone). However, doxazosin versus chlortalidone increased the total number of cardiovascular events after 4 years (25% with doxazosin v 22% with chlortalidone; HR 1.25, 95% CI 1.17 to 1.33) and, in particular, increased congestive heart failure (8% with doxazosin v 4% with chlortalidone; HR 2.04, 95% CI 1.79 to 2.32).[137] **Drug treatment in people with diabetes:** See cardiovascular disease in diabetes, p 46.

Harms: **Quality of life and tolerability:** In the three long term, double blind comparisons of low dose diuretics, β blockers, ACE inhibitors, and calcium channel blockers, tolerability and overall quality of life indicators tended to be more favourable for diuretics and β blockers than for newer drugs.[138–140] One systematic review (search date 1998) of RCTs comparing thiazides versus β blockers found that thiazides were associated with fewer withdrawals because of adverse effects (RR 0.69, 95% CI 0.63 to 0.76).[141] Adverse effects are agent specific. The recent unblinded RCT comparing diuretics, β blockers, calcium channel antagonists, and ACE inhibitors found that after 5 years' follow up, 26% of people receiving felodipine or isradipine (calcium channel antagonists) reported ankle oedema, 30% receiving enalapril or lisinopril (ACE inhibitors) reported cough, and 9% receiving diuretics, β blockers, or both reported cold hands and feet.[142] **Major harm controversies:** Case control, cohort, and randomised studies suggest that short and intermediate acting dihydropyridine calcium channel blockers, such as nifedipine and isradipine, may increase cardiovascular morbidity and mortality.[143]

Comment: None.

QUESTION **What are the effects of lowering cholesterol concentration in asymptomatic people?**

Michael Pignone

Systematic reviews have found that in people with an annual risk of coronary heart disease events 0.6–1.5% a year, cholesterol reduction reduces non-fatal myocardial infarction (see cholesterol reduction under secondary prevention of ischaemic cardiac events for additional information, p 189). RCTs have found that absolute benefit is related to an individual's baseline risk of cardiovascular events and to the degree of cholesterol lowering rather than to the individual's cholesterol concentration.

Benefits: **Cholesterol lowering drug treatment:** We found two systematic reviews of any type of cholesterol lowering drug treatment versus placebo or no treatment in people without a diagnosis of coronary heart disease (CHD).[144,145] Both systematic reviews found similar results. The most recent systematic review (search date 1999) found four RCTs (2 with statins, 1 with fibrates, and 1 with cholestyramine, 21 087 people).[144] It found that cholesterol reduction treatment versus placebo significantly reduced CHD events and CHD mortality, but found no significant effect on overall mortality (OR for treatment v placebo; 0.70, 95% CI 0.62 to 0.79 for CHD events; 0.71, 95% CI 0.56 to 0.91 for CHD mortality; 0.94, 95% CI 0.81 to 1.09 for overall mortality). **Statins:** We found five systematic reviews (search dates 1995,[146] 1997,[147] 1998,[148] 1999,[144] and not stated[145]) and two subsequent RCTs[149,150] that considered the effect of 3-hydroxy-3-methylglutaryl coenzyme A reductase inhibitors (statins) versus placebo on clinical outcomes in people given long term (≥ 6 months) treatment. All the systematic reviews included the same two RCTs of statins in primary prevention (13 200 people).[151,152] All the systematic reviews found similar results. After 4–6 years of treatment for primary prevention, statins compared with placebo did not significantly reduce all cause mortality or CHD mortality, but did reduce major coronary events and cardiovascular mortality (all cause mortality: OR 0.87, 95% CI 0.71 to 1.06; CHD mortality OR 0.73, 95% CI 0.51 to 1.05; major coronary events: OR 0.66, 95% CI 0.57 to 0.76; cardiovascular mortality: OR 0.68, 95% CI 0.50 to 0.93).[148] The absolute risk reduction for CHD events, CHD mortality, and total mortality varied with the baseline risk (see figure 1, p 188). The first subsequent RCT (15 454 men and 5082 women) included 7150 people with no diagnosis of CHD but at high risk (1820 had cerebrovascular disease, 2701 had peripheral arterial disease, and 3982 had diabetes).[149] In people with no diagnosis of CHD, simvastatin versus placebo reduced the risk of a major vascular event (major coronary event, stroke, or revascularisation) after 5 years (risk of major vascular event: event rate ratio 0.75, 95% CI 0.67 to 0.84). The second subsequent RCT (246 men with hyperlipidaemia) compared three treatments: diet alone; diet with pravastatin, and diet and probucol. It found that pravastatin reduced cardiovascular events compared with diet alone after 2 years (AR for any cardiovascular event 4.8% with pravastatin v 13.6% with diet alone, P value and CI not provided).[150] **Low fat diet:** See changing behaviour, p 74.

Harms: Specific harms of statins are discussed under secondary prevention of ischaemic cardiac events, p 189.

Comment: The CHD event rate in the placebo group of the two large primary prevention RCTs using statins was 0.6%[151] and 1.5%[152] a year. If the 17% relative reduction in total mortality observed in the higher risk west of Scotland RCT is real, then about 110 high risk people without known CHD would need to be treated for 5 years to save one life. One regression analysis of all the major statin trials found that mortality benefits of statins outweigh risks in people with a 10 year CHD risk of more than 13%.[156] **Cholesterol lowering treatment in older people:** We found no RCTs specifically evaluating the effect of cholesterol lowering treatment in asymptomatic people aged over 75 years. One large RCT comparing statin with placebo included more than 5000 people over the age of 70 years. It found major vascular events were reduced to a similar extent in people above and below the age of 70 years.[149] **Cholesterol lowering treatment in women:** Subgroup analyses of two RCTs have found conflicting results. One RCT (5608 men, 997 women) compared statins with placebo for primary prevention in women.[151] It found that lovastatin reduced the risk of CHD events in women but this was not statistically significant (RR 0.54, 95% CI 0.22, 1.35). In the second RCT, the reduction in major event rate was similar in men and women (quantitative results not reported).[149] Other treatments are discussed under changing behaviour, p 37, or were performed in people with known CHD (see secondary prevention of ischaemic cardiac events, p 189). We found one systematic review (search date 1996, 59 RCTs, 173 160 people receiving drug treatments, dietary intervention, or ileal bypass), which did not differentiate primary and secondary prevention and included RCTs of any cholesterol lowering intervention, irrespective of duration, as long as mortality data were reported.[157] Overall, baseline risk was similar in people allocated to all interventions. Among non-surgical treatments, the review found that only statins reduced CHD mortality (RR v control: 0.69, 95% CI 0.59 to 0.80 for statins; 0.44, 95% CI 0.18 to 1.07 for n–3 fatty acids; 0.98, 95% CI 0.78 to 1.24 for fibrates; 0.71, 95% CI 0.51 to 0.99 for resins; 1.04, 95% CI 0.93 to 1.17 for hormones; 0.95, 95% CI 0.83 to 1.10 for niacin; 0.91, 95% CI 0.82 to 1.01 for diet), and that only statins and n–3 fatty acids reduced all cause mortality (RR v control: 0.79, 95% CI 0.71 to 0.89 for statins; 0.68, 95% CI 0.53 to 0.88 for n–3 fatty acids; 1.06, 95% CI 0.78 to 1.46 for fibrates; 0.85, 95% CI 0.66 to 1.08 for resins; 1.09, 95% CI 1.00 to 1.20 for hormones; 0.96, 95% CI 0.86 to 1.08 for niacin; 0.97, 95% CI 0.81 to 1.15 for diet).[157]

QUESTION **What is the role of antithrombotic treatment in asymptomatic people?**

Cathie Sudlow

OPTION **ASPIRIN**

We found the role of antiplatelet treatment in individuals without symptoms of cardiovascular disease to be uncertain. We found insufficient evidence from RCTs to identify which individuals would benefit overall and which would be harmed by regular treatment with aspirin, although those at high and intermediate rather than low risk, would be more likely to gain benefit (see table 2, p 186 and table 3, p 187).

Benefits: We found four recent systematic reviews[158–161], which between them included five large RCTs of aspirin versus control among individuals with no prior history of vascular disease, with or without vascular risk factors.[88,129,162–164] The earliest two trials recruited a total of about 30 000 healthy, mainly middle aged, male doctors (5139 in the UK, randomised between aspirin 500 mg/day and control, and 22 071 in the USA, randomised between aspirin 325 mg every other day and placebo).[162,163] Three subsequent RCTs included asymptomatic people with identifiable risk factors for vascular events. All three had a factorial design. The first compared aspirin 75 mg daily versus placebo and low intensity warfarin versus placebo in 5000 middle aged men with coronary heart disease risk score in the top 20–25% of the population distribution.[165] The second compared aspirin 75 mg daily versus placebo in three groups with different intensities of blood pressure reduction in a total of about 19 000 people with hypertension, most of whom had no history of vascular disease.[129] The third compared aspirin 100 mg daily versus placebo and vitamin E versus placebo in about 4500 people aged more than 50 years, with at least one major cardiovascular risk factor (hypertension, hypercholesterolaemia, diabetes, obesity, family history of premature myocardial infarction, or age ≥65 years).[92] The average control group risk of a serious vascular event (myocardial infarction, stroke, or death from a vascular cause) in each of these trials was low (about 1% a year). Data from these five RCTs were pooled in our own meta-analysis (which is updated for each issue of *Clinical Evidence*, and currently includes about 55 000 people low risk individuals). Results are summarised in table 2, p 186 and table 3, p 187. We found that, overall, aspirin slightly reduced the risk of a serious vascular event (OR 0.86, 95% CI 0.80 to 0.00; ARR 1/1000 people/year), reduced the relative risk of myocardial infarction by about a third (OR 0.71, 95% CI 0.60 to 0.80), but had an uncertain effect on stroke (OR 1.05, 95% CI 0.90 to 1.20). The systematic reviews found similar results.[158–161] One of these systematic reviews[158] also included an RCT in about 3000 people with diabetes[164] who were at substantially higher average risk of vascular events (about 4% a year) than the low risk individuals in the primary prevention RCTs included in our meta-analysis.

Harms: Serious, potentially life threatening bleeding is the most important adverse effect of aspirin. **Intracranial haemorrhage:** These are uncommon, but they are often fatal and usually cause substantial disability in survivors. We found one relevant systematic review (search date 1997) in which people were randomised to aspirin or control treatment for at least 1 month. It found that aspirin produced a small increased risk of intracranial haemorrhage of about 1/1000 (0.1%) people treated for 3 years.[167] Our meta-analysis of the primary prevention RCTs found a somewhat smaller absolute overall excess of about 0.1/1000 (0.01%) people treated with aspirin per year (see table 3, p 187). **Extracranial haemorrhage:** Major extracranial bleeds occur mainly in the gastrointestinal tract and may require hospital admission or blood transfusion, but do not generally result in permanent disability and are rarely fatal. We found one relevant systematic review of aspirin versus control with a scheduled treatment duration of at least 1 year. It found the relative excess risk of gastrointestinal bleeding with aspirin to be about 70% (OR 1.7, 95% CI 1.5 to 1.9).[168] A recent overview of 15 observational studies, including over 10 000 cases of upper gastrointestinal bleeding or perforation requiring hospitalisation, found the relative risk with aspirin to be 2.5 (95% CI 2.4 to 2.7). If only those studies that had a prospective (and so methodologically more rigorous) design were considered, the relative risk fell to 1.9 (95% CI 1.7 to 2.1), similar to that found in the RCTs.[169] Meta-analysis of primary prevention RCTs found a similar relative excess risk of major extracranial (mainly gastrointestinal) haemorrhage and an absolute excess of about 0.7 major extracranial haemorrhages per 1000 people treated with aspirin a year (see table 3, p 187).

Comment: Since the average risk of a serious vascular event in the primary prevention RCTs (about 1% a year in the control group) was low, the absolute benefit of aspirin was small and was of similar magnitude to the risks of major haemorrhage. Although there was a small reduction in serious vascular events overall, it therefore seems likely that some asymptomatic individuals would gain net benefit whereas others would experience net harm with regular aspirin treatment. The size and direction of the effects of aspirin in particular individuals may well depend on specific factors, such as age, blood

Primary prevention

pressure, and smoking status. People without symptoms at inter-mediate rather than low risk of vascular disease may benefit overall, but we found insufficient evidence to be certain.[160,161] However, one large overview of randomised trials of antiplatelet treatment among people at high risk of vascular events (> 3% a year), including people with diabetes, found clear evidence of net benefit (see stroke prevention, p 244, secondary prevention of ischaemic cardiac events, p 189, and cardiovascular disease in diabetes, p 046).[170] Further information will soon be available from a detailed overview of individual participant data from the completed primary prevention RCTs (Baigent C, personal communication, 2001); from the Women's Health Study, comparing aspirin 100 mg daily versus placebo among 40 000 healthy postmenopausal women;[171] and from the Aspirin in Asymptomatic Atherosclerosis RCT, comparing low dose aspirin versus placebo in 3300 middle aged people with asymptomatic atherosclerosis, identified by an ankle brachial pressure index ≥ 0.9 (Fowkes G, personal communication, 2000).

OPTION   **ANTICOAGULANT TREATMENT**

We found evidence from one RCT that the benefits and risks of low intensity oral anticoagulation among individuals without evidence of cardiovascular disease are finely balanced, and the net effects are uncertain.

Benefits: We found no systematic review. We found one RCT assessing anticoagulation (with a low target international normalised ratio of 1.5) among people without evidence of cardiovascular disease.[165] It found that the proportional effects of warfarin were similar among people allocated aspirin or placebo, and overall warfarin non-significantly reduced the odds of a vascular event over about 6.5 years compared with placebo (253 events in 2762 people allocated to warfarin, AR 9.2% v 288 events in 2737 people allocated to placebo, AR 10.5%; mean ARR warfarin v placebo about 2 events/ 1000 individuals/year; reduction in odds of vascular event warfarin v placebo +14%, 95% CI –2% to +28%). Compared with placebo, warfarin produced a relative reduction in the rate of all ischaemic heart disease (RRR 21%, 95% CI 4% to 35%), but had no signifi-cant effect on the rate of stroke (increase in RR +15%, 95% CI –22% to +68%) or other causes of vascular death.[165]

Harms: Allocation to warfarin was associated with a non-significant excess of about 0.4 intracranial bleeds per 1000 individuals a year (14/ 2762 [0.5%] with warfarin v 7/2737 [0.3%] with placebo) and a non-significant excess of extracranial bleeds of about 0.5/1000 individuals a year (21/2545 [0.8%] with warfarin v 12/2540 [0.5%] with placebo; RR 1.75, 95% CI 0.86 to 3.5).[165]

Comment: As is the case for aspirin, the benefits and risks of low intensity oral anticoagulation among people without evidence of cardiovascular disease are finely balanced. The number of individuals randomised to date is only about 10% of the number included in primary prevention RCTs of aspirin (see aspirin, p 176), and so the reliable identification of those who may benefit from such treatment will require further large scale randomised evidence.

REFERENCES

1. http://www.who.int/whr/1999/en/report.htm (last accessed 19 Sept 2002).

2. Heller RF, Chinn S, Pedoe HD, et al. How well can we predict coronary heart disease? Findings of the United Kingdom heart disease prevention project. *BMJ* 1984;288:1409–1411.

3. Tunstall Pedoe H, Morrison C, Woodward M, et al. Sex differences in myocardial infarction and coronary deaths in the Scottish MONICA population of Glasgow 1985 to 1991: presentation, diagnosis, treatment, and 28-day case fatality of 3991 events in men and 1551 events in women. *Circulation* 1996;93:1981–1992.

4. Anderson KV, Odell PM, Wilson PWF, et al. Cardiovascular disease risk profiles. *Am Heart J* 1991;121:293–298.

5. National Health Committee. Guidelines for the management of mildly raised blood pressure in New Zealand. Wellington Ministry of Health, 1993. http://www.nzgg.org.nz/library/gl_complete/bloodpressure/table1.cfm (last accessed 19 Sept 2002).

6. Powell KE, Thompson PD, Caspersen CJ, et al. Physical activity and the incidence of coronary heart disease. *Ann Rev Public Health* 1987;8:253–287. Search date 1995; primary sources computerised searches of personal files, *J Chronic Dis* 1983–1985, and *Am J Epidemiol* 1984–1985.

7. Berlin JA, Colditz GA. A meta-analysis of physical activity in the prevention of coronary heart disease. *Am J Epidemiol* 1990;132:612–628. Search date not stated; primary sources review articles and Medline.

8. Eaton CB. Relation of physical activity and cardiovascular fitness to coronary heart disease. Part I: a meta-analysis of the independent relation of physical activity and coronary heart disease. *J Am Board Fam Pract* 1992;5:31–42. Search date not stated; primary source Medline.

9. Fraser GE, Strahan TM, Sabate J, et al. Effects of traditional coronary risk factors on rates of incident coronary events in a low-risk population: the Adventist health study. *Circulation* 1992;86:406–413.

10. Lindsted KD, Tonstad S, Kuzma JW. Self-report of physical activity and patterns of mortality in Seventh-Day Adventist men. *J Clin Epidemiol* 1991;44:355–364.

11. Folsom AR, Arnett DK, Hutchinson RG, et al. Physical activity and incidence of coronary heart disease in middle-aged women and men. *Med Sci Sports Exerc* 1997;29:901–909.

12. Jensen G, Nyboe J, Appleyard M, et al. Risk factors for acute myocardial infarction in Copenhagen. II: smoking, alcohol intake, physical activity, obesity, oral contraception, diabetes, lipids, and blood pressure. *Eur Heart J* 1991;12:298–308.

13. Simonsick EM, Lafferty ME, Phillips CL, et al. Risk due to inactivity in physically capable older adults. *Am J Public Health* 1993;83:1443–1450.

14. Haapanen N, Miilunpalo S, Vuori I, et al. Association of leisure time physical activity with the risk of coronary heart disease, hypertension and diabetes in middle-aged men and women. *Int J Epidemiol* 1997;26:739–747.

15. Sherman SE, D'Agostino RB, Cobb JL, et al. Does exercise reduce mortality rates in the elderly? Experience from the Framingham heart study. *Am Heart J* 1994;128:965–672.

16. Rodriguez BL, Curb JD, Burchfiel CM, et al. Physical activity and 23-year incidence of coronary heart disease morbidity and mortality among middle-aged men: the Honolulu heart program. *Circulation* 1994;89:2540–2544.

17. Eaton CB, Medalie JH, Flocke SA, et al. Self-reported physical activity predicts long-term coronary heart disease and all-cause mortalities: 21-year follow-up of the Israeli ischemic heart disease study. *Arch Fam Med* 1995;4:323–329.

18. Stender M, Hense HW, Doring A, et al. Physical activity at work and cardiovascular disease risk: results from the MONICA Augsburg study. *Int J Epidemiol* 1993;22:644–650.

19. Leon AS, Myers MJ, Connett J. Leisure time physical activity and the 16-year risks of mortality from coronary heart disease and all-causes in the multiple risk factor intervention trial (MRFIT). *Int J Sports Med* 1997;18(suppl 3):208–315.

20. Rosolova H, Simon J, Sefrna F. Impact of cardiovascular risk factors on morbidity and mortality in Czech middle-aged men: Pilsen longitudinal study. *Cardiology* 1994;85:61–68.

21. Luoto R, Prattala R, Uutela A, et al. Impact of unhealthy behaviors on cardiovascular mortality in Finland, 1978–1993. *Prev Med* 1998;27:93–100.

22. Woo J, Ho SC, Yuen YK, et al. Cardiovascular risk factors and 18-month mortality and morbidity in an elderly Chinese population aged 70 years and over. *Gerontology* 1998;44:51–55.

23. Gartside PS, Wang P, Glueck CJ. Prospective assessment of coronary heart disease risk factors: the NHANES I epidemiologic follow-up study (NHEFS) 16-year follow up. *J Am Coll Nutr* 1998;17:263–269.

24. Dorn JP, Cerny FJ, Epstein LH, et al. Work and leisure time physical activity and mortality in men and women from a general population sample. *Ann Epidemiol* 1999;9:366–373.

25. Hakim AA, Curb JD, Petrovitch H, et al. Effects of walking on coronary heart disease in elderly men: the Honolulu heart program. *Circulation* 1999;100:9–13.

26. Pate RR, Pratt M, Blair SN, et al. Physical activity and public health. A recommendation from the Centers for Disease Control and Prevention and the American College of Sports Medicine. *JAMA* 1995;273:402–407.

27. Lee IM, Rexrode KM, Cook NR, et al. Physical activity and coronary heart disease in women: is "no pain, no gain" passe? *JAMA* 2001;285:1447–1454.

28. Eaton CB. Relation of physical activity and cardiovascular fitness to coronary heart disease, part II: cardiovascular fitness and the safety and efficacy of physical activity prescription. *J Am Board Fam Pract* 1992;5:157–165. Search date not stated; primary sources Medline and hand searches.

29. Blair SN, Kohl HW 3rd, Barlow CE, et al. Changes in physical fitness and all-cause mortality: a prospective study of healthy and unhealthy men. *JAMA* 1995;273:1093–1098.

30. Lakka TA, Laukkanen JA, Rauramaa R, et al. Cardiorespiratory fitness and the progression of carotid atherosclerosis in middle-aged men. *Ann Intern Med* 2001;134:12–20.

31. Williams PT. Physical fitness and activity as separate heart disease risk factors: a meta-analysis. *Med Sci Sports Exerc* 2001;33:754–761.

32. Sacco RL, Gan R, Boden-Albala B, et al. Leisure-time physical activity and ischemic stroke risk: the Northern Manhattan stroke study. *Stroke* 1998;29:380–387.

Primary prevention

33. Shinton R. Lifelong exposures and the potential for stroke prevention: the contribution of cigarette smoking, exercise, and body fat. *J Epidemiol Community Health* 1997;51:138–143.

34. Gillum RF, Mussolino ME, Ingram DD. Physical activity and stroke incidence in women and men. The NHANES I epidemiologic follow-up study. *Am J Epidemiol* 1996;143:860–869.

35. Kiely DK, Wolf PA, Cupples LA, et al. Physical activity and stroke risk: the Framingham study [correction appears in *Am J Epidemiol* 1995;141:178]. *Am J Epidemiol* 1994;140:608–620.

36. Abbott RD, Rodriguez BL, Burchfiel CM, et al. Physical activity in older middle-aged men and reduced risk of stroke: the Honolulu heart program. *Am J Epidemiol* 1994;139:881–893.

37. Haheim LL, Holme I, Hjermann I, et al. Risk factors of stroke incidence and mortality: a 12-year follow-up of the Oslo study. *Stroke* 1993;24:1484–1489.

38. Wannamethee G, Shaper AG. Physical activity and stroke in British middle aged men. *BMJ* 1992;304:597–601.

39. Menotti A, Keys A, Blackburn H, et al. Twenty-year stroke mortality and prediction in twelve cohorts of the seven countries study. *Int J Epidemiol* 1990;19:309–315.

40. Lindenstrom E, Boysen G, Nyboe J. Risk factors for stroke in Copenhagen, Denmark. II. Lifestyle factors. *Neuroepidemiology* 1993;12:43–50.

41. Lindenstrom E, Boysen G, Nyboe J. Lifestyle factors and risk of cerebrovascular disease in women: the Copenhagen City heart study. *Stroke* 1993;24:1468–1472.

42. Folsom AR, Prineas RJ, Kaye SA, et al. Incidence of hypertension and stroke in relation to body fat distribution and other risk factors in older women. *Stroke* 1990;21:701–706.

43. Nakayama T, Date C, Yokoyama T, et al. A 15.5-year follow-up study of stroke in a Japanese provincial city: the Shibata study. *Stroke* 1997;28:45–52.

44. Lee IM, Hennekens CH, Berger K, et al. Exercise and risk of stroke in male physicians. *Stroke* 1999;30:1–6.

45. Evenson KR, Rosamond WD, Cai J, et al. Physical activity and ischemic stroke risk: the atherosclerosis in communities study. *Stroke* 1999;30:1333–1339.

46. Mittleman MA, Maclure M, Tofler GH, et al. Triggering of acute myocardial infarction by heavy physical exertion. Protection against triggering by regular exertion: determinants of myocardial infarction onset study investigators. *N Engl J Med* 1993;329:1677–1683.

47. Willich SN, Lewis M, Lowel H, et al. Physical exertion as a trigger of acute myocardial infarction: triggers and mechanisms of myocardial infarction study group. *N Engl J Med* 1993;329:1684–1690.

48. Thompson PD. The cardiovascular complications of vigorous physical activity. *Arch Intern Med* 1996;156:2297–2302.

49. Oberman A. Exercise and the primary prevention of cardiovascular disease. *Am J Cardiol* 1985;55:10–20.

50. Andersen RE, Wadden TA, Bartlett SJ, et al. Effects of lifestyle activity vs structured aerobic exercise in obese women: a randomized trial. *JAMA* 1999;281:335–340.

51. Dunn AL, Marcus BH, Kampert JB, et al. Comparison of lifestyle and structured interventions to increase physical activity and cardiorespiratory fitness: a randomized trial. *JAMA* 1999;281:327–434.

52. Pereira MA, Kriska AM, Day RD, et al. A randomized walking trial in postmenopausal women: effects on physical activity and health 10 years later. *Arch Intern Med* 1998;158:1695–1701.

53. DeBusk RF, Stenestrand U, Sheehan M, et al. Training effects of long versus short bouts of exercise in healthy subjects. *Am J Cardiol* 1990;65:1010–1013.

54. Ness AR, Powles JW. Fruit and vegetables and cardiovascular disease: a review. *Int J Epidemiol* 1997;26:1–13. Search date 1995; primary sources Medline, Embase, and hand searches of personal bibliographies, books, reviews, and citations in located reports.

55. Law MR, Morris JK. By how much does fruit and vegetable consumption reduce the risk of ischaemic heart disease? *Eur J Clin Nutr* 1998;52:549–556. Search date not stated; primary sources Medline, Science Citation Index, and hand searches of review articles.

56. Klerk M, Jansen MCJF, van't Veer P, et al. Fruits and vegetables in chronic disease prevention. Wageningen: Grafisch Bedrijf Ponsen and Looijen, 1998. Search date 1998; primary sources Medline, Current Contents, and Toxline.

57. Knekt P, Isotupa S, Rissanen H, et al. Quercetin intake and the incidence of cerebrovascular disease. *Eur J Clin Nutr* 2000;54:415–417.

58. Key TJA, Thorogood M, Appleby PN, et al. Dietary habits and mortality in 11 000 vegetarians and health conscious people: results of a 17 year follow up. *BMJ* 1996;313:775–779.

59. Pietinen P, Rimm EB, Korhonen P, et al. Intake of dietary fibre and risk of coronary heart disease in a cohort of Finnish men. *Circulation* 1996;94:2720–2727.

60. Mann JI, Appleby PN, Key TJA, et al. Dietary determinants of ischaemic heart disease in health conscious individuals. *Heart* 1997;78:450–455.

61. Geleijnse M. Consumptie van groente en fruit en het risico op myocardinfarct 1997. Basisrapportage. Rotterdam: Erasmus Universiteit (cited in appendix XIII of review by Klerk).

62. Todd S, Woodward M, Tunstall-Pedoe H, et al. Dietary antioxidant vitamins and fiber in the etiology of cardiovascular disease and all-cause mortality: results from the Scottish heart health study. *Am J Epidemiol* 1999;150:1073–1080.

63. Bazzano L, Ogden LG, Vupputuri S, et al. Fruit and vegetable intake reduces cardiovascular mortality: results from the NHANES I epidemiologic follow-up study (NHEFS). Abstract presented at the 40th Annual conference on Cardiovascular Epidemiology and Prevention, San Diego California March 1–4, 2000.

64. Liu S, Lee I-M, Ajani U, et al. Intake of vegetables rich in carotenoids and risk of coronary heart disease in men: the Physicians' Health Study. *Int J Epidemiol* 2001;30:130–135.

65. Lui S, Manson JE, Lee I-M, et al. Fruit and vegetable intake and risk of cardiovascular disease: the Women's Health Study. *Am J Clin Nutr* 2000;72:922–928.

66. Cox BD, Whichelow MJ, Prevost AT. Seasonal consumption of salad vegetables and fresh fruit in relation to the development of cardiovascular disease and cancer. *Public Health Nutr* 2000;3:19–29.

67. van't Veer P, Jansen MCJF, Klerk M, et al. Fruits and vegetables in the prevention of cancer and cardiovascular disease. *Public Health Nutr* 2000;3:103–107.

68. Joshipura KJ, Ascherio A, Manson JE, et al. Fruit and vegetable intake in relation to risk of ischemic stroke. *JAMA* 1999;282:1233–1239.

69. Ness AR, Powles JW. Does eating fruit and vegetables protect against heart attack and stroke? *Chem Indus* 1996;792–794.

70. Ness AR, Powles JW. Dietary habits and mortality in vegetarians and health conscious people: several uncertainties exist. *BMJ* 1997;314:148.

71. Serdula MK, Byers T, Mokhad AH, et al. The association between fruit and vegetable intake and chronic disease risk factors. *Epidemiology* 1996;7:161–165.

72. Lonn EM, Yusuf S, Is there a role for antioxidant vitamins in the prevention of cardiovascular disease? An update on epidemiological and clinical trials data. *Can J Cardiol* 1997;13:957–965. Search date not stated; primary sources Medline, Science Citation Index, and hand searching.

73. Jha P, Flather M, Lonn E, et al. The antioxidant vitamins and cardiovascular disease: a critical review of epidemiologic and clinical trial data. *Ann Intern Med* 1995;123:860–872.

74. Roxrode KM, Manson JE. Antioxidants and coronary heart disease: observational studies. *J Cardiovasc Risk* 1996;3:363–367.

75. Egger M, Schneider M, Davey Smith G. Spurious precision? Meta-analysis of observational studies. *BMJ* 1998;316:140–144.

76. Gaziano JM. Randomized trials of dietary antioxidants in cardiovascular disease prevention and treatment. *J Cardiovasc Risk* 1996;3:368–371.

77. Ness AR, Powles JW, Khaw KT. Vitamin C and cardiovascular disease — a systematic review. *J Cardiovasc Risk* 1997;3:513–521. Search date 1996; primary sources Medline, Embase, and hand searches of personal bibliographies, books, reviews, and citations in located reports.

78. Daviglus ML, Orencia AJ, Dyer AR, et al. Dietary vitamin C, beta-carotene and 30-year risk of stroke: results from the Western Electric study. *Neuroepidemiology* 1997;16:69–77.

79. Hirvonen T, Virtamo J, Korhonen P, et al. Intake of flavonoids, carotenoids, vitamin C and E, and risk of stroke in male smokers. *Stroke* 2000;31:2301–2306.

80. Klipstein-Grobusch K, Geleijnse JM, den Breeijen JH, et al. Dietary antioxidants and risk of myocardial infarction in the elderly: the Rotterdam study. *Am J Clin Nutr* 1999;69:261–266.

81. Ascherio A, Rimm EB, Hernan MA, et al. Relation of consumption of vitamin E, vitamin C, and carotenoids to risk for stroke among men in the United States. *Ann Intern Med* 1999;130:963–970.

82. Yochum L, Folsom AR, Kushi LH. Intake of antioxidant vitamins and risk of death from stroke in postmenopausal women. *Am J Clin Nutr* 2000;72:476–483.

83. Li J, Taylor PR, Li B, et al. Nutrition intervention trials in Linxian, China: multiple vitamin/mineral supplementation, cancer incidence, and disease-specific mortality among adults with esophageal dysplasia. *J Natl Cancer Inst* 1993;85:1492–1498.

84. Mark SD, Wang W, Fraumeni JF, et al. Lowered risks of hypertension and cerebrovascular disease after vitamin/mineral supplementation. *Am J Epidemiol* 1996;143:658–664.

85. Mark SD, Wang W, Fraumeni JFJ, et al. Do nutritional supplements lower the risk of stroke or hypertension? *Epidemiology* 1998;9:9–15.

86. Losonczy KG, Harris TB, Havlik RJ. Vitamin E and vitamin C supplement use and risk of all-cause and coronary mortality in older persons: the established populations for epidemiologic studies of the elderly. *Am J Clin Nutr* 1996;64:190–196.

87. Sahyoun NR, Jacques PF, Russell RM. Carotenoids, vitamin C and E, and mortality in an elderly population. *Am J Epidemiol* 1996;144:501–511.

88. Collaborative group of the Primary Prevention Project (PPP). Low-dose aspirin and vitamin E in people at cardiovascular risk: a randomised trial in general practice. *Lancet* 2001;357:89–95.

89. Keli SO, Hertog MGL, Feskens EJM, et al. Dietary flavonoids, antioxidant vitamins, and incidence of stroke. *Arch Intern Med* 1996;156:637–642.

90. Leppälä JM, Virtamo J, Fogelholm R, et al. Controlled trial of α-tocopherol and β-carotene supplements on stroke incidence and mortality in male smokers *Arterioscler Thromb Vasc Biol* 2000;20:230–235.

91. Houtman JP. Trace elements and cardiovascular disease. *J Cardiovasc Risk* 1996;3:18–25.

92. Nève J. Selenium as a risk factor for cardiovascular disease. *J Cardiovasc Risk* 1996;3:42–47.

93. Hertog MGL, Feskens EJM, Hollman PCH, et al. Dietary antioxidant flavonoids and risk of coronary heart disease: the Zutphen elderly study. *Lancet* 1993;342:1007–1011.

94. Yochum L, Kushi LH, Meyer K, et al. Dietary flavonoid intake and risk of cardiovascular disease in postmenopausal women. *Am J Epidemiol* 1999;149:943–949.

95. Knekt P, Jarvinen R, Reunanen A, et al. Flavonoid intake and coronary mortality in Finland: a cohort study. *BMJ* 1996;312:478–481.

96. Rimm EB, Katan MB, Ascherio A, et al. Relation between intake of flavonoids and risk for coronary heart disease in male health professionals. *Ann Intern Med* 1996;125:384–389.

97. Hertog MGL, Sweetnam PM, Fehily AM. Antioxidant flavonols and ischemic heart disease in a Welsh population of men: the Caerphilly study. *Am J Clin Nutr* 1997;65:1489–1494.

98. Doering WV. Antioxidant vitamins, cancer, and cardiovascular disease. *N Engl J Med* 1996;335:1065.

99. Pietrzik K. Antioxidant vitamins, cancer, and cardiovascular disease. *N Engl J Med* 1996;335:1065–1066.

100. Hennekens CH, Gaziano JM, Manson JE, et al. Antioxidant vitamin cardiovascular disease hypothesis is still promising, but still unproven: the need for randomised trials. *Am J Clin Nutr* 1995;62(suppl):1377–1380.

101. US Department of Health and Human Services. The health benefits of smoking cessation: a report of the Surgeon General. Rockville, Maryland: US Department of Health and Human Services, Public Health Service, Centers for Disease Control, 1990. DHHS Publication (CDC) 90–8416.

102. Royal College of Physicians. *Smoking and health now.* London: Pitman Medical and Scientific Publishing, 1971.

103. Doll R, Peto R, Wheatley K, et al. Mortality in relation to smoking: 40 years' observations on male British doctors. *BMJ* 1994;309:901–911.

104. Kawachi I, Colditz GA, Stampfer MJ, et al. Smoking cessation in relation to total mortality rates in women: a prospective cohort study. *Ann Intern Med* 1993;119:992–1000.

105. Rosenberg L, Kaufman DW, Helmrich SP, et al. The risk of myocardial infarction after quitting smoking in men under 55 years of age. *N Engl J Med* 1985;313:1511–1514.

106. Rosenberg L, Palmer JR, Shapiro S. Decline in the risk of myocardial infarction among women who stop smoking. *N Engl J Med* 1990;322:213–217.

107. Rose G, Hamilton PJ, Colwell L, et al. A randomised controlled trial of anti-smoking advice: 10-year results. *J Epidemiol Community Health* 1982;36:102–108.

108. Shinton R, Beevers G. Meta-analysis of relation between cigarette smoking and stroke. *BMJ* 1989;298:789–794. Search date 1988; primary source index references from three studies on cigarette smoking and stroke on medicine.

109. Rogot E, Murray JL. Smoking and causes of death among US veterans: 16 years of observation. *Public Health Rep* 1980;95:213–222.

110. Wannamethee SG, Shaper AG, Ebrahim S. History of parental death from stroke or heart trouble and the risk of stroke in middle-aged men. *Stroke* 1996;27:1492–1498.

111. Whelton SP, Chin A, Xin X, et al. Effect of aerobic exercise on blood pressure: a meta-analysis of randomized, controlled trials. *Ann Intern Med* 2002;136:493–503.

112. Ebrahim S, Davey Smith G. Lowering blood pressure: a systematic review of sustained non-pharmacological interventions. *J Public Health Med* 1998;20:441–448. Search date 1995; primary source Medline.

113. Engstom G, Hedblad B, Janzon L. Hypertensive men who exercise regularly have lower rate of cardiovascular mortality. *J Hypertens* 1999;17:737–742.

114. Appel LJ, Moore TJ, Obarzanek E, et al. A clinical trial of the effects of dietary patterns on blood pressure. *N Engl J Med* 1997;336:1117–1124.

115. Beilin LJ, Puddey IB, Burke V. Alcohol and hypertension: kill or cure? *J Hum Hypertens* 1996;10(suppl 2):1–5.

116. Xin X, HE J, Frontini MG, et al. Effects of alcohol reduction on blood pressure: a meta-analysis of randomized controlled trials. *Hypertension*. 2001;38:1112–1117. Search date 1999; primary sources Medline and reference lists of retrieved articles.

117. Graudal NA, Galloe AM, Garred P. Effects of sodium restriction on blood pressure, renin, aldosterone, catecholamines, cholesterols, and triglyceride. *JAMA* 1998;279:1383–1391. Search date 1997; primary source Medline.

118. Whelton PK, Appel LJ, Espelland MA, et al. Sodium reduction and weight loss in the treatment of hypertension in older persons: a randomized controlled trial of non pharmacologic interventions in the elderly (TONE). *JAMA* 1998;279:839–846.

119. Sacks FM, Svetkey LP, Vollmer WM, et al. Effects on blood pressure of reduced dietary sodium and the dietary approaches to stop hypertension (DASH) diet. *N Engl J Med* 2001;344:3–10

120. Midgley JP, Matthew AG, Greenwood CMT, et al. Effect of reduced dietary sodium on blood pressure. *JAMA* 1996;275:1590–1597. Search date 1994; primary sources Medline and Current Contents.

121. Mulrow CD, Chiquette E, Angel L, et al. Dieting to reduce body weight for controlling hypertension in adults. In: The Cochrane Library, Issue 2, 2002. Oxford: Update Software. Search date 1998; primary source Cochrane Library, Medline, and contact with experts in the field.

122. Metz JA, Stern JS, Kris-Etherton P, et al. A randomized trial of improved weight loss with a prepared meal plan in overweight and obese patients. *Arch Intern Med* 2000;160:2150–2158.

123. Stevens VJ, Obarzanek E, Cook NR, et al. Long-term weight loss and changes in blood pressure: results of the Trials of Hypertension Prevention, phase II. *Ann Intern Med* 2001;134:1–11.

124. Whelton PK, He J, Cutler JA, et al. Effects of oral potassium on blood pressure: meta-analysis of randomized controlled clinical trials. *JAMA* 1997;277:1624–1632. Search date 1995; primary source Medline.

125. Morris MC, Sacks F, Rosner B. Does fish oil lower blood pressure? A meta-analysis of controlled clinical trials. *Circulation* 1993;88:523–533. Search date not stated; primary source Index Medicus.

126. Griffith LE, Guyatt GH, Cook RJ, et al. The influence of dietary and nondietary calcium supplementation on blood pressure. *Am J Hypertens* 1999;12:84–92. Search date 1994; primary sources Medline and Embase.

127. Gueyffier F, Froment A, Gouton M. New meta-analysis of treatment trials of hypertension: improving the estimate of therapeutic benefit. *J Hum Hypertens* 1996;10:1–8. Search date 1997; primary source Medline.

128. Staessen JA, Gasowski J, Wang JG, et al. Risks of untreated and treated isolated systolic hypertension in the elderly: meta-analysis of outcome trials. *Lancet* 2000;355:865–872. Search date 1999; primary sources other systematic reviews and reports from collaborative trialists.

129. Hansson L, Zanchetti AZ, Carruthers SG, et al. Effects of intensive blood pressure lowering and low-dose aspirin in patients with hypertension: principal results of the hypertension optimal treatment (HOT) trial. *Lancet* 1998;351:1755–1762.

130. Beto JA, Bansal VK. Quality of life in treatment of hypertension: a meta-analysis of clinical trials. *Am J Hypertens* 1992;5:125–133. Search date 1990; primary sources Medline and ERIC.

131. Croog SH, Levine S, Testa MA. The effects of antihypertensive therapy on quality of life. *N Engl J Med* 1986;314:1657–1664.

132. Boutitie F, Gueyffier F, Pocock S, et al. J-Shaped relationship between blood pressure and mortality in hypertensive patients: new insights from a meta-analysis of individual-patient data. *Ann Intern Med* 2002;136:438–448.

133. Psaty BM, Smith NS, Siscovick DS, et al. Health outcomes associated with antihypertensive therapies used as first line agents: a systematic review and meta-analysis. *JAMA* 1997;277:739–745. Search date 1995; primary source Medline.

134. Messerli FH, Grossman E, Goldbourt U. Are beta blockers efficacious as first-line therapy for hypertension in the elderly? A systematic review. *JAMA* 1998;279:1903–1907. Search date 1998; primary source Medline.

135. Blood Pressure Lowering Treatment Trialists' Collaboration. Effects of ACE inhibitors, calcium antagonists, and other blood-pressure-lowering drugs: results of prospectively designed overviews of trials. *Lancet* 2000;356:1955–1964. Search date 2000; primary sources WHO-International Society of Hypertension registry of randomised trials; trials were sought that had not published or presented their results before July 1995.

136. Staessen JA, Wang JG, Thijs L. Cardiovascular protection and blood pressure reduction: a meta-analysis. *Lancet* 2001;358:1305–1315.

137. The ALLHAT Officers and Coordinators for the ALLHAT Collaborative Research Group. Major cardiovascular events in hypertensive patients randomized to doxazosin vs chlorthalidone: the

antihypertensive and lipid-lowering treatment to prevent heart attack trial (ALLHAT). *JAMA* 2000;283:1967–1975.

138. Neaton JD, Grimm RH, Prineas RJ, et al. Treatment of mild hypertension study: final results. *JAMA* 1993;270:713–724.

139. Materson BJ, Reda DJ, Cushman WC, et al. Single drug therapy for hypertension in men. *N Engl J Med* 1993;328:914–921.

140. Philipp T, Anlauf M, Distler A, et al. Randomised, double blind, multicentre comparison of hydrochlorothiazide, atenolol, nitrendipine, and enalapril in antihypertensive treatment: results of the HANE study. *BMJ* 1997;315:154–159.

141. Wright JM, Lee CH, Chambers CK. Systematic review of antihypertensive therapies: does the evidence assist in choosing a first line drug? *Can Med Assoc J* 1999;161:25 32. Search date 1998; primary sources Medline and Cochrane Library.

142. Hansson L, Zanchetti AZ, Carruthers SG, et al. Effects of intensive blood pressure lowering and low-dose aspirin in patients with hypertension. principal results of the hypertension optimal treatment (HOT) trial. *Lancet* 1998;351:1755–1762.

143. Cutler JA. Calcium channel blockers for hypertension — uncertainty continues. *N Engl J Med* 1998;338:679–680.

144. Pignone M, Phillips C, Mulrow C. Use of lipid lowering drugs for primary prevention of coronary heart disease: meta-analysis of randomised trials. *BMJ* 2000;321:983–986. Search date 1999; primary sources Medline, Cochrane Library, and hand searches of bibliographies of systematic reviews and clinical practice guidelines.

145. Cucherat M, Lievre M, Gueyffier F. Clinical benefits of cholesterol lowering treatments. Meta-analysis of randomized therapeutic trials. *Presse Med* 2000 May 13;29:965–976. Search date and primary sources not stated.

146. Katerndahl DA, Lawler WR. Variability in meta-analytic results concerning the value of cholesterol reduction in coronary heart disease: a meta-meta-analysis. *Am J Epidemiol* 1999;149:429–441. Search date 1995; primary sources Medline and meta-analysis bibliographies.

147. Ebrahim S, Davey Smith G, McCabe CCC, et al. What role for statins? A review and economic model. *Health Technol Assess* 1999;3(10):i iv, 1–91. Search dates 1997; primary sources Medline, Cochrane Controlled Trials Register, and personal contact with investigators working in the field of cholesterol lowering.

148. LaRosa JC, He J, Vupputuri S. Effect of statins on risk of coronary disease: a meta-analysis of randomized controlled trials. *JAMA* 1999;282:2340–2346. Search date 1998; primary sources Medline, bibliographies, and authors' reference files.

149. Heart Protection Study Collaborative Group MRC/BHF Heart Protection Study of cholesterol lowering with simvastatin in 20536 high-risk individuals: a randomised placebo-controlled trial. *Lancet* 2002;360:7–22.

150. Sawayama Y, Shimuzu C, Maeda N, et al. Effects of probucol and pravastatin on common carotid atherosclerosis in patients with asymptomatic hypercholesterolemia. Fukuoka Atherosclerosis Trial (FAST). *J Am Coll Cardiol* 2002;39:610 616.

151. Downs JR, Clearfield M, Weis S, et al. Primary prevention of acute coronary events with lovastatin in men and women with average cholesterol levels: results of the AFCAPS/TexCAPS. *JAMA* 1998;279:1615–1622.

152. Shepherd J, Cobbe SM, Ford I, et al. Prevention of coronary heart disease with pravastatin in men with hypercholesterolemia. *N Engl J Med* 1995;333:1301–1307.

153. Scandinavian Simvastatin Survival Study Group. Randomized trial of cholesterol lowering in 4444 patients with coronary heart disease: the Scandinavian simvastatin survival study (4S). *Lancet* 1995;344:1383–1389.

154. Long-term Intervention with Pravastatin in Ischemic Disease (LIPID) Study Program. Prevention of cardiovascular events and death with pravastatin in patients with coronary heart disease and a broad range of initial cholesterol levels. *N Engl J Med* 1998;339:1349–1357.

155. Sacks FM, Pfeffer MA, Moye LA, et al. Effect of pravastatin on coronary events after myocardial infarction in patients with average cholesterol levels. *N Engl J Med* 1996;335:1001–1009.

156. Jackson PR, Wallis EJ, Haq IU, et al. Statins for primary prevention: at what coronary risk is safety assured? *Br J Clin Pharmacol* 2001;52:439–446.

157. Bucher HC, Griffith LE, Guyatt G. Systematic review on the risk and benefit of different cholesterol lowering interventions. *Arterioscler Thromb Vasc Biol* 1999;19;187–195. Search date 1996; primary sources Medline, Embase, and hand searches of bibliographies.

158. Hart RG, Halperin JL, McBride R, et al. Aspirin for the primary prevention of stroke and other major vascular events. Meta-analysis and hypotheses. *Arch Neurol* 2000;57:326 332. Search date 1998; primary sources unspecified computerised medical databases, Cochrane Collaboration Registry, and hand searched references of Antiplatelet Trialists' Collaboration publications.

159. Hebert PR, Hennekens CH. An overview of the 4 randomized trials of aspirin therapy in the primary prevention of vascular disease. *Arch Int Med* 2000;160:3123–3127. Search date and primary sources not stated.

160. Sanmuganathan PS, Ghahramani P, Jackson PR, et al. Aspirin for primary prevention of coronary heart disease: safety and absolute benefit related to coronary risk derived from a meta-analysis of randomised trials. *Heart* 2001;85:265–271. Search date not stated; primary sources Medline and previous meta-analyses and review articles.

161. Hayden M, Pignone M, Phillips C, et al. Aspirin for the primary prevention of cardiovascular events: a summary of the evidence for the US preventive services task force. *Ann Intern Med* 2002;136:161–172.

162. Peto R, Gray R, Collins R, et al. Randomised trial of prophylactic daily aspirin in British male doctors. *BMJ* 1988;296:313–316.

163. Steering Committee of the Physicians' Health Study Research Group. Final report on the aspirin component of the ongoing physicians' health study. *N Engl J Med* 1989;321:129–135.

164. ETDRS Investigators. Aspirin effects on mortality and morbidity in patients with diabetes mellitus. Early treatment diabetic retinopathy study report 14. *JAMA* 1992;268:1292–1300.

165. Medical Research Council's General Practice Research Framework. Thrombosis prevention trial: randomised trial of low-intensity anticoagulation with warfarin and low dose aspirin in the primary prevention of ischaemic heart disease in men at increased risk. *Lancet* 1998;351:233–241.

166. Antiplatelet Trialists' Collaboration. Collaborative overview of randomised trials of antiplatelet

therapy — I: prevention of death, myocardial infarction, and stroke by prolonged antiplatelet therapy in various categories of patients. *BMJ* 1994;308:81–106. Search date 1990; primary sources Medline, Current Contents, hand searches of reference list of trials and review articles, journal abstracts and meeting proceedings, trial register of the International Committee on Thrombosis and Haemostasis, and personal contacts with colleagues and antiplatelet manufacuters.

167. He J, Whelton PK, Vu B, et al. Aspirin and risk of hemorrhagic stroke: a meta-analysis of randomized controlled trials. *JAMA* 1998;280:1930–1935. Search date 1997; primary sources Medline, the authors' reference files, and reference lists from original communications and review articles.

168. Derry S, Loke YK. Risk of gastrointestinal haemorrhage with long term use of aspirin: meta-analysis. *BMJ* 2000;321:1183–1187. Search date not stated; primary sources Medline, Embase, and reference lists from previous review papers and retrieved trials.

169. García Rodríguez LA, Hernández-Díaz S, De Abajo FJ. Association between aspirin and upper gastrointestinal complications: a systematic review of epidemiologic studies. *Br J Clin Pharmacol Zool* 2001;52:563–571.

170. Antithrombotic Trialists' Collaboration. Collaborative meta-analysis of randomised trials of antiplatelet therapy for prevention of death, myocardial infarction, and stroke in high risk patients. *BMJ* 2002;324:71–86.

171. Buring JE, Hennekens CH. Women's health study: summary of the study design. *J Myocard Ischemia* 1992;4:27–29.

Michael Murphy
Director, ICRF General Practice
Research Group

Charles Foster
British Heart Foundation Scientist

University of Oxford
Oxford
UK

Cathie Sudlow
Wellcome Clinician Scientist
Department of Clinical Neurosciences
University of Edinburgh
Edinburgh
UK

Julian Nicholas
Resident Physician
Mayo Clinic
Rochester
USA

Cindy Mulrow
Professor of Medicine
University of Texas Health Science
Center
San Antonio
USA

Andy Ness
Senior Lecturer in Epidemiology
University of Bristol
Bristol
UK

Michael Pignone
Assistant Professor of Medicine
Division of General Internal Medicine
University of North Carolina
Chapel Hill
USA

Competing interests: CM has participated in multicentre research trials evaluating antihypertensive agents that were funded by industry; other authors, none declared.

TABLE 1	Examples of common physical activities by intensity of effort required in multiples of the resting rate of oxygen consumption during physical activity (see text, p 159). Published in *JAMA* 1995;273:402–407.[26]

Activity type	Light activity (< 3.0 METs)	Moderate activity (3.0–6.0 METs)	Vigorous activity (> 6.0 METs)
Walking	Slowly (1–2 mph)	Briskly (3–4 mph)	Briskly uphill or with a load
Swimming	Treading slowly	Moderate effort	Fast treading or swimming
Cycling	NA	For pleasure or transport (≤ 10 mph)	Fast or racing (> 10 mph)
Golf	Power cart	Pulling cart or carrying clubs	NA
Boating	Power boat	Canoeing leisurely	Canoeing rapidly (> 4 mph)
Home care	Carpet sweeping	General cleaning	Moving furniture
Mowing lawn	Riding mower	Power mower	Hand mower
Home repair	Carpentry	Painting	NA

METs, work metabolic rate/resting metabolic rate; 1 MET represents the rate of oxygen consumption of a seated adult at rest; mph, miles per hour; NA, not applicable.

TABLE 2 Effects of aspirin on vascular events (myocardial infarction, stroke, or vascular death) in RCTs among individuals without evidence of cardiovascular disease (see text, p 176).

Trials (duration)	Annual risk of vascular event (control)	Vascular events Antiplatelet, control, and odds ratio* (CI†)	Events avoided per 1000 person-years	Myocardial infarction Antiplatelet, control, and odds ratio* (CI†)	Stroke Antiplatelet, control, and odds ratio* (CI†)
UK doctors[162] (70 months)	1.5%	288/3429, 280/3420‡, 1.03 (0.6 to 2.3)	–0.4	169/3429, 176/3420‡, 0.96 (0.7 to 1.4)	91/3429, 78/3420‡, 1.16 (0.7 to 1.9)
US physicians[163] (60 months)	0.7%	321/11037, 387/11034, 0.82 (0.7 to 1.0)	1.2	139/11037, 239/11034, 0.58 (0.5 to 0.8)	119/11037, 98/11034, 1.22 (0.9 to 1.7)
TPT[165] (76 months)	1.8%	239/2545, 270/2540, 0.87 (0.7 to 1.1)	2.0	154/2545, 190/2540, 0.80 (0.7 to 1.1)	47/2545, 48/2540, 0.98 (0.6 to 1.7)
HOT[142] (46 months)	1.0%	315/9399, 368/9391, 0.85 (0.7 to 1.0)	1.5	82/9399, 127/9391, 0.65 (0.5 to 0.9)	146/9399, 148/9391, 0.99 (0.7 to 1.3)
PPP[88] (44 months)	0.8%	45/2226, 64/2269, 0.71 (0.4 to 1.2)	2.2	19/2226, 28/2269, 0.69 (0.3 to 1.5)	16/2226, 24/2269, 0.68 (0.3 to 1.6)
All trials (56 months)	1.0%	1208/28 636 (4.2%), 1369/28 654 (4.8%), 0.86§ (0.8 to 0.9)	1.2	563/28 636 (2.0%), 760/28 654 (2.4%), 0.71§ (0.6 to 0.8)	419/28 636 (1.5%), 396/28 654 (1.4%), 1.05§ (0.9 to 1.2)

Data from individual trial publications and from the APT overview (1994).[166] The effects of aspirin were similar in the absence or presence of warfarin, so the data presented are not stratified by warfarin allocation. * Odds ratios calculated using the "observed minus expected" method;[166] † 99% CI for individual trials 95% CI for "All trials"; ‡ Number of patients in control group was 1710 (randomisation ratio 2 : 1); numerator and denominator multiplied by 2 to calculate totals for absolute differences between antiplatelet and control group event rates; actual numbers of events used to calculate odds ratios and confidence intervals; ¶ Weighted by study size; § Heterogeneity of odds ratios between five trials not significant (P > 0.05).

TABLE 3 Effects of aspirin on intracranial and major extracranial haemorrhages in RCTs among individuals without evidence of cardiovascular disease (see text, p 176).

Trials	Antiplatelet	Control	Summary odds ratio* (95% CI)	Excess bleeds per 1000 patients treated per year
Intracranial bleeds				
UK doctors[160]	13/3429	12/3420†		
US physicians[161]	23/11037	12/11034		
TPT[164]	12/2545	6/2540		
HOT[132]	14/9399	15/9391		
PPP[96]	2/2226	3/2269		
All trials	**64/28 636** (0.22%)	**48/28654** (0.17%)	1.4(0.9 to 2.0)	0.1 (P = 0.1)
Major extracranial bleeds				
UK Doctors[160]	21/3429	20/3420†		
US Physicians[161]	48/11037	28/11034		
TPT[164]	20/2545	13/2540		
HOT[132]	122/9399	63/9391		
All trials	**211/26 410** (0.8%)	**134/28 095** (0.5%)	1.7(1.4 to 2.1)	0.7 (P < 0.00001)

Data from individual trial publications. *Odds ratios calculated using the "observed minus expected" method.[166]
†Number of patients in control group was 1:10 (randomisation ratio 2 : 1); numerator and denominator multiplied by 2 to calculate totals for absolute differences between antiplatelet and control group event rates; actual numbers of events used to calculate odds ratios and confidence intervals.

Cardiovascular disorders

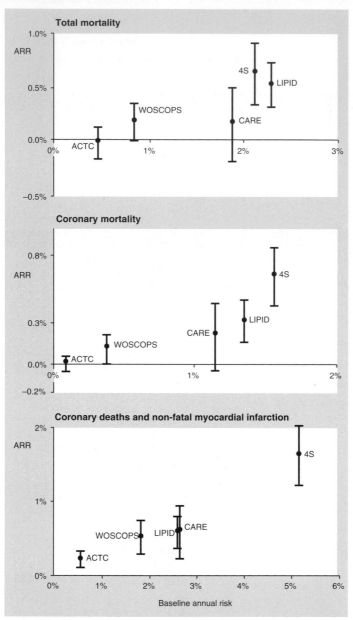

FIGURE 1 Effects of cholesterol lowering: relation between the ARR (for annual total mortality, coronary heart disease mortality, coronary deaths, and non-fatal myocardial infarction) and the baseline risk of those events in the placebo group for five large statin trials (ACTC = AFCAPS/TexCAPS,[151] 4S,[153] LIPID,[154] CARE,[155] WOSCOPS[152]) (see text, p 174).

Search date March 2002

Clinical Evidence writers on secondary prevention of ischaemic cardiac events

Key Messages

Antithrombotic treatment

- **Adding anticoagulants to antiplatelet treatment** One systematic review and one subsequent RCT found no evidence that addition of oral anticoagulation at low (INR < 1.5) or moderate (INR 1.5–3) intensity to aspirin reduced risk of death or recurrent cardiac events, but found an increased risk of major haemorrhage.

- **Anticoagulants in the absence of antiplatelet treatment** One systematic review has found that high or moderate intensity oral anticoagulants given alone significantly reduce the risk of serious vascular events in people with coronary artery disease, but are associated with substantial risk of haemorrhage.

- **Any oral antiplatelet treatment** One systematic review has found that prolonged antiplatelet treatment versus placebo or no antiplatelet treatment reduces the risk of serious vascular events in people at high risk of ischaemic cardiac events.

- **Aspirin** One systematic review has found that, for prolonged use, aspirin 75–150 mg daily is as effective as higher doses, but found insufficient evidence that doses below 75 mg daily are as effective.

- **Oral glycoprotein IIb/IIIa receptor inhibitors** One systematic review in people with acute coronary syndromes or undergoing percutaneous coronary interventions has found that oral glycoprotein IIb/IIIa receptor inhibitors versus placebo increase risk of mortality and bleeding.

- **Thienopyridines** One systematic review has found that clopidogrel is at least as safe and effective as aspirin in people at high risk of vascular events.

Other drug treatments

- **Angiotensin converting enzyme inhibitors in high risk people without left ventricular dysfunction** One large RCT in people without left ventricular dysfunction found that ramipril versus placebo significantly reduced the combined outcome of cardiovascular death, stroke, and myocardial infarction after about 5 years (NNT 27, 95% CI 20 to 45).

- **Angiotensin converting enzyme inhibitors in people with left ventricular dysfunction** One systematic review has found that in people who have had a myocardial infarction and have left ventricular dysfunction, angiotensin converting enzyme inhibitors versus placebo significantly reduce mortality (NNT 17, CI not available), admission to hospital for congestive heart failure (NNT 28, CI not available), and recurrent non-fatal myocardial infarction (NNT 43, CI not available) after 2 years' treatment.

- **Amiodarone in selected high risk people** Two systematic reviews have found that amiodarone versus placebo significantly reduces the risk of sudden cardiac death, and reduces mortality at 1 year in people at high risk of death after myocardial infarction.

- **β Blockers** Systematic reviews in people after myocardial infarction have found that long term β blockers reduce all cause mortality, coronary mortality, recurrent non-fatal myocardial infarction, and sudden death. One RCT found that about 25% of people suffer adverse effects.

- **Calcium channel blockers (dihydropyridines)** One systematic review found non-significantly higher mortality with dihydropyridines compared with placebo.

- **Calcium channel blockers (diltiazem and verapamil)** One systematic review found no benefit from calcium channel blockers in people after myocardial infarction or with chronic coronary heart disease. Diltiazem and verapamil may reduce rates of reinfarction and refractory angina in people after myocardial infarction who do not have heart failure.

- **Class I antiarrhythmic agents** One systematic review has found that class I antiarrhythmic agents versus placebo given after myocardial infarction significantly increase the risk of cardiovascular mortality and sudden death.

- **Hormone replacement therapy** One large RCT found no evidence that hormone replacement therapy versus placebo reduces major cardiovascular events in postmenopausal women with established coronary artery disease.

- **Sotalol** One RCT found limited evidence that sotalol versus placebo significantly increased mortality within 1 year.

Cholesterol reduction

- **Cholesterol lowering drugs** Systematic reviews and large subsequent RCTs have found that lowering cholesterol in people at high risk of ischaemic coronary events substantially reduces the risk of overall mortality, cardiovascular mortality, and non-fatal cardiovascular events. One systematic review of primary and secondary prevention trials found that statins, in people also given dietary advice, were the only non-surgical treatment for cholesterol reduction to significantly reduce mortality. One systematic review found that the absolute benefits increase as baseline risk increases, but are not additionally influenced by the person's absolute cholesterol concentration.

Blood pressure reduction

- **Blood pressure lowering in people at high risk of ischaemic coronary events** We found no direct evidence of the effects of blood pressure lowering in people with established coronary heart disease. Observational studies, and extrapolation of primary prevention trials of blood pressure reduction, support the lowering of blood pressure in those at high risk of ischaemic coronary events. The evidence for benefit is strongest for β blockers, although not specifically in people with hypertension. The target blood pressure in these people is not clear. Angiotensin converting enzyme inhibitors, calcium channel blockers, and β blockers are discussed separately.

Non-drug treatments

- **Advice to eat less fat** RCTs found no strong evidence that low fat diets reduced mortality at 2 years.

- **β Carotene** Large RCTs found no evidence of benefit with β carotene, and one RCT found evidence of a significant increase in mortality. Four large RCTs of β carotene supplementation in primary prevention found no cardiovascular benefits, and two of the RCTs raised concerns about increased mortality.

- **Cardiac rehabilitation** One systematic review has found that cardiac rehabilitation including exercise reduces the risk of major cardiac events.

- **Eating more fish (particularly oily fish)** One RCT has found that advising people with coronary heart disease to eat more fish (particularly oily fish) significantly reduces mortality at 2 years (NNT 29, 95% CI 17 to 129). A second RCT found that fish oil capsules significantly reduced mortality at 3.5 years.

- **Exercise without cardiac rehabilitation** One systematic review has found that exercise alone versus usual care significantly reduces mortality.

- **Mediterranean diet** One RCT has found that advising people with coronary artery disease to eat more bread, fruit, vegetables, and fish, and less meat, and to replace butter and cream with rapeseed margarine significantly reduces mortality at 27 months (NNT 26, 95% CI 14 to 299).

- **Psychosocial treatment** One systematic review of mainly poor quality RCTs found that psychological treatments versus usual treatment may decrease rates of myocardial infarction or cardiac death in people with coronary heart disease.

- **Smoking cessation** We found no RCTs of the effects of smoking cessation on cardiovascular events in people with coronary heart disease. Moderate evidence from epidemiological studies indicates that people with coronary heart disease who stop smoking, rapidly reduce their risk of recurrent coronary events or death. Treatment with nicotine patches seems safe in people with coronary heart disease.

- **Stress management** One systematic review of mainly poor quality RCTs found that stress management may decrease rates of myocardial infarction or cardiac death in people with coronary heart disease.

- **Vitamin C** Pooled analysis of three small RCTs found no evidence that vitamin C versus placebo provided any substantial benefit.

- **Vitamin E** Pooled analysis of four large RCTs found no evidence that vitamin E versus placebo given for 1.3–4.5 years altered cardiovascular events and all cause mortality.

Surgical treatments

- **Coronary artery bypass grafting versus coronary percutaneous transluminal angioplasty for multi vessel disease** One systematic review has found that coronary artery bypass grafting versus percutaneous transluminal angioplasty has no significant effect on death, myocardial infarction, or quality of life. Percutaneous transluminal angioplasty is less invasive but increased the number of repeat procedures.

- **Coronary artery bypass grafting versus medical treatment alone** One systematic review found that coronary artery bypass grafting reduced the risk of death from coronary artery disease at 5 and 10 years compared with medical treatment alone. Greater benefit occurred in people with poor left ventricular function. One subsequent RCT in people with asymptomatic disease found that revascularisation with coronary artery bypass grafting or coronary percutaneous transluminal angioplasty versus medical treatment alone reduced mortality at 2 years.

- **Coronary percutaneous transluminal angioplasty versus medical treatment alone** One systematic review found that coronary percutaneous transluminal angioplasty versus medical treatment alone improved angina, but was associated with a higher rate of coronary artery bypass grafting. The review found higher mortality and rates of myocardial infarction with percutaneous transluminal angioplasty versus medical treatment but the difference was not significant. RCTs have found that percutaneous transluminal angioplasty is associated with increased risk of emergency coronary artery bypass grafting and myocardial infarction during and soon after the procedure. One RCT found that percutaneous transluminal angioplasty reduced cardiac events and improved angina severity compared with medical treatment alone in people over the age of 75 years.

■ **Intracoronary stents versus coronary percutaneous transluminal angioplasty alone** One systematic review found that intracoronary stents versus coronary percutaneous transluminal angioplasty alone significantly reduce the need for repeat vascularisation. It found no significant difference in mortality or myocardial infarction, but crossover rates from percutaneous transluminal angioplasty alone to stent were high. RCTs found that intracoronary stents improved outcomes after 4–9 months compared with percutaneous transluminal angioplasty alone in people with previous coronary artery bypass grafting, chronic total occlusions, and for treatment of restenosis after initial percutaneous transluminal angioplasty.

DEFINITION   Secondary prevention in this context is the long term management of people with a prior acute myocardial infarction, and of people at high risk of ischaemic cardiac events for other reasons, such as a history of angina or coronary surgical procedures.

INCIDENCE/   Coronary artery disease is the leading cause of mortality in devel-
PREVALENCE oped countries and is becoming a major cause of morbidity and mortality in developing countries. There are pronounced international, regional, and temporal differences in death rates. In the USA, the prevalence of overt coronary artery disease approaches 4%.[1]

AETIOLOGY/   Most ischaemic cardiac events are associated with atheromatous
RISK FACTORS plaques that can cause acute obstruction of coronary vessels. Atheroma is more likely in elderly people, in those with established coronary artery disease, and in those with risk factors (such as smoking, hypertension, high cholesterol, and diabetes mellitus).

PROGNOSIS   Almost 50% of those who suffer an acute myocardial infarction die before they reach hospital. Of those admitted to hospital, 7–15% die in hospital and another 7–15% die during the following year. People who survive the acute stage of myocardial infarction fall into three prognostic groups, based on their baseline risk (see table 1, p 226);[2–4] high (20% of all survivors), moderate (55%), and low (25%) risk. Long term prognosis depends on the degree of left ventricular dysfunction, the presence of residual ischaemia, and the extent of any electrical instability. Further risk stratification procedures include assessment of left ventricular function (by echocardiography or nuclear ventriculography) and of myocardial ischaemia (by non-invasive stress testing).[4–8] Those with low left ventricular ejection fraction, ischaemia, or poor functional status can be assessed further by cardiac catheterisation.[9]

AIMS   To improve long term survival and quality of life; to prevent (recurrent) myocardial infarction, unstable angina, left ventricular dysfunction, heart failure, and sudden cardiac death; and to restore and maintain normal activities.

OUTCOMES   Mortality (total, cardiovascular, coronary, sudden death, non-cardiovascular); morbidity (myocardial infarction, severe angina, stroke); quality of life.

METHODS   *Clinical Evidence* update search and appraisal March 2002.

Cardiovascular disorders

Secondary prevention of ischaemic cardiac events

Cathie Sudlow

OPTION ANY ORAL ANTIPLATELET TREATMENT

One systematic review has found that prolonged antiplatelet treatment reduces the risk of serious vascular events in people at high risk of ischaemic cardiac events.

Benefits:
Oral antiplatelet treatment versus no antiplatelet treatment: We found one systematic review (search date 1997, 195 RCTs, > 140 000 high risk people) comparing an antiplatelet regimen (mostly aspirin) versus no antiplatelet treatment (including placebo).[10] It found that antiplatelet treatment reduced the odds of a serious vascular event (myocardial infarction, stroke, or vascular death) by 25% among all types of high risk people (OR 0.75, 95% CI 0.72 to 0.78), excluding those with acute ischaemic stroke (among whom the proportional benefits were smaller).[10] The proportional effects of antiplatelet treatment were similar regardless of whether the people were included on the basis of a prior or acute myocardial infarction, prior stroke or transient ischaemic attack, stable or unstable angina, peripheral arterial disease, atrial fibrillation, or other high risk condition. Most of these people were at high risk of ischaemic cardiac events, and some (including those with a history of myocardial infarction, those with stable angina, and those who had undergone coronary revascularisation procedures) were at particularly high risk. Among the 20 000 people with a prior myocardial infarction it was estimated that antiplatelet treatment prevented 18 non-fatal recurrent myocardial infarctions, five non-fatal strokes, and 14 vascular deaths per 1000 people treated for about 2 years. The review also found that antiplatelet treatment reduced the risk of all cause mortality (see figure 1, p 227).

Harms:
Oral antiplatelet treatment: The most important adverse effect of antiplatelet treatment is haemorrhage, particularly intracranial haemorrhage because it is frequently fatal or disabling. The systematic review (search date 1997) found a proportional increase in the risk of intracranial haemorrhage of about a quarter (OR 1.22, 95% CI 1.03 to 1.44). However, the absolute excess risk was no more than one or two events per 1000 people a year.[10] Antiplatelet treatment was associated with about a 60% increased odds of extracranial haemorrhage (mainly from the gastrointestinal tract) (OR 1.6, 95% CI 1.4 to 1.8) corresponding to an absolute excess risk of about 1–2/1000 people treated a year with a prior myocardial infarction. Most of the extracranial haemorrhages were non-fatal.[10]

Comment:
Among people at high risk of cardiac events, the large absolute reductions in serious vascular events associated with antiplatelet treatment far outweigh any absolute risks.

OPTION   ASPIRIN

One systematic review has found that for prolonged use, aspirin
75–150 mg daily is as effective as higher doses, but found insufficient
evidence that doses below 75 mg daily are as effective. It found no clear
evidence that any alternative antiplatelet regimen is superior to aspirin in
the long term secondary prevention of vascular events, but found that
clopidogrel is at least as effective and as safe as aspirin.

Benefits: **Versus no aspirin:** We found one systematic review (search date
1997, 195 RCTs, > 140 000 high risk people) comparing an
antiplatelet regimen versus no antiplatelet treatment (including
placebo).[10] Aspirin was by far the most widely studied antiplatelet
drug in the systematic review. Among almost 60 000 people,
excluding those with acute ischaemic stroke, aspirin reduced the
odds of a serious vascular event by about a quarter compared with
control (OR 0.77, 95% CI 0.73 to 0.81).[10] **Different daily doses:**
Direct comparisons (3197 high risk people) between daily doses of
500–1500 mg versus 75–325 mg found no significant difference in
effect (OR higher versus lower dose 0.97, 95% CI 0.79 to 1.19).[10]
A subsequent RCT (2849 high risk people) compared four doses of
aspirin, two lower doses (81 or 325 mg/day), and two higher doses
(650 or 1300 mg/day). It found that the combined rate of myocardial infarction, stroke, or death was slightly lower in the lower dose
than in the higher dose groups at 3 months (AR 6.2% with lower
doses v 8.4% with higher doses; P = 0.03).[11] Direct comparisons
(3570 people in the review) between daily doses greater than or
equal to 75 mg and less than 75 mg daily found no significant
difference, but the confidence intervals included a potentially clinically important difference (OR higher v lower doses 1.08, 95%
CI 0.90 to 1.31).[10] Indirect comparisons of trials in the review
comparing different daily aspirin doses versus control among people
at high risk (excluding those with acute ischaemic stroke) found
similar reductions in serious vascular events for the higher daily
doses 500–1500 mg daily (OR 0.81, 95% CI 0.75 to 0.87),
160–325 mg daily (OR 0.74, 95% CI 0.69 to 0.80), 75–150 mg
daily (OR 0.68, 95% CI 0.59 to 0.79), but somewhat smaller effect
with less than 75 mg daily (OR 0.87, 95% CI 0.74 to 1.03)(see
figure 2, p 228).[10] **Versus or with thienopyridines:** See benefits
of thienopyridines, p 196. **Versus or with anticoagulants:** See
benefits of oral anticoagulants in absence of antiplatelet treatment,
p 198. See benefits of oral anticoagulants in addition to antiplatelet
treatment, p 198.

Harms: **Intracranial haemorrhage:** A systematic review of aspirin versus
control for at least 1 month found that aspirin produced a small
increased risk of intracranial haemorrhage of about 1/1000 (0.1%)
people treated for 3 years.[12] There was no clear variation in risk with
the dose of aspirin used. In RCTs directly comparing different daily
doses there was no significant difference in the risk of intracranial
haemorrhage, but the number of events was small and the confidence intervals wide.[11,13,14] Two observational studies (1 case
control and 1 cohort study) found a dose dependent association
between aspirin and intracranial haemorrhage, but the methods of

these studies prevent firm conclusions being drawn.[15,16] **Extracranial haemorrhage:** The systematic review (search date 1997) found that aspirin slightly increased the risk of major extracranial haemorrhage, similar to the risk for antiplatelet treatment in general (see harms of antiplatelet treatment, p 194). It found that the risk of major extracranial haemorrhage was similar with different daily doses (numerical results not presented).[10] **Gastrointestinal haemorrhage:** A systematic review (search date 1999) of aspirin versus control found an increased risk of gastrointestinal haemorrhage with aspirin (OR 1.68, 95% CI 1.51 to 1.88), with no definite variation in risk between doses or different formulations.[17] RCTs directly comparing different doses of aspirin found a trend towards more gastrointestinal haemorrhages with high (500–1500 mg/day) versus medium (75–325 mg/day) doses (OR 1.7, 95% CI 0.9 to 2.1), but no difference between medium (283 mg/day) and low (30 mg/day) doses (OR 1.2, 95% CI 0.7 to 2.0).[11,13,14] A recent overview of 15 observational studies including over 10 000 cases of upper gastrointestinal haemorrhage or perforation requiring admission to hospital, found a more than doubled increased risk with aspirin (RR 2.5, 95% CI 2.4 to 2.7).[18] Restricting the analysis to prospective studies gave a lower risk (RR 1.9, 95% CI 1.7 to 2.1), similar to that found in the RCTs.[17,18] **Upper gastrointestinal symptoms:** RCTs directly comparing different doses of aspirin found that high dose (500–1500 mg/day) significantly increased the odds of upper gastrointestinal symptoms compared with medium dose (75–325 mg/day; OR 1.3, 95% CI 1.1 to 1.5),[11,13] and that medium dose (283 mg/day) aspirin was associated with non-significantly higher odds of upper gastrointestinal upset compared with low dose (30 mg/day) (OR 1.1, 95% CI 0.9 to 1.4).[14]

Comment: Among people at high risk of cardiac events, the large absolute reductions in serious vascular events associated with aspirin far outweigh any absolute risks.

OPTION   THIENOPYRIDINES (CLOPIDOGREL OR TICLOPIDINE)

One RCT has found that clopidogrel is at least as effective at preventing vascular events and is at least as safe as aspirin in people with a history of cardiovascular disease.

Benefits: **Versus aspirin:** One RCT (19 185 people with a history of myocardial infarction, stroke, or peripheral arterial disease) compared clopidogrel (75 mg/day) versus aspirin (325 mg/day).[19] It found that clopidogrel reduced the odds of a serious vascular event by 10% (OR 0.9, 95% CI 0.82 to 0.99). One systematic review found similar, but non-significant results for ticlopidine (a thienopyridine similar to clopidogrel) versus aspirin (4 RCTs, 3791 high risk people, RR 0.88, 95% CI 0.75 to 1.03).[10] We found one subsequent RCT comparing ticlopidine versus aspirin.[20] It found a non-significant lower risk of a vascular event (OR 0.69, 95% 0.31 to 1.48). A separate systematic review comparing ticlopidine or clopidogrel versus aspirin (search date 1999, 4 RCTs, 22 656 people at high risk of vascular disease, most of whom were included in the trial comparing clopidogrel with aspirin[20]) found that ticlopidine or clopidogrel reduced the odds of a vascular event compared with aspirin (OR 0.91, 95% CI 0.84 to 0.98).[21] However, there was substantial uncertainty about the absolute size of any additional benefit (average 11 events prevented/1000 people treated for 2 years, 95% CI 2 to 19). **Thienopyridines plus aspirin versus aspirin alone:** We found no completed long term trials of the effects of adding clopidogrel to aspirin among people at high risk of occlusive arterial disease but without an acute cardiovascular event. We found one RCT in people with acute coronary syndromes (see comment below).

Harms: One systematic review of randomised trials of the thienopyridine derivatives versus aspirin found that the thienopyridines produced significantly less gastrointestinal haemorrhage and upper gastrointestinal upset than aspirin.[21] However, the odds of skin rash and diarrhoea were doubled with ticlopidine and increased by about a third with clopidogrel. Ticlopidine (but not clopidogrel) increased the odds of neutropenia. Observational studies have also found that ticlopidine is associated with thrombocytopenia and thrombotic thrombocytopenic purpura.[22,23] However, we found no clear evidence of an excess of haematological adverse effects with clopidogrel.[24,25] Three RCTs (about 2700 people undergoing coronary artery stenting) of clopidogrel plus aspirin versus ticlopidine plus aspirin suggested better safety and tolerability with clopidogrel versus ticlopidine.[26–28]

Comment: One RCT (about 12 500 people within 24 h of onset of an acute coronary syndrome without ST segment elevation) compared clopidogrel plus aspirin versus placebo plus aspirin.[29] After 3–12 months' treatment, it found that adding clopidogrel to aspirin significantly reduced the risk of a major vascular event (RR 0.88, 95% CI 0.72 to 0.90).[29] See antiplatelets under unstable angina, p 285. The trial found that combined treatment increased risk of major haemorrhages (mainly gastrointestinal) and bleeding at sites of arterial punctures (RR 1.38, 95% CI 1.13 to 1.67), but did not increase intracranial, life-threatening, or fatal haemorrhages compared with aspirin alone.[29] An RCT of the effects of adding clopidogrel to aspirin in people with acute myocardial infarction is under way.[30]

OPTION   ORAL GLYCOPROTEIN IIB/IIIA RECEPTOR INHIBITORS

One systematic review in people with acute coronary syndromes or undergoing percutaneous coronary interventions has found that oral glycoprotein IIb/IIIa receptor inhibitors versus placebo increase risk of mortality and bleeding.

Benefits: One systematic review in people with acute coronary syndrome or undergoing percutaneous coronary intervention (search date 2000, 4 RCTs, 33 326 people) found that oral glycoprotein IIb/IIIa receptor inhibitors versus placebo increased mortality but did not significantly affect the risk of myocardial infarction after 3–10 months (mortality: pooled OR 1.37, 95% CI 1.13 to 1.66; myocardial infarction: pooled OR 1.04, 95% CI 0.93 to 1.16).[31]

Harms: The review found that oral glycoprotein IIb/IIIa receptor inhibitors increased all cause mortality and major bleeding compared with placebo. One subsequent RCT (9200 people with a recent myocardial infarction, unstable angina, ischaemic stroke/transient ischaemic attack, or peripheral arterial disease) assessing the effects of adding an oral glycoprotein IIb/IIIa receptor inhibitor to aspirin was stopped early because of safety concerns.[32]

Comment: None.

OPTION	ORAL ANTICOAGULANTS IN THE ABSENCE OF ANTIPLATELET TREATMENT

One systematic review has found that high or moderate intensity oral anticoagulants given alone reduce the risk of serious vascular events in people with coronary artery disease, but are associated with substantial risks of haemorrhage. Oral anticoagulants require regular monitoring for intensity of anticoagulant effect.

Benefits: We found one systematic review (search date 1999) of the effects of oral anticoagulation in people with coronary artery disease.[33] It identified 16 RCTs of high intensity anticoagulation (international normalised ratio [see glossary, p 221] > 2.8) versus control (either no anticoagulation or placebo) in 10 056 people, and four RCTs of moderate intensity anticoagulation (INR 2–3) versus control in 1365 people. Antiplatelet treatment was not routinely given in any of these 20 trials. The review found that high intensity anticoagulation reduced the odds of the combined outcome of mortality, myocardial infarction, or stroke compared with control (OR 0.57, 95% CI 0.51 to 0.63; about 98 events avoided/1000 people treated). Compared with control, moderate intensity anticoagulation was associated with a smaller non-significant reduction.[33] In direct comparisons of high or moderate intensity oral anticoagulation with aspirin, the effects on mortality, myocardial infarction, or stroke were similar (OR 1.04, 95% CI 0.80 to 1.34).[33]

Harms: Compared with control, high intensity anticoagulation increased the odds of major (mainly extracranial) haemorrhage by about sixfold (OR 6.0, 95% CI 4.4 to 8.2; absolute increase of 39 events/1000 people treated), and moderate intensity anticoagulation also increased the odds of major haemorrhage by about eightfold (OR 7.7, 95% CI 3.3 to 17.6).[33] Compared with aspirin, high or moderate intensity oral anticoagulation increased the odds of major haemorrhage more than twofold (OR 2.4, 95% CI 1.6 to 3.6).[33]

Comment: Oral anticoagulants provide substantial protection against vascular events in the absence of antiplatelet treatment, but the risks of serious haemorrhage are higher than for antiplatelet treatment and regular monitoring is required. Aspirin provides similar protection, but is safer and easier to use (see harms under antiplatelet treatment, p 194).

OPTION	ORAL ANTICOAGULANTS IN ADDITION TO ANTIPLATELET TREATMENT

One systematic review found no evidence that the addition of low intensity oral anticoagulation (target international normalised ratio < 1.5) to aspirin reduced mortality, myocardial infarction, and stroke. One

Cardiovascular disorders

systematic review and subsequent RCTs found that adding moderate intensity oral anticoagulation (target international normalised ratio 1.5–3.0) to aspirin did not reduce the risk of recurrent cardiovascular events or mortality compared with aspirin alone, although it increased the risk of major haemorrhage.

Benefits: We found one systematic review (search date 1999, 6 RCTs, 8915 people with coronary artery disease) of adding an oral anticoagulant regimen to aspirin.[33] Three of these RCTs assessed the addition of a low intensity (target international normalised ratio [see glossary, p 221] < 1.5) regimen to aspirin in a total of 8435 people, and found no significant reduction in the odds of mortality, myocardial infarction, or stroke (OR 0.91, 95% CI 0.79 to 1.06).[33] Trials assessing the addition of a moderate intensity (INR 2–3) oral anticoagulant regimen to aspirin were too small (480 people) to produce reliable estimates of efficacy and safety.[33] We found one subsequent RCT (3712 people with unstable angina) of 5 months' oral anticoagulant treatment (target INR 2.0–2.5) plus standard treatment (usually including aspirin) versus standard treatment alone.[34] When this trial was included in a meta-analysis with the previous trials assessing the addition of moderate intensity oral anticoagulation to aspirin, oral anticoagulation was associated with a non-significant reduction in mortality, myocardial infarction, or stroke (OR 0.83; 95% CI 0.66 to 1.03).[33] We found one subsequent unblinded RCT (5059 people with myocardial infarction in the previous 14 days), that compared warfarin (target INR 1.5–2.5) plus aspirin (81 mg/day) versus aspirin alone (162 mg/day).[35] It found no significant differences between treatments in mortality, recurrent myocardial infarction, or stroke after a median of 2.7 years (mortality 17.6% with warfarin plus aspirin v 17.3% with aspirin alone, P = 0.8; AR for recurrent myocardial infarction 13.3% with warfarin plus aspirin v 13.1% with aspirin alone, P = 0.8; AR for stroke 3.1% with warfarin plus aspirin v 3.5% with aspirin alone, P = 0.5).

Harms: The systematic review found a non-significant excess of major haemorrhage with the addition of low intensity oral anticoagulation to aspirin (OR 1.29, 95% CI 0.96 to 1.75).[33] An updated meta-analysis assessing the addition of moderate intensity oral anticoagulation to aspirin included the RCTs from the systematic review[33] and one subsequent trial[34] (total of 4192 people with coronary artery disease). It found a clear excess of major haemorrhage in people allocated oral anticoagulation (OR 1.95, 95% CI 1.27 to 2.98).[34] One of the more recent RCTs (5059 people) examining the addition to aspirin of moderate intensity anticoagulation also found that combined treatment increased risk of major haemorrhage (RR 1.78, 95% CI 1.27 to 2.72).[35]

Comment: The issue of whether adding a moderately intense oral anticoagulant regimen to aspirin provides additional net benefit to people at high risk of ischaemic cardiac events is being assessed in several ongoing RCTs. One RCT (135 people with unstable angina or non-ST segment myocardial infarction, with prior coronary artery bypass grafting) compared three treatments: aspirin alone (80 mg/day) plus placebo; warfarin (target INR 2.0–2.5) plus placebo, and aspirin plus warfarin.[36] It found no significant difference among treatments for rates of primary end point (death or myocardial infarction or unstable angina requiring admission to hospital at 1 year; AR 14.6% with warfarin alone v 11.5% with aspirin alone v 11.3% with combination, P = 0.76).[36] However, it found no significant difference for major haemorrhage among people taking warfarin compared with those who were not. Event rates were low and the study may have lacked power to detect a clinically important difference for adverse effects.[36]

QUESTION   What are the effects of other drug treatments?

Eva Lonn

OPTION   β BLOCKERS

Systematic reviews have found strong evidence that β blockers reduce the risk of all cause mortality, coronary mortality, recurrent non-fatal myocardial infarction, and sudden death in people after myocardial infarction. Most benefit was seen in those at highest risk of mortality after a myocardial infarction (> 50 years old; previous myocardial infarction, angina pectoris, hypertension, or treatment with digitalis; transient mechanical or electrical failure; higher heart rate at study entry). About 25% of people suffered adverse effects.

Benefits: **Survival and reinfarction:** One systematic review (search date 1993, 26 RCTs, > 24 000 people) compared oral β blockers versus placebo within days or weeks of an acute myocardial infarction (late intervention trials) and continued for between 6 weeks to 3 years.[37] Most RCTs followed people for 1 year. The review found improved survival in people given β blockers (RR 0.77, 95% CI 0.70 to 0.86).[37] One prior systematic review (search date not stated, 24 RCTs) found that long term use of β blockers versus placebo after myocardial infarction reduced total mortality (RR about 0.80; NNT 48), sudden death (RR about 0.70; NNT 63), and non-fatal reinfarction (RR about 0.75; NNT 56).[38] **Anginal symptoms:** We found no good RCTs assessing the antianginal effects of β blockers in people after myocardial infarction. One trial found atenolol more effective than placebo in people with chronic stable effort angina or silent ischaemia.[39] **Different types of β blockers:** The earlier review found no differences between β blockers with and without cardioselectivity or membrane stabilising properties, but it raised concerns about the lack of efficacy of β blockers with intrinsic sympathomimetic activity in long term management after myocardial infarction.[38] One RCT (607 people after myocardial infarction) found that acebutolol, a β blocker with moderate partial agonist activity, decreased 1 year mortality compared with placebo (AR of death: 11% with placebo v 6% with acebutolol; RR 0.52, 95% CI 0.29 to 0.91).[40] **Effects in different subgroups:** One systematic review (search date 1983, 9 RCTs) compared β blockers versus placebo started more than 24 hours after onset of symptoms of acute myocardial infarction and continued for 9–24 months.[41] Pooled analysis of individual data (13 679 people) found that the benefits of β blockers versus placebo on mortality seemed comparable in men and women. The highest absolute benefit from β blockers was found in subgroups with the highest baseline risks (i.e. those with the highest mortality on placebo), those over 50 years of age; those with a history of previous myocardial infarction, angina pectoris, hypertension, or treatment with digitalis; those with transient signs or symptoms of mechanical or electrical failure in the early phases of myocardial infarction; and those with a higher heart rate at study entry. Low risk subgroups had smaller mean absolute benefit.

Harms: Adverse effects include shortness of breath, bronchospasm, bradycardia, hypotension, heart block, cold hands and feet, diarrhoea, fatigue, reduced sexual activity, depression, nightmares, faintness, insomnia, syncope, and hallucinations. Rates vary in different studies. One RCT reported an absolute risk increase for any adverse effect on propranolol compared with placebo of 24% (no CI available; NNH 4). Serious adverse effects were uncommon and only a small proportion of people withdrew from the study as a result.[42]

Comment: Continued benefit from β blockers has been reported up to 6 years after myocardial infarction (ARR for mortality: 5.9%, P = 0.003; RR 0.82, no CI available). However, the study was not blinded after 33 months.

OPTION   ANGIOTENSIN CONVERTING ENZYME INHIBITORS

One systematic review has found that in people who have had a myocardial infarction and have left ventricular dysfunction, angiotensin converting enzyme inhibitors versus placebo reduce mortality, admission to hospital for congestive heart failure, and recurrent non-fatal myocardial infarction. One large RCT in people without left ventricular dysfunction found that ramipril versus placebo reduced cardiovascular death, stroke, and myocardial infarction.

Benefits: **In people with left ventricular dysfunction:** One systematic review (search date not stated, 3 RCTs, 5966 people)[43] compared angiotensin converting enzyme (ACE) inhibitors (captopril, ramipril, or trandolapril) versus placebo started 3–16 days after acute myocardial infarction and continued for 15–42 months. It analysed individual data from 5966 people with a recent myocardial infarction and with clinical manifestations of congestive heart failure or moderate left ventricular dysfunction (left ventricular ejection fraction ≥ 35–40%). ACE inhibitors versus placebo significantly reduced mortality (702/2995 [23.4%] with ACE v 866/2971 [29.1%] with control; OR 0.74, 95% CI 0.66 to 0.83; NNT 17 people treated for about 2 years to prevent 1 death, CI not provided), admission to hospital for congestive heart failure (355/2995 [11.9%] with ACE v 460/2971 [15.5%] with control; OR 0.73, 95% CI 0.63 to 0.85; NNT 28, CI not available), and recurrent non-fatal myocardial infarction (324/2995 [10.8%] with ACE v 391/2971 [13.1%] with control; OR 0.80, 95% CI 0.69 to 0.94; NNT 43, CI not available). **In people without impaired ventricular function or evidence of congestive heart failure:** We found no systematic review but found one large RCT (9297 people at high risk of cardiovascular events).[44] It found that ramipril (10 mg/day) versus placebo reduced the composite primary outcome of cardiovascular death, myocardial infarction, or stroke over an average of 4.7 years (RR for composite outcome: 0.78, 95% CI 0.70 to 0.86, NNT 27, 95% CI 20 to 45; RR for cardiovascular death: 0.74, 95% CI 0.64 to 0.87, NNT 50, CI not available; RR for myocardial infarction: 0.80, 95% CI 0.70 to 0.90, NNT 42, CI not available; RR for stroke: 0.68, 95% CI 0.56 to 0.84, NNT 67, CI not available; RR for death from all causes: 0.84, 95% CI 0.75 to 0.95, NNT 56, CI not available). The RCT found that ramipril reduced the need for revascularisation procedures and reduced heart failure related outcomes (need for revascularisation: RR 0.85, no CI available; heart failure related outcomes: RR 0.77, no CI available). Ramipril versus placebo produced benefit in all subgroups examined, including women and men; people aged over and under 65 years; those with and without a history of coronary artery disease, hypertension, diabetes, peripheral vascular disease, cerebrovascular disease, and those with and without microalbuminuria at study entry.[44] **In people with diabetes:** See antihypertensive treatment under cardiovascular disease in diabetes, p 46.[45]

Harms: The major adverse effects reported in these trials were cough (ARI 5–10% with ACE inhibitors v placebo), dizziness, hypotension (ARI with 5–10% ACE inhibitors v placebo), renal failure (ARI < 3% with ACE inhibitors v placebo), hyperkalaemia (ARI < 3% with ACE inhibitors v placebo), angina, syncope, diarrhoea (ARI 2% with ACE inhibitors v placebo), and, for captopril, alteration in taste (2% of captopril users).[43]

Comment: There are several other ongoing large RCTs assessing ACE inhibitors in people without clinical manifestations of heart failure and with no or with mild impairment in left ventricular systolic function. These include one trial of trandolapril in 8000 people with coronary artery disease, and one trial of perindopril in 10 500 people with stable coronary artery disease.[46]

OPTION	CLASS I ANTIARRHYTHMIC AGENTS (QUINIDINE, PROCAINAMIDE, DISOPYRIMIDE, ENCAINIDE, FLECAINIDE, AND MORACIZINE)

One systematic review has found that class I antiarrhythmic agents after myocardial infarction increase the risk of cardiovascular mortality and sudden death.

Benefits: None (see harms below).

Harms: One systematic review (search date 1993, 51 RCTs, 23 229 people) compared class I antiarrhythmic drugs versus placebo given acutely and later in the management of myocardial infarction.[37] The review found that the antiarrhythmic agents increased mortality (AR of death 5.6% with class I antiarrhythmic v 5.0% with placebo; OR 1.14, 95% CI 1.01 to 1.28). One RCT (1498 people with myocardial infarction and asymptomatic or mildly symptomatic ventricular arrhythmia) found that encainide or flecainide versus placebo increased the risk of death or cardiac arrest after 10 months (RR 2.38, 95% CI 1.59 to 3.57; NNH 17).[47]

Comment: The evidence implies that class I antiarrhythmic drugs should not be used in people after myocardial infarction or with significant coronary artery disease.

| OPTION | CLASS III ANTIARRHYTHMIC AGENTS (AMIODARONE, SOTALOL) |

Systematic reviews have found that amiodarone versus placebo reduces the risk of sudden death and marginally reduces mortality in people at high risk of death after myocardial infarction. One RCT found limited evidence that sotalol versus placebo significantly increased mortality within 1 year.

Benefits: **Amiodarone:** We found two systematic reviews.[48,49] The first systematic review (search date not stated, individual data from 6553 high risk people in 13 RCTs) compared amiodarone versus control treatments.[48] People were selected with a recent myocardial infarction and a high risk of death from cardiac arrhythmia (based on low left ventricular ejection fraction, frequent ventricular premature depolarisation, or non-sustained ventricular tachycardia, but no history of sustained symptomatic ventricular tachycardia or ventricular fibrillation); 78% of people from eight RCTs had a recent myocardial infarction, and 22% of people from five RCTs had congestive heart failure.[48] Most trials were placebo controlled with a mean follow up of about 1.5 years. The people with congestive heart failure were symptomatic but stable and did not have a recent myocardial infarction, although in most cases the heart failure was ischaemic in origin. All RCTs used a loading dose of amiodarone (400 mg/day for 28 days or 800 mg/day for 14 days) followed by a maintenance dose (200–400 mg/day). Amiodarone versus placebo significantly reduced total mortality: 10.9% a year with amiodarone v 12.3% a year with placebo; RR 0.87, 95% CI 0.78 to 0.99; NNT 71 a year to avoid 1 additional death) and rates of sudden cardiac death (RR 0.71, 95% CI 0.59 to 0.85; NNT 59). Amiodarone had similar effects in the studies after myocardial infarction and congestive heart failure. The second systematic review (search date 1997, 5864 people with myocardial infarction, congestive heart failure, left ventricular dysfunction, or cardiac arrest) found similar results.[49] **Sotalol:** We found one RCT (3121 people with myocardial infarction and left ventricular dysfunction), which found increased mortality with the class III antiarrhythmic agent sotalol versus placebo (AR for death: 5.0% with sotalol v 3.1% with placebo; RR 1.65, 95% CI 1.15 to 2.36). The trial was terminated prematurely after less than 1 year.[50]

Harms: Adverse events leading to discontinuation of amiodarone were hypothyroidism (expressed as events per 100 person-years: 7.0 with amiodarone v 1.1 with placebo; OR 7.3), hyperthyroidism (1.4 with amiodarone v 0.5 with placebo; OR 2.5), peripheral neuropathy (0.5 with amiodarone v 0.2 with placebo; OR 2.8), lung infiltrates (1.6 with amiodarone v 0.5 with placebo; OR 3.1), bradycardia (2.4 with amiodarone v 0.8 with placebo; OR 2.6), and liver dysfunction (1.0 with amiodarone v 0.4 with placebo; OR 2.7).[48]

Comment: The conclusions of the review are probably specific to amiodarone.[48,49] The two largest RCTs of amiodarone after myocardial infarction found a favourable interaction between β blockers and amiodarone, with additional reduction in cardiac mortality.[51,52]

OPTION	CALCIUM CHANNEL BLOCKERS

One systematic review found no benefit from calcium channel blockers in people after myocardial infarction or with chronic coronary heart disease. Diltiazem and verapamil may reduce rates of reinfarction and refractory angina in people after myocardial infarction who do not have heart failure. The review found non-significantly higher mortality with dihydropyridines compared with placebo.

Benefits: One systematic review (search date 1993, 24 RCTs) compared calcium channel blockers (including dihydropyridines, diltiazem, and verapamil) versus placebo given early or late during the course of acute myocardial infarction or unstable angina and continued in the intermediate or long term.[37] Two of the RCTs used angiographic regression of coronary stenosis as an outcome in people with stable coronary heart disease treated with calcium channel blockers. The review found no significant difference in the absolute risk of death compared with placebo (AR 9.7% with calcium channel blockers v 9.3% with placebo; ARI with calcium channel blockers versus placebo +0.4%, 95% CI −0.4% to +1.2%; OR 1.04, 95% CI 0.95 to 1.14). **Diltiazem and verapamil:** The review found no significant effect compared with placebo (OR 0.95, 95% CI 0.82 to 1.09).[37] Three RCTs comparing diltiazem or verapamil versus placebo found decreased rates of recurrent infarction and refractory angina with active treatment but only for those people without signs or symptoms of heart failure. For those with clinical manifestations of heart failure, the trends were towards harm.[53–55] **Dihydropyridines:** The review found non-significantly higher mortality with dihydropyridines compared with placebo (OR 1.16, 95% CI 0.99 to 1.35). Several individual RCTs of dihydropyridines found increased mortality, particularly when these agents were started early in the course of acute myocardial infarction and in the absence of β blockers.

Harms: Adverse effects reported of verapamil and diltiazem include atrioventricular block, atrial bradycardia, new onset heart failure, hypotension, dizziness, oedema, rash, constipation, and pruritus.

Comment: We found little good evidence on newer generation dihydropyridines, such as amlodipine and felodipine, in people after myocardial infarction but these have been found to be safe in people with heart failure, including heart failure of ischaemic origin.

OPTION	HORMONE REPLACEMENT THERAPY

One large, well designed RCT of hormone replacement therapy versus placebo found no reduction of major cardiovascular events in postmenopausal women with established coronary artery disease, despite evidence from RCTs that hormone replacement therapy improves some cardiovascular risk factors.

Benefits: **Combined oestrogen and progestins:** We found no systematic review. One large RCT (2763 postmenopausal women with coronary heart disease) found that conjugated equine oestrogen (0.625 mg/day) plus medroxyprogesterone acetate (2.5 mg/day) versus placebo for an average of 4.1 years produced no significant difference in the risk of non-fatal myocardial infarction or deaths caused by coronary heart disease (172/1380 [12.5%] with hormone replacement therapy v 176/1383 [12.7%] with placebo; ARR +0.3%, 95% CI −2.2% to +2.7%; RR 0.98, 95% CI 0.80 to 1.19).[56] It also found no significant difference in secondary cardiovascular outcomes (coronary revascularisation, unstable angina, congestive heart failure, resuscitated cardiac arrest, stroke or transient ischaemic attack, and peripheral arterial disease) or in all cause mortality. **Oestrogen alone:** We found no good RCTs of oestrogen alone in the secondary prevention of coronary heart disease in postmenopausal women. One RCT found that high dose oestrogen (5 mg/day conjugated equine oestrogen) increased the risk of myocardial infarction and thromboembolic events in men with pre-existing coronary heart disease.[57]

Harms: Pooled estimates from observational studies found an increased risk of endometrial cancer (RR > 8) and of breast cancer (RR 1.25–1.46) when oestrogen was used for more than 8 years. In most observational studies, the addition of progestins prevented endometrial cancer but not breast cancer. The risk of venous thromboembolism, including pulmonary embolism and deep vein thrombosis, was three to four times higher with hormone replacement therapy than without. However, because the incidence of venous thromboembolism is low in postmenopausal women, the absolute increase in risk was only about one to two additional cases of venous thromboembolism in 5000 users a year.[58] In one RCT,[56] more women in the HRT group than in the placebo group experienced venous thromboembolism (34/1380 [2.5%] with HRT v 12/1383 [0.9%] with placebo; OR 2.65, 95% CI 1.48 to 4.75) and gall bladder disease (84/1380 [6.1%] with HRT v 62/1383 [4.5%] with placebo; OR 1.38, 95% CI 0.99 to 1.92).

Comment: Many observational studies have found reduced rates of clinical events caused by coronary heart disease in postmenopausal women using HRT, especially in women with pre-existing coronary heart disease. Hormone users experienced 35–80% fewer recurrent events than non-users.[59,60] Several RCTs have found that HRT improves cardiovascular risk factors.[61] It is not known whether studies longer than 4 years would show a benefit.

QUESTION What are the effects of cholesterol reduction?

Michael Pignone

Systematic reviews and large subsequent RCTs have found that lowering cholesterol in people at high risk of ischaemic coronary events substantially reduces overall mortality, cardiovascular mortality, and non-fatal cardiovascular events. One systematic review of primary and secondary prevention trials found that statins, in people also given dietary advice, were the only non-surgical treatment for cholesterol reduction to significantly reduce mortality. One systematic review found that the absolute benefits increase as baseline risk increases, but are not additionally influenced by the person's absolute cholesterol concentration.

Benefits: **All cholesterol treatments:** We found one systematic review (search date 1996, 59 RCTs, 173 160 people), which did not differentiate primary and secondary prevention, and included RCTs of any cholesterol lowering intervention, irrespective of duration, as long as mortality data were reported.[62] It included drug treatments (statins, n–3 fatty acids, fibrates, resins, hormones, or niacin), dietary intervention alone, or surgery (ileal bypass) alone. Overall, baseline risk was similar among all intervention groups. Among non-surgical treatments, the review found that only statins reduced coronary heart disease mortality, and that only statins and n–3 fatty acids significantly reduced all cause mortality (RR of coronary heart disease mortality: statins v control 0.69, 95% CI 0.59 to 0.80; n–3 fatty acids v control 0.44, 95% CI 0.18 to 1.07; fibrates v control 0.98, 95% CI 0.78 to 1.24; resins v control 0.71, 95% CI 0.51 to 0.99; hormones v control 1.04, 95% CI 0.93 to 1.17; niacin v control 0.95, 95% CI 0.83 to 1.10; diet v control 0.91, 95% CI 0.82 to 1.01. RR of all cause mortality: statins v control 0.79, 95% CI 0.71 to 0.89; n–3 fatty acids v control 0.68, 95% CI 0.53 to 0.88; fibrates v control 1.06, 95% CI 0.78 to 1.46; resins v control 0.85, 95% CI 0.66 to 1.08; hormone v control 1.09, 95% CI 1.00 to 1.20; niacin v control 0.96, 95% CI 0.86 to 1.08; diet v control 0.97, 95% CI 0.81 to 1.15).[62] **Statins:** We found one systematic review (search date 1998, 5 RCTs, 30 817 people) that compared long term (≥ 4 years) treatment with statins versus placebo.[63] Combining the three secondary prevention trials, the review found that statins reduced coronary heart disease mortality, cardiovascular mortality, and all cause mortality compared with placebo over a mean of 5.4 years (coronary heart disease mortality: OR 0.71, 95% CI 0.63 to 0.80; cardiovascular mortality: OR 0.73, 95% CI 0.66 to 0.82; all cause mortality: OR 0.77, 95% CI 0.70 to 0.85). One subsequent RCT (20 536 adults with total cholesterol > 3.5 mmol/L [an inclusion threshold lower than previous statin trials], including > 5000 women and > 5000 people over 70 years of age) compared simvastatin (40 mg) versus placebo. The study included both primary and secondary prevention populations.[64] After a mean of 5.5 years follow up, simvastatin reduced total mortality and major vascular events compared with placebo (all cause mortality: 12.9% with simvastatin v 14.7% with placebo, RR 0.87, 95% CI 0.81 to 0.94; major vascular events 19.8% with simvastatin v 25.2% with placebo, RR 0.76, 95% CI 0.72 to 0.81). **Effects of statins in different groups of people:** Combining results from primary and secondary prevention trials, the review found that, compared with placebo, statins reduced coronary events by a similar proportion in men (OR 0.69, 95% CI 0.65 to 0.74; ARR 3.7%, 95% CI 2.9% to 4.4%), in women (OR 0.71, 95% CI 0.64 to 0.76; ARR 3.3%, 95% CI 1.3% to 5.2%), in people under 65 years (OR 0.69, 95% CI 0.64 to 0.76; ARR 3.2%, 95% CI 2.4% to 4.0%), and in people over 65 years (OR 0.68, 95% CI 0.61 to 0.77; ARR 4.4%, 95% CI 3.0% to 5.8%). The reduction of coronary heart disease events in women involved more non-fatal and fewer fatal events than in men. One large RCT found no significant difference in mortality with statins versus placebo for the subgroup of women, but the confidence interval was wide (28/407 [6.9%] with simvastatin v 25/420 [6.0%], RR 1.16, 95% CI 0.68 to 1.99).[65] One recent RCT that was not included in the review found that relative risk reductions were similar for people with initial total cholesterol levels of under 5.0 mmol/L compared with people with levels over 5.0 mmol/L and for women and the elderly compared with younger men.[61] One RCT compared early initiation of atorvastatin (80 mg/day started 1–4 days after admission) versus placebo in people with unstable angina or non-Q wave myocardial infarction.[66] After 3 months, it found no significant difference between treatments for coronary event rates, although atorvastatin reduced readmission rate for recurrent ischaemia compared with placebo (AR for readmission for ischaemia: 6.2% with atorvastatin v 8.4% with placebo, RR 0.74, 95% CI 0.57 to 0.95). **Intensity of statin treatment:** We found one RCT (1351 people with a history of saphenous vein coronary artery bypass grafting) that compared aggressive reduction of cholesterol with lovastatin and, if necessary, colestyramine (cholestyramine) (aiming for target low density lipoprotein cholesterol 1.6–2.2 mmol/L [60–85 mg/dL]) with more moderate reduction (target low density lipoprotein cholesterol 3.4–3.7 mmol/L [130–140 mg/dL]) with the same drugs.[67] The trial found that aggressive treatment reduced the risk of needing repeat revascularisation at 4 years (6.5% with aggressive treatment v 9.2% with moderate treatment, P = 0.03). After an additional 3 years, aggressive treatment reduced the risk of revascularisation and cardiovascular death compared with moderate treatment (AR of revascularisation 19% with aggressive treatment v 27% with moderate treatment, P = 0.0006; AR for cardiovascular death, 7.4% with aggressive treatment v 11.3% with moderate treatment, P = 0.03).[67] **Fibrates:** We found one systematic review (search date not stated, 4 RCTs)[68] and two additional RCTs.[69,70] The systematic review compared fibrates versus placebo in people with known coronary heart disease. The review identified one RCT (2531 men with coronary heart disease and a level of high density lipoprotein cholesterol > 1 mmol/L) that found gemfibrozil versus placebo reduced the composite outcome of non-fatal myocardial infarction plus death from coronary heart disease after a median of 5.1 years (AR 219/1264 [17%] for gemfibrozil v 275/1267 [22%] for placebo; ARR 4.4%, 95% CI 1.4% to 7.0%; RR 0.80, 95% CI 0.68 to 0.94; NNT 23, 95% CI 14 to 73). The review identified three trials comparing clofibrate versus placebo, which found no consistent difference between groups. The two additional RCTs[69,70] both compared bezafibrate versus placebo. The larger RCT (3090 people selected with previous myocardial infarction or stable angina, high density lipoprotein cholesterol < 45 mg/dL, and low density lipoprotein cholesterol < 180 mg/dL) found that bezafibrate versus placebo did not significantly reduce all cause mortality or the composite end point of myocardial infarction plus sudden death (AR for myocardial infarction or sudden death: 13.6% with bezafibrate v 15.0% with placebo; cumulative RR 0.91; P = 0.26).[69] The smaller RCT (92 young male survivors of myocardial infarction) found that bezafibrate versus placebo significantly reduced the combined outcome of death, reinfarction, plus revascularisation (3/47 [6%] with bezafibrate v 11/45 [24%], RR 0.26, 95% CI 0.08 to 0.88).[70] **Cholesterol lowering versus angioplasty:** We found no systematic review. One RCT found that aggressive lipid lowering

Cardiovascular disorders

treatment was as effective as percutaneous transluminal angioplasty for reducing ischaemic events, although anginal symptoms were reduced more by percutaneous transluminal angioplasty (see percutaneous transluminal angioplasty versus medical treatment, p 216).

Harms: Total non-cardiovascular events, total and tissue specific cancers, and accident and violent deaths have been reported in statin trials. However, the systematic review of long term statin trials found no significant difference between statins and placebo in terms of non-cardiovascular mortality, cancer incidence, asymptomatic elevation of creatine kinase (> 10 times upper reference limit), or elevation of transaminases (> 3 times upper reference limit) during a mean of 5.4 years of treatment (OR of event, statin v placebo for non-cardiovascular mortality 0.93, 95% CI 0.81 to 1.07; for cancer 0.99, 95% CI 0.90 to 1.08; for creatine kinase increase 1.25, 95% CI 0.83 to 1.89; for transaminase increase 1.13, 95% CI 0.95 to 1.33).[65] We found no evidence of additional harm associated with cholesterol lowering in elderly people, or in people after acute myocardial infarction.

Comment: Multivariate analysis in one systematic review (search date 1996) indicates that in a wide range of clinical contexts the relative risk reduction depends on the percent reduction in total or low density lipoprotein cholesterol and is not otherwise dependent on the method by which cholesterol is lowered. The absolute benefit over several years of lowering cholesterol will therefore be greatest in people with the highest baseline risk of an ischaemic cardiac event. Even if the relative risk reduction attenuates at older age, the absolute risk reduction for ischaemic cardiac events may be higher in elderly people than in younger people. The Women's Health Initiative (48 000 people, completion 2007, diet, up to age 79 years),[71] and the Antihypertensive and Lipid Lowering Treatment to Prevent Heart Disease Trial (10 000 people, completion 2002, pravastatin, no upper age limit) are ongoing.[72] We found no large direct comparisons of cholesterol modifying drugs; it remains unclear whether any one drug has advantages over others in subgroups of high risk people with particular lipid abnormalities. Because the main aim of treatment is to reduce absolute risk (rather than to reduce the cholesterol to any particular concentration), treatments aimed at lowering cholesterol need assessing for effectiveness in comparison and in combination with other possible risk factor interventions in each individual. People in the large statin trials in both treatment and placebo groups were given dietary advice aimed at lowering cholesterol.

QUESTION   What are the effects of blood pressure reduction?

Eva Lonn

We found no direct evidence of the effects of blood pressure lowering in people with established coronary heart disease. Observational studies, and extrapolation of primary prevention trials of blood pressure reduction, support the lowering of blood pressure in those at high risk of ischaemic coronary events. The evidence for benefit is strongest for β blockers, although not specifically in people with hypertension. The target blood pressure in these people is not clear.

Benefits: We found no systematic review and no RCTs designed specifically to examine blood pressure reduction in those with established coronary heart disease. Prospective epidemiological studies have established that blood pressure continues to be a risk factor for cardiovascular events in people who have already experienced myocardial infarction. Prospective follow up of 5362 men who reported prior myocardial infarction during screening for one large RCT found no detectable association between systolic blood pressure and coronary heart disease mortality, and increased coronary heart disease mortality for those with lowest diastolic blood pressure in the first 2 years.[73] After 15 years there were highly significant linear associations between both systolic and diastolic blood pressure and increased risk of coronary heart disease mortality (stronger relation for systolic blood pressure), with apparent benefit for men with blood pressure maintained at levels lower than the arbitrarily defined "normal" levels. Experimental evidence of benefit from lowering of blood pressure in those with coronary heart disease requires extrapolation from primary prevention trials, because trials of antihypertensive treatment in elderly people[74-76] are likely to have included those with preclinical coronary heart disease. Mortality benefit has been established for β blockers after myocardial infarction (see beta blockers, p 200), for verapamil and diltiazem after myocardial infarction in those without heart failure (see calcium channel blockers, p 204), and for angiotensin converting enzyme inhibitors after myocardial infarction, especially in those with heart failure (see angiotensin converting enzyme inhibitors, p 201).

Harms: Some observational studies have found increased mortality among those with low diastolic blood pressure.[77] Trials in elderly people of blood pressure lowering for hypertension or while treating heart failure[78] found no evidence of a J-shaped relation between blood pressure and death.

Comment: Without specific studies comparing different antihypertensive treatments, the available evidence is strongest for a beneficial effect of β blockers when treating survivors of a myocardial infarction who have hypertension. We found no specific evidence about the target level of blood pressure.

QUESTION What are the effects of non-drug treatments?

Andy Ness and Eva Lonn

OPTION DIETARY INTERVENTIONS

One RCT found that advising people with coronary heart disease to eat more fruit and vegetables, bread, pasta, potatoes, olive oil, and rapeseed margarine (i.e. a Mediterranean diet) may result in a substantial survival benefit. We found no strong evidence from RCTs for a beneficial effect of low fat or high fibre diets on major non-fatal coronary heart disease events or coronary heart disease mortality. One RCT has found that advising people with coronary heart disease to eat more fish (particularly oily fish) significantly reduces mortality at 2 years. A second RCT found that fish oil capsules significantly reduced mortality at 3.5 years.

Secondary prevention of ischaemic cardiac events

Benefits: **Low fat diets:** One systematic review (search date not stated) found no evidence that allocation to a low fat diet reduced mortality from coronary heart disease in people after myocardial infarction (RR 0.94, 95% CI 0.84 to 1.06).[79] One large RCT included in the review (2033 middle aged men with a recent myocardial infarction) compared three dietary options: fat advice (to eat less fat), fibre advice (to eat more cereal fibre), and fish advice (to eat at least 2 portions of oily fish a week).[80] Advice to reduce fat was complicated and, though fat intake reduced only slightly in the fat advice group, fruit and vegetable intake increased by about 40 g daily.[81] However, there was no significant reduction in mortality (unadjusted RR at 2 years for death from any cause 0.97, 95% CI 0.75 to 1.27). **High fibre diets:** In the RCT, people advised to eat more fibre doubled their intake, but survival was non-significantly worse (unadjusted RR at 2 years for death from any cause 1.23, 95% CI 0.95 to 1.60).[80] **High fish diets:** In the RCT, those advised to eat more fish ate three times as much fish, although about 14% could not tolerate the fish and were given fish oil capsules. Those given fish advice were significantly less likely to die within 2 years (94/1015 [9.3%] with fish advice v 130/1018 [12.8%] with no fish advice, NNT 29, 95% CI 17 to 129, RR 0.71, 95% CI 0.54 to 0.93).[80] In a second trial, 11 324 people who had survived a recent myocardial infarction were randomised to receive 1 g daily of n–3 polyunsaturated fatty acids (fish oil) or no fish oil. Those given fish oil were less likely to die within 3.5 years (RR 0.86, 95% CI 0.76 to 0.97).[82] **Mediterranean diet:** One RCT (605 middle aged people with a recent myocardial infarction) compared advice to eat a Mediterranean diet (more bread, fruit and vegetables, fish, and less meat, and to replace butter and cream with rapeseed margarine) versus usual dietary advice.[83] There were several dietary differences between the groups. Fruit intake, for example, was about 50 g daily higher in the intervention group than the control group. After 27 months, the trial was stopped prematurely because of significantly better outcomes in the intervention group (mortality: 8/302 [2.6%] with intervention v 20/303 [6.6%] with usual dietary advice, adjusted RR of death 0.24, 97% CI 0.15 to 0.91 [97% CI to allow for early stopping]; NNT 25, 95% CI 14 to 299 over 27 months).[83]

Harms: No major adverse effects have been reported.

Comment: Diets low in saturated fat and cholesterol can lead to 10–15% reductions in cholesterol concentrations in highly controlled settings, such as in metabolic wards.[84] In people in the community the effects are smaller: 3–5% reductions in cholesterol concentrations in general population studies and 9% reductions in people after myocardial infarction.[79,85–87] Several RCTs of intensive dietary intervention in conjunction with multifactorial risk reduction treatment found decreased progression of anatomic extent of coronary heart disease on angiography.[88] A trial of advice to eat more fruit and vegetables in men with angina is underway (Burr M, personal communication, 2001) **Effect on cardiovascular risk factors:** Other studies have investigated the effects of dietary interventions on cardiovascular risk factors rather than the effect on cardiovascular morbidity and mortality. One systematic review (search date 1992) suggested that garlic may reduce cholesterol by about

10%.[89] Some trials in this review had problems with their methods. More recent reports (published in 1998) found no effects of garlic powder or garlic oil on cholesterol concentrations.[90,91] One systematic review (search date 1991) reported modest reductions in cholesterol levels of 2–5% from oats and psyllium enriched cereals (high fibre diets), although we found no evidence that high fibre diets reduce mortality in people with coronary heart disease.[92] One systematic review (search date 1991) of soy protein also reported modest reductions in cholesterol concentrations.[92]

OPTION	ANTIOXIDANT VITAMINS (VITAMIN E, β CAROTENE, VITAMIN C)

Pooled analysis from four large RCTs found no evidence that vitamin E altered cardiovascular events and all cause mortality compared with placebo when given for 1.3–4.5 years. Pooled analysis from three small RCTs found no evidence that vitamin C provided any substantial benefit. Large RCTs found no evidence of benefit with β carotene, and one RCT found evidence of a significant increase in mortality. Four large RCTs of β carotene supplementation in primary prevention found no cardiovascular benefits, and two of the RCTs raised concerns about increased mortality.

Benefits: We found no systematic review. **Vitamin E and β carotene:** We found four large RCTs of vitamin E in people with coronary artery disease.[82,93–95] The first RCT (2002 people with angiographically proved ischaemic heart disease)[93] used a high dose of vitamin E (400 or 800 IU) and follow up was brief (median 510 days). The RCT found that vitamin E reduced non-fatal coronary events (RR 0.23, 95% CI 0.11 to 0.47), but also found a non-significant increase in coronary death (RR 1.18, 95% CI 0.62 to 2.27) and all cause mortality. The second RCT (29 133 male Finnish smokers) compared β carotene supplements versus vitamin E supplements versus both versus placebo.[94] The dose of vitamin E (50 mg/day) was smaller than that used in the first trial. In the subgroup analysis of data from the 1862 men with prior myocardial infarction, the trial found that vitamin E reduced non fatal myocardial infarction (RR 0.62, 95% CI 0.41 to 0.96) but non-significantly increased coronary death (RR 1.33, 95% CI 0.86 to 2.05).[94] There were significantly more deaths from coronary heart disease on β carotene and β carotene plus vitamin E than placebo. There was no significant difference between vitamin E alone and placebo. The third RCT (11 324 people ≤ 3 months after myocardial infarction)[82] used a factorial design to compare vitamin E (300 mg/day) versus no vitamin E (as well as fish oil v no fish oil). After 3.5 years there was a small and non-significant reduction in the risk of cardiovascular death and deaths from all causes in those who received vitamin E compared with those who did not (all cause mortality: RR 0.92, 95% CI 0.82 to 1.04). There was no significant change in the rate of non-fatal coronary events in those who received vitamin E (RR 1.04, 95% CI 0.88 to 1.22).[82] The fourth RCT (9541 people at high cardiovascular risk, 80% with prior clinical coronary artery disease, remainder with other atherosclerotic disease or diabetes with ≥ 1 additional cardiovascular risk factor) compared natural source vitamin E (D-α tocopherol acetate, 400 IU/day) versus placebo and followed people for an average of 4.7 years.[95] It found no significant differences in any cardiovascular outcomes between vitamin E and placebo (AR for major fatal or non-fatal cardiovascular event 16.2% with vitamin E v 15.5% with placebo, P > 0.05; AR for cardiovascular death 7.2% with vitamin E v 6.9% with placebo, P > 0.05; AR for non-fatal myocardial infarction 11.2% v 11.0% with placebo, P > 0.05; AR for stroke 4.4% with vitamin E v 3.8% with placebo, P > 0.05; AR for death from any cause 11.2% with vitamin E v 11.2% with placebo, P > 0.05). Pooled analysis from all four of these major RCTs found no evidence that vitamin E altered cardiovascular events and all cause mortality compared with placebo when given for 1.3–4.5 years. One additional smaller RCT (196 people on haemodialysis, aged 40–75 years) compared high dose vitamin E (800 IU/day) versus placebo.[96] After a median of 519 days, it found that vitamin E reduced the rate of combined cardiovascular end points but found no significant effect for all cause mortality (cardiovascular end points: vitamin E v placebo RR 0.54, 95% CI 0.23 to 0.89; mortality: vitamin E v placebo RR 1.09, 95% CI 0.70 to 1.70).[96] **Vitamin C:** We found four small RCTs comparing vitamin C with placebo.[97–100] The first RCT (538 people admitted to an acute geriatric unit) compared vitamin C (200 mg/day) versus placebo for 6 months.[97] The second RCT (297 elderly people with low vitamin C levels) compared vitamin C (150 mg/day for 12 wks, then 50 mg/day) versus placebo for 2 years.[98] The third RCT (199 elderly people) compared vitamin C (200 mg/day) versus placebo for 6 months.[99] The three RCTs were small and brief, and their combined results provide no evidence of any substantial early benefit of vitamin C supplementation (mortality: vitamin v placebo RR 1.08, 95% CI 0.93 to 1.26). The fourth small RCT (160 people) found no significant difference in the rate of cardiovascular events between antioxidants vitamins (vitamin E, vitamin C, β carotene, and selenium) versus placebo.[100]

Harms: Two of the trials of vitamin E found non-significant increases in the risk of coronary death (see benefits above).[93,97] Four large RCTs of β carotene supplementation in primary prevention found no cardiovascular benefits, and two of the trials raised concerns about increased mortality (cardiovascular death: β carotene v placebo RR 1.12, 95% CI 1.04 to 1.22) and cancer rates.[101]

Comment: One systematic review (search date 1996) of epidemiological studies found consistent associations between increased dietary intake, supplemental intake of vitamin E, or both, and lower cardiovascular risk and less consistent associations for β carotene and vitamin C.[101] Most observational studies of antioxidants have excluded people with pre-existing disease.[102,103] The results of the trial in people on haemodialysis raises the possibility that high dose vitamin E supplementation may be beneficial in those at high absolute risk of coronary events.[96] Further trials in such groups are required to confirm or refute this finding. The Heart Protection Study (results not fully published at time of search, 20 536 people aged 40–80 years with prior cardiovascular events or at high risk for vascular disease) compared a combination of antioxidant vitamins (vitamin C 250 mg, vitamin E 600 mg, and β carotene 20 mg) versus placebo. After 5.5 years, the antioxidant treatment had no significant effect on total mortality and major cardiovascular events.[104]

| OPTION | CARDIAC REHABILITATION INCLUDING EXERCISE |

One systematic review has found that cardiac rehabilitation including exercise reduces the risk of major cardiac events in people after myocardial infarction. It found that exercise alone reduced the risk of a major cardiac event, and probably reduced mortality.

Benefits: We found one systematic review (search date 1998).[105] **Cardiac rehabilitation:** The review identified 42 RCTs of cardiac rehabilitation including exercise versus usual care (7683 people, who have had myocardial infarction, coronary artery bypass grafting [CABG], or percutaneous transluminal coronary angioplasty, or who have angina pectoris or coronary artery disease defined by angiography). It found that cardiac rehabilitation including exercise reduced the composite end point of mortality, non-fatal myocardial infarction, CABG, percutaneous transluminal angioplasty (636/3863 [16.5%] with cardiac rehabilitation v 734/3820 [19.2%] with usual care, RR 0.85, 95% CI 0.77 to 0.93). It found limited evidence of a reduction in mortality but significance was sensitive to the quality of the trials.[105] **Exercise alone:** The review identified 12 RCTs of exercise alone versus usual care (2582 people, who have had myocardial infarction, CABG, or percutaneous transluminal angioplasty, or who have angina pectoris or coronary artery disease defined by angiography). It found that exercise significantly reduced mortality (93/1297 [7.2%] with exercise v 122/1285 [9.5%] with usual care, RR 0.76, 95% CI 0.59 to 0.98). It was associated with a reduction in the composite end point of mortality, non-fatal myocardial infarction, CABG, and percutaneous transluminal angioplasty, but the difference was not significant (183/1297 [14.1%] with exercise v 216/1285 [16.8%] with usual care, RR 0.85, 95% CI 0.71 to 1.01).[105]

Harms: Rates of adverse cardiovascular outcomes (syncope, arrhythmia, myocardial infarction, or sudden death) were low (2–3/100 000 person h) in supervised rehabilitation programmes, and rates of fatal cardiac events during or immediately after exercise training, were reported in two older surveys as ranging from 1/116 400 to 1/784 000 person hours.[106]

Comment: The review included some RCTs performed before the widespread use of thrombolytic agents and β blockers after myocardial infarction.[105] Most people were white men, without comorbidity, and under 70 years of age. Other interventions aimed at risk factor modification were often provided in the intervention groups (including nutritional education, counselling in behavioural modification, and, in some trials, lipid lowering medications). We found no strong evidence that exercise training and cardiac rehabilitation programmes increased the proportion of people returning to work after myocardial infarction.

Secondary prevention of ischaemic cardiac events

| OPTION | SMOKING CESSATION |

We found no RCTs of the effects of smoking cessation on cardiovascular events in people with coronary heart disease. Moderate quality evidence from epidemiological studies indicates that people with coronary heart disease who stop smoking, rapidly reduce their risk of recurrent coronary events or death. Treatment with nicotine patches seems safe in people with coronary heart disease.

Benefits: We found no RCTs assessing the effects of smoking cessation on coronary morbidity and mortality. Many observational studies have found that people with coronary heart disease who stop smoking, rapidly reduce their risk of cardiac death and myocardial infarction (recurrent coronary events or premature death compared with continuing smokers: RR about 0.50).[107] See smoking cessation under primary prevention for more details, p 155. The studies found that about 50% of the benefits occur in the first year of stopping smoking, followed by a more gradual decrease in risk, reaching the risk of never smokers after several years of abstinence.[107] Among people with peripheral arterial disease and stroke, smoking cessation has been shown in observational studies to be associated with improved exercise tolerance, decreased risk of amputation, improved survival, and reduced risk of recurrent stroke.

Harms: Two recent RCTs found no evidence that nicotine replacement using transdermal patches in people with stable coronary heart disease increased cardiovascular events.[108,109]

Comment: One RCT compared the impact of firm and detailed advice to stop smoking (125 survivors of acute myocardial infarction) versus conventional advice (85 people).[110] Allocation to the intervention or control group was determined by day of admission. At over 1 year after admission, 62% of the intervention group and 28% of the control group were non-smokers. Morbidity and mortality were not reported.

| OPTION | PSYCHOLOGICAL AND STRESS MANAGEMENT |

One systematic review of mainly poor quality RCTs found that psychosocial treatments may decrease rates of myocardial infarction or cardiac death in people with coronary heart disease.

Benefits: One systematic review (search date not stated, 23 RCTs, 3180 people with coronary artery disease) compared a diverse range of psychosocial treatments (2024 people) versus usual treatment (1156 people).[111] Mortality results were available in only 12 RCTs. Psychosocial interventions versus control interventions significantly reduced mortality (OR survival 1.70, 95% CI 1.09 to 2.64) and non-fatal events in the first 2 years after myocardial infarction (OR for no event 1.84, 95% CI 1.12 to 2.99).[111]

Harms: No specific harms were reported.

Comment: These results should be interpreted with caution because of limits of the methods of the individual RCTs and the diversity of interventions (relaxation, stress management, counselling). The RCTs were generally small, with short follow up, and used non-uniform outcome measures. Methods of concealment allocation were not assessed. The authors of the review acknowledged the strong possibility of publication bias but made no attempt to measure it. The results were inconsistent across trials.[112] Several observational studies have found that depression and social isolation (lack of social and emotional support) are independent predictors of mortality and non-fatal coronary heart disease events in people after myocardial infarction.[113]

| QUESTION | What are the effects of surgical treatments? |

Charanjit Rihal

| OPTION | CORONARY ARTERY BYPASS GRAFTING VERSUS MEDICAL TREATMENT ALONE |

One systematic review found that coronary artery bypass grafts reduced the risk of death from coronary artery disease at 5 and 10 years compared with medical treatment alone. Greater benefit occurred in people with poor left ventricular function. One subsequent RCT in people with asymptomatic disease found that revascularisation with coronary artery bypass grafting or coronary percutaneous transluminal angioplasty versus medical treatment alone reduced mortality at 2 years.

Benefits: We found one systematic review comparing coronary artery bypass grafting (CABG) with medical treatment alone[114] and one subsequent RCT in asymptomatic people of revascularisation with CABG or coronary percutaneous transluminal angioplasty versus medical treatment alone.[115] In the systematic review (search date not stated, 7 RCTs, individual results from 2649 people with coronary heart disease) most people were middle aged men with multivessel disease but good left ventricular function who were enrolled from 1972–1984 (97% were male; 82% 41–60 years old; 80% with ejection fraction > 50%; 60% with prior myocardial infarction; and 83% with 2 or 3 vessel disease).[114] People assigned to CABG also received medical treatment, and 40% initially assigned to medical treatment underwent CABG in the following 10 years. The systematic review found that CABG versus medical treatment reduced deaths at 5 and 10 years (death at 5 years: RR 0.61 95% CI 0.48 to 0.77; death at 10 years: RR 0.83, 95% CI 0.70 to 0.98).[114] Most trials did not collect data on recurrent angina or quality of life. **Effects in people with reduced versus normal left ventricular function:** The systematic review found that the relative benefits were similar in people with normal versus reduced left ventricular function (death: OR 0.61, 95% CI 0.46 to 0.81 if left ventricular function was normal; OR 0.59. 95% CI 0.39 to 0.91 if left ventricular function was reduced).[114] The absolute benefit of CABG was greater in people with a reduced left ventricular function because the baseline risk of death was higher. **Effects in people with different numbers of diseased vessels:** The systematic review found lower mortality with CABG versus medical treatment in people with single vessel, two vessel, three vessel, and left main stem disease, but for single vessel and two vessel disease the difference was not statistically significant, possibly because the number of deaths was small (RR with single vessel disease 0.54, 95% CI 0.22

to 1.33; with two vessel disease 0.84, 95% CI 0.54 to 1.32; with three vessel disease 0.58, 95% CI 0.42 to 0.80; with left main stem disease 0.32, 95% CI 0.15 to 0.70).[114] **Effects in asymptomatic people:** We found one RCT (558 people) of revascularisation with CABG or percutaneous transluminal angioplasty versus symptom guided treatment versus electrocardiogram and symptom guided treatment in people with asymptomatic ischaemia identified by exercise test or ambulatory electrocardiogram.[115] It found that revascularisation versus medical treatment alone reduced death or myocardial infarction at 2 years (death or myocardial infarction: AR 4.7% with revascularisation v 8.8% with symptom guided treatment v 12.1% with symptom plus electrocardiogram guided treatment; P < 0.04).

Harms: In the systematic review, of the 1240 people who underwent CABG, 40 (3.2%) died and 88 (7.1%) had documented non-fatal myocardial infarction within 30 days of the procedure. At 1 year, the estimated incidence of death or myocardial infarction was significantly higher with CABG versus medical treatment (11.6% with CABG v 8% with medical treatment, RR 1.45, 95% CI 1.18 to 2.03).[114] The diagnosis of myocardial infarction after CABG is difficult, and true incidence may be higher.

Comment: The results of the systematic review may not be easily generalised to current practice. People were 65 years or younger, but more than 50% of CABG procedures are now performed on people over 65 years of age. Almost all people were male. High risk people, such as those with severe angina and left main coronary artery stenosis, were under-represented. Internal thoracic artery grafts were used in fewer than 5% of people. Lipid lowering agents (particularly statins) and aspirin were used infrequently (aspirin used in 3% of people at enrolment). Only about 50% of people were taking β blockers. The systematic review may underestimate the real benefits of CABG in comparison with medical treatment alone because medical and surgical treatment for coronary artery disease were not mutually exclusive; by 5 years, 25% of people receiving medical treatment had undergone CABG surgery and by 10 years, 41% had undergone CABG surgery. The underestimate of effect would be greatest among people at high risk. People with previous CABG have not been studied in RCTs, although they now represent a growing proportion of those undergoing CABG.

OPTION	CORONARY PERCUTANEOUS TRANSLUMINAL ANGIOPLASTY VERSUS MEDICAL TREATMENT ALONE

One systematic review found that coronary percutaneous transluminal angioplasty versus medical treatment alone improved angina, but was associated with a higher rate of coronary artery bypass grafting. The review found higher mortality and rates of myocardial infarction with percutaneous transluminal angioplasty versus medical treatment but the difference was not significant. RCTs have found that percutaneous transluminal angioplasty was associated with increased risk of emergency coronary artery bypass grafting and myocardial infarction

during and soon after the procedure. One RCT found that percutaneous transluminal angioplasty reduced cardiac events and improved angina severity compared with medical treatment alone in people over the age of 75 years.

Benefits: We found one systematic review (search date 1998, 6 RCTs, 1904 people with stable coronary artery disease) comparing coronary percutaneous transluminal angioplasty (PTA) versus medical treatment alone.[116] Follow up varied from 6–57 months. It found that PTA versus medical treatment alone reduced angina, but increased subsequent coronary artery bypass grafting (CABG) (angina: RR 0.70, 95% CI 0.50 to 0.98; CABG: RR 1.59, 95% CI 1.09 to 2.32). It found higher mortality and myocardial infarction with PTA versus medical treatment alone but the difference was not significant (death: RR 1.32, 95% CI 0.65 to 2.70; myocardial infarction: RR 1.42, 95% CI 0.90 to 2.25). The review found significant heterogencity between trials. The largest RCT identified by the review (1018 people) found that PTA versus medical treatment improved physical functioning, vitality, and general health at 1 year (proportion of people rating their health "much improved": 33% of people treated with PTA v 22% with medical treatment alone; P = 0.008), but found no significant difference at 3 years.[117] The improvements were related to breathlessness, angina, and treadmill tolerance. High transfer (27%) from the medical to PTA group may partly explain the lack of difference between groups at 3 years. **Effects in elderly people:** One RCT (305 people aged > 75 years with chronic refractory angina) compared PTA versus medical treatment alone.[118] It found that PTA reduced all adverse cardiac events and decreased anginal severity compared with medical treatment, but had no significant effect on deaths or non-fatal myocardial infarctions after 6 months (adverse cardiac events: AR 19% with PTA v 49% with medical treatment alone, P < 0.0001; change in angina class: –2.0 with PTA v –1.6 with medical treatment alone, P < 0.0001; deaths: AR 8.5% with PTA v 4.1% with medical treatment alone, P = 0.15; non-fatal infarctions: AR 7.8% with PTA v 11.5% with medical treatment alone, P = 0.46). **Effects in people with different angina severity:** One of the RCTs in the systematic review found that antianginal benefit from PTA was limited to people with moderate to severe (grade 2 or worse) angina (20% lower incidence of angina and 1 min longer treadmill exercise times compared with medical treatment).[119] People with mild symptoms at enrolment derived no significant improvement in symptoms. **Effects in asymptomatic people:** We found one RCT (558 people) of revascularisation with CABG or PTA versus symptom guided treatment versus electrocardiogram and symptom guided treatment in people with asymptomatic ischaemic identified by exercise test or ambulatory electrocardiogram[115] (see benefits of coronary artery bypass grafting versus medical treatment alone, p 215).

Harms: Procedural death and myocardial infarction, as well as repeat procedures for restenosis, are the main hazards of PTA. Four RCTs included in the review reported complications of PTA. In the first RCT, two (1.9%) emergency CABG operations and five (4.8%) myocardial infarctions occurred at the time of the procedure. By 6 months, the PTA group had higher rates of CABG surgery (7% with PTA *v* 0% with medical treatment alone) and non-protocol PTA (15.2% with PTA *v* 10.3% with medical treatment alone).[119,120] In the second RCT, the higher mortality or rate of myocardial infarction with PTA was attributable to one death and seven procedure related myocardial infarctions.[118] The third RCT found a procedure related CABG rate and myocardial infarction rate of 2.8% each, and the fourth found rates of 2.0% for CABG and 3.0% for myocardial infarction.[115]

Comment: We found good evidence that PTA treats the symptoms of angina, but we found no evidence that it reduces the overall incidence of death or myocardial infarction in people with stable angina. This could be because of the risk of complications during and soon after the procedure, and because most PTAs are performed for single vessel disease.

OPTION	CORONARY PERCUTANEOUS TRANSLUMINAL ANGIOPLASTY VERSUS CORONARY ARTERY BYPASS GRAFTING

One systematic review has found that percutaneous transluminal angioplasty versus coronary artery bypass grafting has no significant effect on mortality, the risk of myocardial infarction, or quality of life. Percutaneous transluminal angioplasty is less invasive but increased the number of repeat procedures. The relevant RCTs were too small to exclude a 20–30% relative difference in mortality.

Benefits: We found one systematic review (search date not stated, 8 RCTs, 3371 people)[122], one subsequent RCT[123], one subsequent non-systematic review, (including the subsequent RCT),[124] which compared percutaneous transluminal angioplasty (PTA) versus coronary artery bypass grafting (CABG). **Angina:** The systematic review found that the prevalence of moderate to severe angina (grade 2 or worse) was significantly higher after PTA than after CABG at 1 year (RR 1.6, 95% CI 1.3 to 1.9).[122] After 3 years this difference had decreased (RR 1.2, 95% CI 1.0 to 1.5). **Mortality:** The systematic review found that PTA did not reduce deaths compared with CABG after 1 year (RR 1.08, 95% CI 0.79 to 1.50),[122] the subsequent RCT (392 people) found no significant difference in deaths between CABG versus PTA after 8 years, although the trial was too small to exclude a clinically important difference (AR for survival 83% with CABG *v* 79% with PTA; P = 0.40).[124] The subsequent non-systematic review found that mortality was not significantly different between PTA versus CABG (OR 1.09, 95% CI 0.88 to 1.35).[123] **Repeat procedures:** The systematic review found that PTA increased subsequent procedures compared with CABG (subsequent CABG: RR 1.59, 95% CI 1.09 to 2.32; subsequent PTA: RR 1.29, 95% CI 0.71 to 3.36).[122] **Quality of life:** Two of the RCTs included in the systematic review found no difference in quality of life between people who had PTA and people who had CABG over 3–5 years.[125,126]

Harms: See harms under percutaneous transluminal angioplasty versus medical treatment, p 217. CABG is more invasive than PTA, but PTA is associated with a greater need for repeat procedures.

Comment: Although no major differences in death or myocardial infarction were observed in the systematic review[122] these trials enrolled people at relatively low risk of cardiac events, so it is premature to conclude that PTA and CABG are equivalent for people with multi-vessel disease. Fewer than 20% of people had left ventricular dysfunction, almost 70% had one or two vessel disease, and observed mortality was only 2.6% for the first year and 1.1% for the second year. People enrolled in the largest trial more closely approximated to moderate risk people, but this was caused primarily by the higher proportion of people with diabetes mellitus.[127] Even in that trial nearly 60% of people had two vessel coronary artery disease. The total number of people enrolled in the nine trials so far is not adequate to show anything less than a 20–30% difference in mortality between PTA and CABG. Subgroup analysis of one RCT (1829 people) found that in people with diabetes (353 people) CABG reduced deaths compared with PTA after 7 years[127] (see coronary artery bypass grafting v percutaneous transluminal angioplasty in cardiovascular disease in diabetes, p 46). This difference was not found in people without diabetes or any other subgroup (deaths in people without diabetes: AR 13.6% with CABG v 13.2% with PTA; P = 0.72).[127]

OPTION **INTRACORONARY STENTS VERSUS CORONARY PERCUTANEOUS TRANSLUMINAL ANGIOPLASTY ALONE**

One systematic review has found that intracoronary stents versus coronary percutaneous transluminal angioplasty alone significantly reduce the need for repeat vascularisation. It found no significant difference in mortality or myocardial infarction, but crossover rates from percutaneous transluminal angioplasty alone to stent were high. RCTs found that intracoronary stents improved outcomes after 4–9 months compared with percutaneous transluminal angioplasty alone in people with previous coronary artery bypass grafting, chronic total occlusions, and for treatment of restenosis after initial percutaneous transluminal angioplasty.

Benefits: We found one systematic review (search date 1999, 11 RCTs with 4–11 months' follow up, 4815 people) of stents versus percutaneous transluminal angioplasty (PTA) alone.[129] It found a significant reduction in cardiac event rates after 4–11 months with stents compared with PTA alone (composite of death, myocardial infarction, or repeat vascularisation; 17.9% with stent v 24.1% with PTA; OR 0.68, 95% CI 0.59 to 0.78). Stents reduced repeat vascularisation compared with PTA alone (12.4% with stent v 20.6% with PTA alone; OR 0.54, 95% CI 0.45 to 0.65), whereas there was no significant difference in deaths (0.9% with stent v 1.3% with PTA alone; OR 0.68, 95% CI 0.40 to 1.14) or myocardial infarctions (4.4% with stent v 3.6% with PTA alone; OR 1.23, 95% CI 0.88 to 1.72). Seven RCTs with follow up over 1 year found a significant reduction in cardiac events with stents compared with PTA alone (19.5% with stent v 28.1% with PTA alone, OR 0.62, 95% CI 0.52 to 0.74). **In saphenous vein graft lesions in people with prior coronary artery bypass grafting:** We found one RCT (220 people) comparing stents with PTA alone for stenosed saphenous vein grafts.[130] There was no significant difference in rates of restenosis

(37% with stent *v* 46% with PTA alone; P = 0.24) after 6 months, but stents compared with PTA alone reduced death, myocardial infarction, coronary artery bypass grafting, or repeat PTA (27% with stent *v* 42% with PTA alone; P = 0.03). **In people with total occlusions:** We found three RCTs comparing stents with PTA alone in people with chronic totally occluded coronary arteries.[131–133] The first RCT (119 people) found that stent compared with PTA alone reduced angina, angiographic restenosis, and repeat procedures (angina free at 6 months: 57% with stent *v* 24% with PTA alone; P < 0.001; > 50% stenosis on follow up angiography: 32% with stent *v* 74% with PTA alone; P < 0.001; repeat procedures: 22% with stent *v* 42% with PTA alone; P = 0.03).[131] The second RCT (110 people) found that stents compared with PTA alone reduced restenosis and repeat procedures after 9 months (restenosis: 32% with stent *v* 68%; with PTA alone; P < 0.001; repeat procedures: 5% with stent *v* 22% with PTA alone; P = 0.04).[132] The third RCT (110 people) found that stents versus PTA alone reduced restenosis and repeat PTA after 4 months (restenosis: 26% with stent *v* 62% with PTA alone; P = 0.01; repeat PTA: 24% with stent *v* 55% with PTA alone; P = 0.05). No deaths or coronary artery bypass grafting operations occurred in either group. The incidence of myocardial infarction was low in both groups (0% with stent *v* 2% with PTA alone, P > 0.05).[133] **For treatment of restenosis after initial percutaneous transluminal angioplasty:** We found one RCT (383 people) of coronary stent versus PTA alone for treatment of restenosis. It found that stents versus PTA alone reduced restenosis and repeat procedures, and increased survival free of myocardial infarction and repeat revascularisation after 6 months (restenosis: 18% with stent *v* 32% with PTA alone; P = 0.03; repeat procedures: 10% with stent *v* 27% with PTA alone; P = 0.001; survival free of myocardial infarction or repeat revascularisation: 84% with stent *v* 72% with PTA alone; P = 0.04).[134]

Harms: Initially, aggressive combination antithrombotic and anticoagulant regimens were used after stenting because of a high incidence of stent thrombosis and myocardial infarction. These regimens led to a high incidence of arterial access site haemorrhage.[124] More recently, improved stent techniques and use of aspirin and ticlopidine have reduced both stent thrombosis and arterial access site haemorrhage.[130,134] Currently, the risk of stent thrombosis is less than 1%.[135–137] Haemorrhage (particularly femoral artery haemorrhage) was more frequent after stenting than PTA alone,[138] but occurred in less than 3% after stenting when antiplatelet drugs were used without long term anticoagulants.

Comment: It is unclear whether stenting influences the relative benefits and harms of percutaneous procedures compared with coronary artery bypass grafting. Coronary stents are associated with fewer repeat revascularisation procedures and less angiographic restenosis than PTA. Rates of death and myocardial infarction are low in the RCTs and are not significantly different between stents and PTA. However, any potential differences may be masked by the crossover to stents after poor results (such as dissection) immediately after PTA.

GLOSSARY

International normalised ratio (INR) A value derived from a standardised laboratory test that measures the effect of an anticoagulant. The laboratory materials used in the test are calibrated against internationally accepted standard reference preparations, so that variability between laboratories and different reagents is minimised. Normal blood has an INR of 1. Therapeutic anticoagulation often aims to achieve an INR value of 2.0–3.5.

REFERENCES

1. Greaves EJ, Gillum BS. 1994 Summary: national hospital discharge survey. Advance data from Vital and Health Statistics, no. 278. Hyattsville, Maryland, USA: National Center for Health Statistics, 1996.

2. Shaw LJ, Peterson ED, Kesler K, et al. A meta-analysis of predischarge risk stratification after acute myocardial infarction with stress electrocardiographic, myocardial perfusion, and ventricular function imaging. Am J Cardiol 1996;78:1327–1337. Search date 1995; primary sources Medline and hand searches of bibliographies of review articles.

3. Kudenchuk PJ, Maynard C, Martin JS, et al. Comparison, presentation, treatment and outcome of acute myocardial infarction in men versus women (the myocardial infarction triage and intervention registry). Am J Cardiol 1996;78:9–14.

4. The Task Force on the Management of Acute Myocardial Infarction of the European Society of Cardiology. Acute myocardial infarction: pre-hospital and in-hospital management. Eur Heart J 1996;17:43–63.

5. Peterson ED, Shaw LJ, Califf RM. Clinical guideline: part II. Risk stratification after myocardial infarction. Ann Intern Med 1997;126:561–582.

6. The Multicenter Postinfarction Research Group. Risk stratification and survival after myocardial infarction. N Engl J Med 1983;309:331–336.

7. American College of Cardiology/American Heart Association Task Force on Practice Guidelines (Committee on Exercise Testing). ACC/AHA guidelines for exercise testing. J Am Coll Cardiol 1997;30:260–315.

8. Fallen E, Cairns J, Dafoe W, et al. Management of the postmyocardial infarction patient: a consensus report — revision of the 1991 CCS guidelines. Can J Cardiol 1995;11:477–486.

9. Madsen JK, Grande P, Saunamaki K, et al. Danish multicenter randomized study of invasive versus conservative treatment in patients with inducible ischemia after thrombolysis in acute myocardial infarction (DANAMI). DANish trial in Acute Myocardial Infarction. Circulation 1997;96:748–755.

10. Antithrombotic Trialists' Collaboration. Collaborative meta-analysis of randomised trials of antiplatelet therapy for prevention of death, myocardial infarction and stroke in high risk patients. BMJ 2002;324:71–86. Search date 1997; primary sources Medline, Embase, Derwent, Scisearch, and Biosis, in additional trials registers of Cochrane Stroke and Peripheral Vascular Diseases Group, hand searches of journals, abstracts, and conference proceedings, and contact with experts.

11. Taylor DW, Barnett HJM, Haynes RB, et al. Low-dose and high-dose acetylsalicylic acid for patients undergoing carotid endarterectomy: a randomised controlled trial. Lancet 1999;353:2179–2184.

12. He J, Whelton PK, Vu B, et al. Aspirin and risk of hemorrhagic stroke. A meta-analysis of randomised controlled trials. JAMA 1998;280:1930–1935.

13. Farrell B, Godwin J, Richards S, et al. The United Kingdom transient ischaemic attack (UK TIA) aspirin trial: final results. J Neurol Neurosurg Psychiatry 1991;54:1044–1054.

14. Dutch TIA Trial Study Group. A comparison of two doses of aspirin (30 mg vs 283 mg a day) in patients after a transient ischemic attack or minor ischemic stroke. N Engl J Med 1991;325:1261–1266.

15. Thrift AG, McNeil JJ, Forbes A, et al. Risk factors for cerebral hemorrhage in the era of well-controlled hypertension. Melbourne Risk Factor Study (MERFS) Group. Stroke 1996;27:2020–2025.

16. Iso H, Hennekens CH, Stampfer MJ, et al. Prospective study of aspirin use and risk of stroke in women. Stroke 1999;30:1764–1771.

17. Derry S, Loke YK. Risk of gastrointestinal haemorrhage with long term use of aspirin: meta-analysis. BMJ 2000;321:1183–1187. Search date 1999; primary sources Medline, Embase, and reference lists of existing systematic reviews.

18. García Rodríguez LA, Hernández–Díaz S, de Abajo FJ. Association between aspirin and upper gastrointestinal complications. Systematic review of epidemiologic studies. Br J Clin Pharmacol 2001;52:563–571.

19. CAPRIE Steering Committee. A randomised, blinded, trial of clopidogrel versus aspirin in patients at risk of ischaemic events. Lancet 1996;348:1329–1339.

20. Scrutinio D, Cimminiello C, Marubini E, et al. Ticlopidine versus aspirin after myocardial infarction (STAMI) trial. J Am Coll Cardiol 2001;37:1259–1265.

21. Hankey GJ, Sudlow CLM, Dunbabin DW. Thienopyridine derivatives (ticlopidine, clopidogrel) versus aspirin for preventing stroke and other serious vascular events in high vascular risk patients. In: The Cochrane Library, Issue 2, 2002. Oxford: Update Software. Search date 1999; primary sources Medline, Embase, Cochrane Stroke Group Register, Antithrombotics Trialists' database, authors of trials, and drug manufacturers.

22. Moloney BA. An analysis of the side effects of ticlopidine. In: Hass WK, Easton JD, eds. Ticlopidine, platelets and vascular disease. New York: Springer, 1993:117–139.

23. Bennett CL, Davidson CJ, Raisch DW, et al. Thrombotic thrombocytopenic purpura associated with ticlopidine in the setting of coronary artery stents and stroke prevention. Arch Int Med 1999;159:2524–2528.

24. Bennett CL, Connors JM, Carwile JM, et al. Thrombotic thrombocytopenic purpura associated with clopidogrel. N Engl J Med 2000;342:1773–1777.

25. Hankey GJ. Clopidogrel and thrombotic thrombocytopenic purpura. *Lancet* 2000;356:269–270.

26. Müller C, Büttner HJ, Petersen J, et al. A randomized comparison of clopidogrel and aspirin versus ticlopidine and aspirin after the placement of coronary-artery stents. *Circulation* 2000;101:590–593.

27. Bertrand ME, Rupprecht H-J, Urban P, et al, for the CLASSICS Investigators. Double-blind study of the safety of clopidogrel with and without a loading dose in combination with aspirin compared with ticlopidine in combination with aspirin after coronary stenting. The Clopidogrel Aspirin Stent International Cooperative Study (CLASSICS). *Circulation* 2000;102:624–629.

28. Taniuchi M, Kurz HI, Lasala JM. Randomized comparison of ticlopidine and clopidogrel after intracoronary stent implantation in a broad patient population. *Circulation* 2001;104:539–543.

29. The Clopidogrel in Unstable Angina to Prevent Recurrent Events (CURE) Trial Investigators. Effects of clopidogrel in addition to aspirin in patients with acute coronary syndromes without ST-segment elevation. *N Engl J Med* 2001;345:494–502.

30. Second Chinese Cardiac Study (CCS-2) Collaborative Group. Rationale, design and organisation of the Second Chinese Cardiac Study (CCS-2): a randomised trial of clopidogrel plus aspirin, and of metoprolol, among patients with suspected acute myocardial infarction. *J Cardiovasc Risk* 2000;7:435–441.

31. Chew DP, Bhatt DL, Sapp S, et al. Increased mortality with oral platelet glycoprotein IIb/IIIa antagonists. *Circulation* 2001;103:201–206. Search date 2000; primary source Medline.

32. SoRelle R. SmithKline Beecham halts tests of lotrafiban, an oral glycoprotein IIb/IIIa inhibitor. *Circulation* 2001;103:E9001–9002.

33. Anand SS, Yusuf S. Oral anticoagulant therapy in patients with coronary artery disease: a meta-analysis. *JAMA* 1999;282:2058–2067. Search date 1999; primary sources Medline, Embase, Current Contents, hand searches of reference lists, experts, and pharmaceutical companies.

34. The Organization to Assess Strategies for Ischemic Syndromes (OASIS) Investigators. Effects of long-term, moderate intensity oral anticoagulation in addition to aspirin in unstable angina. *J Am Coll Cardiol* 2001;37:475–484.

35. Fiore LD, Ezekowitz MD, Brophy MT, et al, for the Combination Hemotherapy and Mortality Prevention (CHAMP) Study Group. Department of Veterans Affairs Cooperative Studies Program clinical trial comparing combined warfarin and aspirin alone in survivors of acute myocardial infarction. Primary results of the CHAMP study. *Circulation* 2002;105:557–563.

36. Huynh T, Theroux P, Bogaty P, et al. Aspirin, warfarin, or the combination for secondary prevention of coronary events in patients with acute coronary syndromes and prior coronary artery bypass surgery. *Circulation* 2001;103:3069–3074.

37. Teo KK, Yusuf S, Furberg CD. Effects of prophylactic antiarrhythmic drug therapy in acute myocardial infarction. *JAMA* 1993;270:1589–1595. Search date 1993; primary sources Medline, hand searches of reference lists, and details of unpublished trials sought from pharmaceutical industry/other investigators.

38. Yusuf S, Peto R, Lewis J, et al. Beta blockade during and after myocardial infarction: an overview of the randomized trials. *Prog Cardiovasc Dis* 1985;27:335–371. Search date and primary sources not stated.

39. Pepine CJ, Cohn PF, Deedwania PC, et al. Effects of treatment on outcome in mildly symptomatic patients with ischemia during daily life: the atenolol silent ischemia study (ASIST). *Circulation* 1994;90:762–768.

40. Boissel J-P, Leizerovicz A, Picolet H, et al. Secondary prevention after high-risk acute myocardial infarction with low-dose acebutolol. *Am J Cardiol* 1990;66:251–260.

41. The Beta-Blocker Pooling Project Research Group. The Beta-Blocker Pooling Project (BBPP): subgroup findings from randomized trials in post infarction patients. *Eur Heart J* 1988;9:8–16. Search date 1983; primary sources not stated.

42. Beta-blocker Heart Attack Trial Research Group. A randomized trial of propranolol in patients with acute myocardial infarction: I. mortality results. *JAMA* 1982;247:1707–1714.

43. Flather MD, Yusuf S, Kober L, et al. Long-term ACE-inhibitor therapy in patients with heart failure or left-ventricular dysfunction: a systematic overview of data from individual patients. ACE-Inhibitor Myocardial Infarction Collaborative Group. *Lancet* 2000 6;355:1575–81. Search date not stated; primary sources Medline, hand searches of reference lists, and contact with experts.

44. The Heart Outcomes Prevention Evaluation (HOPE) Investigators. Effects of an angiotensin-converting enzyme inhibitor, ramipril, on cardiovascular events in high-risk patients. *N Engl J Med* 2000;342:145–153.

45. Heart Outcomes Prevention Evaluation (HOPE) Investigators. Effects of ramipril on cardiovascular and microvascular outcomes on people with diabetes mellitus: results of the hope study and MICRO-HOPE substudy. *Lancet* 2000;355:253–259.

46. Yusuf S, Lonn E. Anti-ischaemic effects of ACE inhibitors: review of current clinical evidence and ongoing clinical trials. *Eur Heart J* 1998;19:J36–J44.

47. Echt DS, Liebson PR, Mitchell LB, et al. Mortality and morbidity in patients receiving encainide, flecainide, or placebo. The Cardiac Arrhythmia Suppression Trial. *N Engl J Med* 1991;324:781–788.

48. Amiodarone Trials Meta-Analysis Investigators. Effect of prophylactic amiodarone on mortality after acute myocardial infarction and in congestive heart failure: meta-analysis of individual data from 6500 patients in randomised trials. *Lancet* 1997;350:1417–1424. Search date and primary sources not stated.

49. Sim I, McDonald KM, Lavori PW, et al. Quantitative overview of randomized trials of amiodarone to prevent sudden cardiac death. *Circulation* 1997;96:2823–2829. Search date 1997; primary sources Medline and Biosis.

50. Waldo AL, Camm AJ, de Ruyter H, et al, for the SWORD Investigators. Effect of d-sotalol on mortality in patients with left ventricular dysfunction after recent and remote myocardial infarction. *Lancet* 1996;348:7–12.

51. Cairns JA, Connolly SJ, Roberts R, et al, for the Canadian Amiodarone Myocardial Infarction Arrhythmia Trial Investigators. Randomized trial of outcome after myocardial infarction in patients with frequent or repetitive ventricular premature depolarisations: CAMIAT. *Lancet* 1997;349:675–682.

52. Julian DG, Camm AJ, Janse MJ, et al, for the European Myocardial Infarct Amiodarone Trial Investigators. Randomised trial of effect of

amiodarone on mortality in patients with left-ventricular dysfunction after recent myocardial infarction: EMIAT. *Lancet* 1997;349:667–674.

53. Gibson R, Boden WE, Theroux P, et al. Diltiazem and reinfarction in patients with non-Q-wave myocardial infarction. Results of a double-blind, randomized, multicenter trial. *N Engl J Med* 1986;315:423–429.

54. The Multicenter Diltiazem Postinfarction Trial Research Group. The effect of diltiazem on mortality and reinfarction after myocardial infarction. *N Engl J Med* 1988;319:385–392.

55. The Danish Study Group on Verapamil in Myocardial Infarction. Effect of verapamil on mortality and major events after acute myocardial infarction: the Danish verapamil infarction trial II (DAVIT II). *Am J Cardiol* 1990;66:779–785.

56. Hulley S, Grady D, Bush T, et al. Randomized trial of estrogen plus progestin for secondary prevention of coronary heart disease in postmenopausal women. *JAMA* 1998;280:605–613.

57. Coronary Drug Project Research Group. The coronary drug project: initial findings leading to modifications of its research protocol. *JAMA* 1970;214:1303–1313.

58. Daly E, Vessey MP, Hawkins MM, et al. Risk of venous thromboembolism in users of hormone replacement therapy. *Lancet* 1996;348:977–980.

59. Newton KM, LaCroix AZ, McKnight B, et al. Estrogen replacement therapy and prognosis after first myocardial infarction. *Am J Epidemiol* 1997;145:269–277.

60. Sullivan JM, El-Zeky F, Vander Zwaag R, et al. Effect on survival of estrogen replacement therapy after coronary artery bypass grafting. *Am J Cardiol* 1997;79:847–850.

61. The Writing Group for the PEPI Trial. Effects of estrogen or estrogen/progestin regimens on heart disease risk factors in postmenopausal women. *JAMA* 1995;273:199–208.

62. Bucher HC, Griffith LE, Guyatt G. Systematic review on the risk and benefit of different cholesterol-lowering interventions. *Arterioscler Thromb Vasc Biol* 1999;19:187–195. Search date 1996; primary sources Medline, Embase, and bibliographic searches.

63. Miettinen TA, Pyorala K, Olsson AG, et al. Cholesterol-lowering therapy in women and elderly patients with myocardial infarction or angina pectoris: findings from the Scandinavian Simvastatin Survival Study (4S). *Circulation* 1997;96:4211–4218.

64. Heart Protection Study Collaborative Group. MRC/BHF Heart Protection Study of cholesterol lowering with simvastatin in 20 536 high-risk individuals: a randomised placebo-controlled trial. *Lancet* 2002;360:7M–22M.

65. LaRosa JC, He J, Vupputuri S. Effect of statins on risk of coronary disease: a meta-analysis of randomized controlled trials. *JAMA* 1999;282:2340–2346. Search date 1998; primary sources Medline, bibliographies, and authors' reference files.

66. Schwartz GG, Olsson AG, Ezekowitz MD, et al. Effects of atorvastatin on early recurrent ischemic events in acute coronary syndromes: the MIRACL study: a randomized controlled trial. *JAMA* 2001;285:1711–1718.

67. Knatterud GL, Rosenberg Y, Campeau L, et al. Long-term effects on clinical outcomes of aggressive lowering of low-density lipoprotein cholesterol levels and low-dose anticoagulation in the post coronary artery bypass graft trial. Post CABG Investigators. *Circulation* 2000;102:157–165.

68. Montagne O, Vedel I, Durand-Zaleski I. Assessment of the impact of fibrates and diet on survival and their cost-effectiveness: evidence from randomized, controlled trials in coronary heart disease and health economic evaluations. *Clin Ther* 1999;21:2027–2035. Search date not stated; primary sources Medline, hand searches of reference lists, and systematic reviews.

69. Schlesinger Z, Vered Z, Friedenson A, et al. Secondary prevention by raising HDL cholesterol and reducing triglycerides in patients with coronary artery disease: the Bezafibrate Infarction Prevention (BIP) study. *Circulation* 2000;102:21–27.

70. Ericsson CG, Hamsten A, Nilsson J, et al. Angiographic assessment of effects of bezafibrate on progression of coronary artery disease in young male postinfarction patients. *Lancet* 1996;347:849–853.

71. The Women's Health Initiative Study Group. Design of the women's health initiative clinical trial and observational study. *Control Clin Trials* 1998;19:61–109.

72. Davis BR, Cutler JA Gordon DJ, et al, for the ALLHAT Research Group. Rationale and design for the antihypertensive and lipid lowering treatment to prevent heart attack trial (ALLHAT). *Am J Hypertens* 1996;9:342–360.

73. Flack JM, Neaton J, Grimm R, et al. Blood pressure and mortality among men with prior myocardial infarction. *Circulation* 1995;92:2437–2445.

74. Dahlof B, Lindholm LH, Hansson L, et al. Morbidity and mortality in the Swedish trial in old patients with hypertension (STOP-hypertension). *Lancet* 1991;338:1281–1285.

75. Medical Research Council Working Party. MRC trial on treatment of hypertension in older adults: principal results. *BMJ* 1992;304:405–412.

76. Systolic Hypertension in Elderly Patients (SHEP) Cooperative Research Group. Prevention of stroke by antihypertensive treatment in older persons with isolated systolic hypertension. *JAMA* 1991;265:3255–3264.

77. D'Agostini RB, Belanger AJ, Kannel WB, et al. Relationship of low diastolic blood pressure to coronary heart disease death in presence of myocardial infarction: the Framingham study. *BMJ* 1991;303:385–389.

78. Pfeffer MA, Braunwald E, Moye LA, et al. Effect of captopril on mortality and morbidity in patients with left ventricular dysfunction after myocardial infarction: results of the survival and ventricular enlargement trial. *N Engl J Med* 1992;327:669–677.

79. NHS Centre for Reviews and Dissemination, University of York. Cholesterol and coronary heart disease: screening and treatment. *Eff Health Care* 1998;4:1. Search date and primary sources not stated.

80. Burr ML, Fehily AM, Gilbert JF, et al. Effects of changes in fat, fish, and fibre intakes on death and myocardial reinfarction: Diet And Reinfarction Trial (DART). *Lancet* 1989;2:757–761.

81. Fehily AM, Vaughan-Williams E, Shiels K, et al. The effect of dietary advice on nutrient intakes: evidence from the Diet And Reinfarction Trial (DART). *J Hum Nutr Diet* 1989;2:225–235.

82. GISSI-Prevenzione Investigators. Dietary supplementation with n–3 polyunsaturated fatty acids and vitamin E after myocardial infarction: results of the GISSI-Prevenzione. *Lancet* 1999;354:447–455.

83. De Lorgeril M, Renaud S, Mamelle N, et al. Mediterranean alpha-linolenic acid-rich diet in secondary prevention of coronary heart disease. *Lancet* 1994;343:1454–1459.

84. Clarke R, Frost C, Collins R, et al. Dietary lipids and blood cholesterol: quantitative meta-analysis of metabolic ward studies. *BMJ* 1997;314:112–117. Search date 1995; primary sources Medline, and hand searches of reference lists and nutrition journals.

85. Tang JL, Armitage JM, Lancaster T, et al. Systematic review of dietary intervention trials to lower blood total cholesterol in free-living subjects. *BMJ* 1998;316:1213–1220. Search date 1997; primary sources Medline, Human Nutrition, Embase, and Allied and Alternative Medicine, hand searches the *Am J Clin Nutr*, and references of review articles.

86. Brunner E, White I, Thorogood M, et al. Can dietary interventions change diet and cardiovascular risk factors? A meta-analysis of randomized controlled trials. *Am J Public Health* 1997;87:1415–1422. Search date 1993; primary sources Medline and hand searches of selected journals.

87. Ebrahim S, Davey SG. *Health promotion in older people for the prevention of coronary heart disease and stroke.* London: Health Education Authority, 1996.

88. Waters D. Lessons from coronary atherosclerosis "regression" trials. *Cardiol Clin* 1996;14:31–50.

89. Silagy C, Neil A. Garlic as a lipid lowering agent: a meta-analysis. *J R Coll Physicians Lond* 1994;28:39–45. Search date 1992; primary sources Medline, Alternative Medicine database, contact with authors of published studies, manufacturers, and hand searches of references.

90. Isaacson JL, Moser M, Stein EA, et al. Garlic powder and plasma lipids and lipoproteins. *Arch Intern Med* 1998;158:1189–119.

91. Berthold HK, Sudhop T, von Bergmann K. Effect of a garlic oil preparation on serum lipoproteins and cholesterol metabolism. *JAMA* 1998;279:1900–1902.

92. Ripsin CM, Keenan JM, Jacobs DR Jr, et al. Oat products and lipid lowering: a meta-analysis. *JAMA* 1992;267:3317–3325. Search date 1991; primary sources Medline and unpublished trials solicited from all known investigators of lipid–oats association.

93. Stephens NG, Parsons A, Schofield PM, et al. Randomised controlled trial of vitamin E in patients with coronary disease: Cambridge Heart Antioxidant Study (CHAOS). *Lancet* 1996;347:781–786.

94. Rapola JM, Virtamo J, Ripatti S, et al. Randomised trial of alpha-tocopherol and beta-carotene supplements on incidence of major coronary events in men with previous myocardial infarction. *Lancet* 1997;349:1715–1720.

95. The Heart Outcomes Prevention Evaluation Study Investigators. Vitamin E supplementation and cardiovascular events in high-risk patients. The Heart Outcomes Prevention Evaluation Study Investigators. *N Engl J Med* 2000;342:154–160.

96. Boaz M, Smetana S, Weinstein T, et al. Secondary prevention with antioxidants of cardiovascular disease in endstage renal disease (SPACE): randomised placebo-controlled trial. *Lancet* 2000;356:1213–1218.

97. Wilson TS, Datta SB, Murrell JS, et al. Relation of vitamin C levels to mortality in a geriatric hospital: a study of the effect of vitamin C administration. *Age Aging* 1973;2:163–170.

98. Burr ML, Hurley RJ, Sweetnam PM. Vitamin C supplementation of old people with low blood levels. *Gerontol Clin* 1975;17:236–243.

99. Hunt C, Chakkravorty NK, Annan G. The clinical and biochemical effects of vitamin C supplementation in short-stay hospitalized geriatric patients. *Int J Vitam Nutr Res* 1984;54:65–74.

100. Brown BG, Zhao X-Q, Chait A, et al. Simvastatin and niacin, antioxidant vitamins, or the combination for the prevention of coronary disease. *N Engl J Med* 2001;345:1583–1592.

101. Lonn EM, Yusuf S. Is there a role for antioxidant vitamins in the prevention of cardiovascular diseases? An update on epidemiological and clinical trials data. *Can J Cardiol* 1997;13:957–965. Search date 1996; primary sources Medline and one reference from 1997.

102. Jha P, Flather M, Lonn E, et al. The antioxidant vitamins and cardiovascular disease: a critical review of epidemiologic and clinical trial data. *Ann Intern Med* 1995;123:860–872.

103. Ness AR, Powles JW, Khaw KT. Vitamin C and cardiovascular disease: a systematic review. *J Cardiovasc Risk* 1997;3:513–521. Search date not stated; primary sources Medline, experts, and hand searches of references.

104. Collins R, Peto R, Armitage J. The MRC/BHF heart protection study: preliminary results. *Int J Clin Pract* 2002;56:53.

105. Jolliffe JA, Rees K, Taylor RS, et al. Exercise-based rehabilitation for coronary heart disease. In: The Cochrane Library, Issue 2, 2002. Oxford: Update Software. Search date 1998; primary sources Cardiovascular RCT register at McMaster University, Cochrane Controlled Trials Register, Medline, Embase, Cinahl, Amed, Bids, ISI, and Sportsdiscus, hand searches of reference lists, conference proceedings, and contact with experts.

106. Wenger NK, Froelicher NS, Smith LK, et al. *Cardiac rehabilitation and secondary prevention.* Rockville, Maryland: Agency for Health Care Policy and Research and National Heart, Lung and Blood Institute, 1995. Search date and primary source not stated.

107. US Department of Health and Human Services. *The health benefits of smoking cessation: a report of the surgeon general.* Bethesda, Maryland: US DHSS, 1990.

108. Working Group for the Study of Transdermal Nicotine in Patients with Coronary Artery Disease. Nicotine replacement therapy for patients with coronary artery disease. *Arch Intern Med* 1994;154:989–995.

109. Joseph AM, Norman SM, Ferry LH, et al. The safety of transdermal nicotine as an aid to smoking cessation in patients with cardiac disease. *N Engl J Med* 1996;335:1792–1798.

110. Burt A, Thornley P, Illingworth D, et al. Stopping smoking after myocardial infarction. *Lancet* 1974;1:304–306.

111. Linden W, Stossel C, Maurice J. Psychosocial interventions in patients with coronary artery disease: a meta-analysis. *Arch Intern Med* 1996;156:745–752. Search date and primary sources not stated.

112. US Department of Health and Human Services. Cardiac rehabilitation. AHCPR Publication No 96–0672, 1995;121–128.

113. Hemingway H, Marmot M. Psychosocial factors in the primary and secondary prevention of coronary heart disease: a systematic review. In: Yusuf S, Cairns JA, Camm AJ, et al, eds. *Evidence based cardiology.* London: BMJ Books, 1998. Search date 1996; primary sources Medline, and manual searches of bibliographies of retrieved articles and review articles.

114. Yusuf S, Zucker D, Peduzzi P, et al. Effect of coronary artery bypass graft surgery on survival: overview of 10-year results from randomized trials by the Coronary Artery Bypass Graft Surgery Trialists Collaboration. *Lancet* 1994;344:563–570. Search date and primary sources not stated.

115. Davies RF, Goldberg AD, Forman S, et al. Asymptomatic Cardiac Ischemia Pilot (ACIP) study two year follow up: outcomes of patients randomized to initial strategies of medical therapy versus revascularization. *Circulation* 1997;95:2037–2043.

116. Bucher HC, Hengstler P, Schindler C, et al. Percutaneous transluminal coronary angioplasty versus medical treatment for non-acute coronary heart disease: meta-analysis of randomised controlled trials. *BMJ* 2000;321:73–77. Search date 1998; primary sources Medline, Embase, Cochrane Library, Biological Abstracts, Health Periodicals Database, Pascal, and hand searches of references.

117. Pocock SJ, Henderson RA, Clayton T, et al. Quality of life after coronary angioplasty or continued medical treatment for angina: three-year follow-up in the RITA-2 trial. Randomized Intervention Treatment of Angina. *J Am Coll Cardiol* 2000;35:907–914.

118. TIME investigators. Trial of invasive versus medical therapy in elderly patients with chronic symptomatic coronary-artery disease (TIME): a randomised trial. *Lancet* 2001;358:951–957.

119. RITA-2 Trial Participants. Coronary angioplasty versus medical therapy for angina: the second randomized intervention treatment of angina (RITA-2) trial. *Lancet* 1997;350:461–468.

120. Parisi AF, Folland ED, Hartigan P. A comparison of angioplasty with medical therapy in the treatment of single-vessel coronary artery disease. *N Engl J Med* 1992;326:10–16.

121. Morris KG, Folland ED, Hartigan PM, et al. Unstable angina in late follow-up of the ACME trial. *Circulation* 1995;92(suppl S):3484.

122. Pocock SJ, Henderson RA, Rickards AF, et al. Meta-analysis of randomized trials comparing coronary angioplasty with bypass surgery. *Lancet* 1995;346:1184–1189. Search date and primary sources not stated.

123. Rihal CS, Gersh BJ, Yusuf S. Chronic coronary artery disease: coronary artery bypass surgery vs percutaneous transluminal coronary angioplasty vs medical therapy. In: Yusuf S, Cairns JA, Camm JA, et al. eds. *Evidence based cardiology.* London: BMJ Books, 1998.

124. King SB, Kosinski AS, Guyton RA, et al. Eight-year mortality in the Emory Angioplasty versus Surgery Trial (EAST). *J Am Coll Cardiol* 2000;35:1116–1121.

125. Hlatky MA, Rogers WJ, Johnstone I, et al. Medical care costs and quality of life after randomization to coronary angioplasty or coronary bypass surgery. *N Engl J Med* 1997;336:92–99.

126. Währborg P. Quality of life after coronary angioplasty or bypass surgery. *Eur Heart J* 1999;20:653–658.

127. Bypass Angioplasty Revascularization Investigation (BARI) Investigators. Comparison of coronary bypass surgery with angioplasty in patients with multivessel disease. *N Engl J Med* 1996;335:217–225.

128. The BARI Investigators. Seven-year outcome in the Bypass Angioplasty Revascularization Investigation (BARI) by treatment and diabetic status. *J Am Coll Cardiol* 2000;35:1122–1129.

129. National Institute of Clinical Excellence http://www.nice.org.uk/pdf/HTAReport-Stents.pdf (last accessed 19 September 2002). Search date 1999; primary sources Medline, Embase, Bids, Cochrane Library, and York HTA.

130. Savage MP, Douglas JS Jr, Fischman DL, et al. Stent placement compared with balloon angioplasty for obstructed coronary bypass grafts. *N Engl J Med* 1997;337:740–747.

131. Sirnes P, Golf S, Yngvar M, et al. Stenting In Chronic Coronary Occlusion (SICCO): a randomized controlled trial of adding stent implantation after successful angioplasty. *J Am Coll Cardiol* 1996;28:1444–1451.

132. Rubartelli P, Niccoli L, Verna E, et al. Stent implantation versus balloon angioplasty in chronic coronary occlusions: results from the GISSOC trial. Gruppo Italiano di Studio sullo Stent nelle Occlusioni Coronariche. *J Am Coll Cardiol* 1998;32:90–96.

133. Sievert H, Rohde S, Utech A, et al. Stent or Angioplasty after Recanalization of Chronic Coronary Occlusions? (The SARECCO trial). *Am J Cardiol* 1999;84:386–390.

134. Erbel R, Haude M, Hopp HW, et al. Coronary artery stenting compared with balloon angioplasty for restenosis after initial balloon angioplasty. *N Engl J Med* 1998;23:1672–1688.

135. Versaci F, Gaspardone A, Tomai F, et al. A comparison of coronary-artery stenting with angioplasty for isolated stenosis of the proximal left anterior descending coronary artery. *N Engl J Med* 1997;336:817–822.

136. Schomig A, Neumann FJ, Kastrati A, et al. A randomized comparison of antiplatelet and anticoagulation therapy after the placement of intracoronary stents. *N Engl J Med* 1996;334:1084–1089.

137. Leon MB, Baim DS, Gordon P, et al. Clinical and angiographic results from the Stent Anticoagulation Regimen Study (STARS). *Circulation* 1996;94(suppl S):4002.

138. Witkowski A, Ruzyllo W, Gil R, et al. A randomized comparison of elective high pressure stenting with balloon angioplasty: six-month angiographic and two-year clinical follow-up. *Am Heart J* 2000;140:264–271.

Cathie Sudlow
Wellcome Clinician Scientist
Western General Hospital
University of Edinburgh
Edinburgh, UK

Eva Lonn
Associate Professor of Medicine
Hamilton General Hospital
Hamilton, Canada

Secondary prevention of ischaemic cardiac events

Michael Pignone
Division of General Internal Medicine
University of North Carolina
Chapel Hill, USA

Andrew Ness
Senior Lecturer in Epidemiology
University of Bristol
Bristol, UK

Charanjit Rihal
Consultant Cardiologist
Mayo Clinic and Mayo Foundation
Rochester, USA

Competing interests: CR none declared. AN none declared. EL has reveived reimbursement for participating at symposiums, presentations of lectures and organising education activities for different pharmaceutical companies. CR none declared. CS on one occasion received fee from Sanofi-Synthelabo for giving a talk at a GP meeting.

| TABLE 1 | Prognostic groups for people who survive the acute stage of myocardial infarction (see text, p 193). |

Baseline risk	1 year mortality	Clinical markers[2-4]
High	10–50%	Older age; history or previous myocardial infarction; reduced exercise tolerance (New York Heart Association functional classes II–IV) before admission; clinical signs of heart failure in the first 2 days (Killip classes IIb, III, and IV) or persistent heart failure on days 3–5 after infarction; early increased heart rate; persistent or early appearance of angina at rest or with minimal exertion; and multiple or complex ventricular arrhythmias during monitoring in hospital.
Moderate	10%	ND
Low	2–5%	Younger age (< 55 years), no previous myocardial infarction, an event free course during the first 5 days after myocardial infarction.[2]

ND, no data.

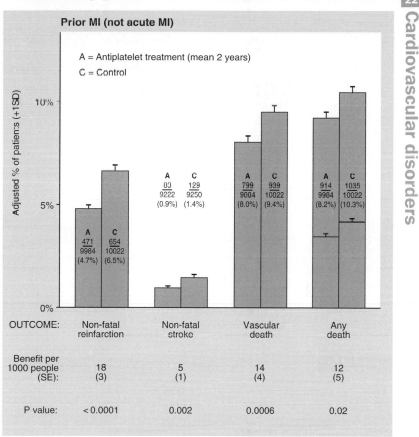

Prior MI (not acute MI)

A = Antiplatelet treatment (mean 2 years)
C = Control

OUTCOME:	Non-fatal reinfarction	Non-fatal stroke	Vascular death	Any death
Benefit per 1000 people (SE):	18 (3)	5 (1)	14 (4)	12 (5)
P value:	< 0.0001	0.002	0.0006	0.02

FIGURE 1 The absolute effects of antiplatelet treatment on various outcomes in people with prior myocardial infarction: results of a systematic review.[10] The columns show the absolute risks over 2 years for each outcome. The error bars represent standard deviations. In the "any death" column, non-vascular deaths are represented by lower horizontal lines (see text, p 194).

Secondary prevention of ischaemic cardiac events

Cardiovascular disorders

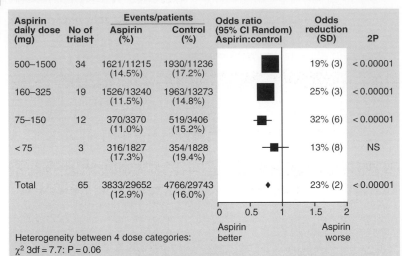

Aspirin daily dose (mg)	No of trials†	Events/patients		Odds ratio (95% CI Random) Aspirin:control	Odds reduction (SD)	2P
		Aspirin (%)	Control (%)			
500–1500	34	1621/11215 (14.5%)	1930/11236 (17.2%)		19% (3)	< 0.00001
160–325	19	1526/13240 (11.5%)	1963/13273 (14.8%)		25% (3)	< 0.00001
75–150	12	370/3370 (11.0%)	519/3406 (15.2%)		32% (6)	< 0.00001
< 75	3	316/1827 (17.3%)	354/1828 (19.4%)		13% (8)	NS
Total	65	3833/29652 (12.9%)	4766/29743 (16.0%)		23% (2)	< 0.00001

Heterogeneity between 4 dose categories:
χ^2 3df = 7.7: P = 0.06

† Some trials contributed to more than one daily dose category.

Typical odds ratio for each category shown as square (with area proportional to the variance of observed - expected) together with its 99% confidence interval (horizontal line). Typical odds ratio for the total shown as diamond with its 95% confidence interval (horizontal line = width of diamond). Vertical dotted line passes through point estimate of typical odds ratio for total.

FIGURE 2 Effects of different doses of aspirin (see text, p 194).

Key Messages

Acute ischaemic stroke

- **Acute reduction in blood pressure** One systematic review found insufficient evidence about the effects of antihypertensives versus placebo, but RCTs have suggested that people treated with antihypertensive agents may have a worse clinical outcome and increased mortality.

- **Aspirin** One systematic review in people with ischaemic stroke confirmed by computerised tomography scan has found that aspirin versus placebo within 48 hours of stroke onset significantly reduces death or dependency at 6 months (NNT 77, 95% CI 43 to 333) and significantly increases the number of people making a complete recovery (NNT 91, 95% CI 50 to 500). We found indirect evidence that aspirin should not be delayed if a computerised tomography scan is not available within 48 hours: results from two large RCTs found no significant difference in further stroke or death with aspirin versus placebo in people who were subsequently found to have haemorrhagic rather than ischaemic stroke.

- **Immediate systemic anticoagulation** One systematic review comparing systemic anticoagulants (unfractionated heparin, low molecular weight heparin, heparinoids, oral anticoagulants, or specific thrombin inhibitors) versus usual care without systemic anticoagulants found no significant difference in death or dependence after 3–6 months. One systematic review has found that immediate systemic anticoagulation significantly reduces the risk of deep venous thrombosis (NNT 3, 95% CI 2 to 4) and symptomatic pulmonary embolus (NNT 333, 95% CI 167 to 1000), but increases the risk of intracranial haemorrhage (NNH 108, 95% CI 85 to 147) or extracranial haemorrhage (NNH 109, 95% CI 87 to 149). One RCT in people with acute ischaemic stroke and atrial fibrillation found no significant difference with low molecular weight heparin versus aspirin in recurrent ischaemic stroke within 14 days. One RCT in people within 48 hours of stroke onset found no significant difference with high or low dose tinzaparin versus aspirin in people achieving functional independence at 6 months.

■ **Neuroprotective agents (calcium channel antagonists, γ-aminobutyric acid agonists, lubeluzole, glycine antagonists, tirilazad, N-methyl-D-aspartate antagonists)** RCTs found no evidence that, compared with placebo, calcium channel antagonists, tirilazad, lubeluzole, γ-aminobutyric acid agonists, glycine antagonists, or N-methyl-D-aspartate antagonists significantly improve clinical outcomes. One systematic review found that lubeluzole versus placebo was associated with a significant increase in the risk of having Q-T prolongation to more than 450 ms on electrocardiography (NNH 45, 95% CI 23 to 1000).

■ **Specialised care** One systematic review has found that specialist stroke rehabilitation units versus alternate (less organised) care significantly reduce death or dependency after 1 year (NNT 21, 95% CI 13 to 63).

■ **Thrombolysis** One systematic review has found that thrombolysis versus placebo significantly reduces the risk of death or dependency in the long term (NNT 24, 95% CI 14 to 83), but significantly increases the risk of death from intracranial haemorrhage measured in the first 7–10 days (NNH 23, 95% CI 19 to 29).

Intracerebral haematomas

■ **Evacuation** We found that the balance between benefits and harms has not been clearly established for the evacuation of supratentorial haematomas. We found no evidence from RCTs on the role of evacuation or ventricular shunting in people with infratentorial haematoma whose consciousness level is declining.

DEFINITION   Stroke is characterised by rapidly developing clinical symptoms and signs of focal, and at times global, loss of cerebral function lasting more than 24 hours or leading to death, with no apparent cause other than that of vascular origin.[1] Ischaemic stroke is stroke caused by vascular insufficiency (such as cerebrovascular thromboembolism) rather than haemorrhage.

INCIDENCE/ PREVALENCE   Stroke is the third most common cause of death in most developed countries.[2] It is a worldwide problem; about 4.5 million people die from stroke a year. Stroke can occur at any age, but half of all strokes occur in people over 70 years old.[3]

AETIOLOGY/ RISK FACTORS   About 80% of all acute strokes are caused by cerebral infarction, usually resulting from thrombotic or embolic occlusion of a cerebral artery.[4] The remainder are caused either by intracerebral or subarachnoid haemorrhage.

PROGNOSIS   About 10% of all people with acute ischaemic strokes will die within 30 days of stroke onset.[5] Of those who survive the acute event, about 50% will experience some level of disability after 6 months.[6]

AIMS	To minimise impairment, disability, secondary complications, and adverse effects from treatment.
OUTCOMES	Risk of death or dependency (generally assessed as the proportion of people dead or requiring physical assistance for transfers, mobility, dressing, feeding, or toileting 3–6 months after stroke onset);[6] quality of life.
METHODS	*Clinical Evidence* search and appraisal January 2002.

QUESTION What are the effects of specialised care in people with stroke?

One systematic review has found that specialist stroke rehabilitation units versus alternate (less organised) care significantly reduces death or dependency after 1 year. Prospective observational data suggest these findings may be reproducible in routine clinical settings.

Benefits: We found one systematic review (search date 2001, 23 RCTs, 4911 people with stroke) comparing specialised stroke rehabilitation versus conventional care.[7] In most trials, the specialised stroke rehabilitation unit consisted of a designated area or ward, although some trials used a mobile "stroke team". People in these trials were usually transferred to stroke unit care within the first or second week after stroke onset. It found people cared for in a stroke rehabilitation unit had lower rates of death or dependency after a median follow up of 1 year (AR 60.5% without stroke unit v 55.8% with stroke unit, ARR 4.7%, 95% CI 1.6% to 7.8%; NNT 21, 95% CI 13 to 63; OR 0.78, 95% CI 0.68 to 0.89) (see figure 1, p 243).[7] The duration of stay was calculated differently for many of the trials, so the consequent heterogeneity between results limits generalisability. However, overall, duration of stay in the stroke unit was about 6 days (95% CI 2 to 10 days) shorter than duration of stay in a non-stroke unit setting. The review found that organised stroke unit care versus alternate service significantly reduced death or dependency at 5 years' follow up (223/286 [78%] with organised stroke unit care v 214/249 [86%] with alternate care; RR 0.91, 95% CI 0.84 to 0.99).[7] One RCT (220 people) included in the review found that care in a combined acute and rehabilitation unit compared with care in general wards increased the proportion of people able to live at home 10 years after their stroke (ARI 11%, 95% CI 1.9% to 20%; NNT 9, 95% CI 5 to 52).[11] We found one additional RCT, which randomised 76 people 2–10 days after their stroke to either an integrated care pathway (see glossary, p 240) or to conventional multidisciplinary care on a stroke rehabilitation unit in the UK.[12] All received similar occupational and physical therapy. Conventional treatment versus the integrated care pathway produced more improvement in the Barthel Index from 4–12 weeks (CI not provided; $P < 0.01$), and higher scores on the Euroquol (Quality of Life Scale) after 6 months ($P < 0.05$). It found no significant difference between the two treatments in mortality, duration of hospital stay, or the proportion of people requiring long term institutional care.

Harms: No detrimental effects attributable to stroke units were reported.[7]

Stroke management

Cardiovascular disorders

Comment: Although the proportional reduction in death or dependency seems larger with thrombolysis (see thrombolysis option, p 232), stroke unit care is applicable to most people with stroke whereas thrombolysis is applicable only to a small proportion. The systematic review did not provide evidence about which aspects of the multidisciplinary approach led to improved outcome,[7] although one limited retrospective analysis of one of the RCTs found that several factors, including early mobilisation, increased use of oxygen, intravenous saline solutions, and antipyretics, might have been responsible.[13] Most of the trials excluded the most mild and severe strokes. After publication of the systematic review,[7] prospective observational data have been collected in one large series of over 14 000 people in 80 Swedish hospitals.[14] In this series, people admitted to stroke units had reduced dependence at 3 months (RRR 6%, 95% CI 1% to 11%). Although biases are inherent in such observational data, the findings suggest that the results of the meta-analysis may be reproducible in routine clinical settings.

QUESTION **What are the effects of medical treatment in acute ischaemic stroke?**

OPTION **THROMBOLYSIS**

One systematic review has found that thrombolysis versus placebo significantly reduces the risk of death or dependency in the long term, but significantly increases the risk of death from intracranial haemorrhage measured in the first 7–10 days.

Benefits: We found one systematic review (search date 1999, 17 RCTs, 5216 highly selected people) comparing thrombolysis with placebo given soon after the onset of stroke.[8] All trials used computerised tomography or magnetic resonance scanning before randomisation to exclude intracranial haemorrhage or other non-stroke disorders. Results for three different thrombolytic agents (streptokinase, urokinase, and recombinant tissue plasminogen activator) were included, but direct comparison of different thrombolytic drugs was not possible. Two trials used intra-arterial administration and the rest used the intravenous route. Thrombolysis significantly reduced the risk of death or dependency at the end of the studies (ARR 4.2%, 95% CI 1.2% to 7.2%; RRR 7%, 95% CI 3% to 12%; NNT 24, 95% CI 14 to 83) (see figure 1, p 243 and figure 2, p 243).[8] In the subset of trials that assessed intravenous recombinant tissue plasminogen activator, the findings were similar (ARR 5.7%, 95% CI 2.0% to 9.4%; RRR 10%, 95% CI 4% to 16%; NNT 18, 95% CI 11 to 50). One meta-analysis (4 RCTs, individual results of 1292 people with acute ischaemic stroke treated with streptokinase or placebo) found that streptokinase versus placebo had no clear effect on the proportion of people dead or dependent at 3 months, and included the possibility of both substantial benefit or substantial harm (RRR +1%, 95% CI –6% to +8%).[15] People allocated to streptokinase were more likely to be dead after 3 months (RRI 46%, 95% CI 24% to 73%). The combination of aspirin plus streptokinase significantly increased mortality at 3 months (P = 0.005), but this did not affect the combined risk of death or severe disability (CI not provided; P = 0.28).

Harms: **Fatal intracranial haemorrhage:** In the systematic review, thrombolysis increased fatal intracranial haemorrhage compared with placebo measured in the first 7–10 days (ARI 4.4%, 95% CI 3.4% to 5.4%; RRI 396%, 95% CI 220% to 668%; NNH 23, 95% CI 19 to 29).[8] In the subset of trials that assessed intravenous recombinant tissue plasminogen activator, the findings were similar (ARI 2.9%, 95% CI 1.7% to 4.1%; RRI 259%, 95% CI 102% to 536%; NNH 34, 95% CI 24 to 59). **Death:** In the systematic review, thrombolysis compared with placebo increased the risk of death by the end of the follow up (ARI 3.3%, 95% CI 1.2% to 5.4%; RRI 23%, 95% CI 10% to 38%; NNH 30, 95% CI 19 to 83).[8] This excess of deaths was offset by fewer people being alive but dependent 6 months after stroke onset. The net effect was a reduction in the number of people who were dead or dependent.

Comment: There was no significant heterogeneity of treatment effect overall, but heterogeneity of results was noted for the outcomes of death, and death or dependency at final follow up among the eight trials of intravenous recombinant tissue plasminogen activator.[8] Explanations may include the combined use of antithrombotic agents (aspirin or heparin within the first 24 h of thrombolysis), stroke severity, the presence of early ischaemic changes on computerised tomography scan, and the time from stroke onset to randomisation. A subgroup analysis suggested that thrombolysis may be more beneficial if given within 3 hours of symptom onset, but the duration of the "therapeutic time window" could not be determined reliably. Most of the trial results were of outcome at 3 months; only one trial reported 1 year outcome data.[16] We found little evidence about which people are most and least likely to benefit from thrombolysis. A number of trials of different thrombolytic regimens are underway.[17] In addition, preliminary information from a meta-analysis of individual patient data from the recombinant tissue plasminogen activator trials by the ECASS, NINDS, and ATLANTIS investigators was recently reported at a platform session of the 27th International Stroke Conference; full publication is awaited, and will be presented in future *Clinical Evidence* updates (B Thomas, personal communication, 2002).

OPTION	ASPIRIN

One systematic review in people with ischaemic stroke confirmed by computerised tomography scan has found that aspirin versus placebo within 48 hours of stroke onset significantly reduces death or dependency at 6 months and significantly increases the number of people making a complete recovery. We found indirect evidence that aspirin should not be delayed if a computerised tomography scan is not available within 48 hours; results from two large RCTs found no significant difference in further stroke or death with aspirin versus placebo in people who were subsequently found to have haemorrhagic rather than ischaemic stroke.

Cardiovascular disorders

Stroke management

Benefits: **Early use of aspirin:** We found one systematic review (search date 1999, 8 RCTs, 41 325 people with definite or presumed ischaemic stroke), which compared antiplatelet treatment started within 14 days of the stroke versus placebo.[18] Of the data in the systematic review, 98% came from two large RCTs of aspirin (160–300 mg daily) started within 48 hours of stroke onset.[9,10] Most people had an ischaemic stroke confirmed by computerised tomography scan before randomisation, but people who were conscious could be randomised before computerised tomography scan if the stroke was very likely to be ischaemic on clinical grounds. Treatment duration varied from 10–28 days. Aspirin started within the first 48 hours of acute ischaemic stroke reduced death or dependency at 6 months' follow up (RRR 3%, 95% CI 1% to 5%; NNT 77, 95% CI 43 to 333) (see figure 1, p 243) and increased the number of people making a complete recovery (NNT 91, 95% CI 50 to 500). A prospective combined analysis[19] of the two large RCTs[9,10] found a significant reduction in the outcome of further stroke or death with aspirin versus placebo (ARR 0.9%, 95% CI 0.75% to 1.85%; NNT 111, 95% CI 54 to 133). The effect was similar across subgroups (older *v* younger; male *v* female; impaired consciousness or not; atrial fibrillation or not; blood pressure; stroke subtype; timing of computerised tomography scanning). For the 773 people subsequently found to have had a haemorrhagic stroke rather than an ischaemic stroke, the subgroup analysis found no difference in the outcome of further stroke or death between those who were randomised to aspirin versus placebo (16% *v* 18%; ARR +2.0%, 95% CI −4.0% to +6.6%).[19] **Long term treatment:** See aspirin under stroke prevention, p 244.

Harms: Aspirin caused an excess of about two intracranial and four extracranial haemorrhages per 1000 people treated, but these small risks were more than offset by the reductions in death and disability from other causes both in the short term[18] and in the long term.[20] Common adverse effects of aspirin (such as dyspepsia and constipation) were dose related.[21]

Comment: We found no clear evidence that any one dose of aspirin is more effective than any other in the treatment of acute ischaemic stroke. One recent meta-regression analysis of the dose–response effect of aspirin on stroke found a uniform effect of aspirin in a range of doses from 50–1500 mg daily.[22] People unable to swallow safely after a stroke may be given aspirin as a suppository.

| OPTION | IMMEDIATE SYSTEMIC ANTICOAGULATION |

One systematic review comparing systemic anticoagulants (unfractionated heparin, low molecular weight heparin, heparinoids, oral anticoagulants, or specific thrombin inhibitors) versus usual care without systemic anticoagulants has found no significant difference in death or dependence after 3–6 months. One systematic review has found that immediate systemic anticoagulation significantly reduces the risk of deep venous thrombosis and symptomatic pulmonary embolus, but increases the risk of intracranial haemorrhage or extracranial haemorrhage. One RCT in people with acute ischaemic stroke and atrial fibrillation found no significant difference with low molecular weight heparin versus aspirin in

recurrent ischaemic stroke within 14 days. One RCT in people within 48 hours of stroke onset found no significant difference with high or low dose tinzaparin versus aspirin in people achieving functional independence at 6 months.

Benefits:

Death or dependency: We found one systematic review (search date 1999, 21 RCTs, 23 427 people)[23] and three subsequent RCTs.[24–26] The systematic review compared unfractionated heparin, low molecular weight heparin, heparinoids, oral anticoagulants, or specific thrombin inhibitors versus usual care without systemic anticoagulants.[23] Over 80% of the data came from one trial, which randomised people with any severity of stroke to either subcutaneous heparin or placebo, usually after exclusion of haemorrhage by computerised tomography scan.[10] The systematic review found no significant difference in the proportion of people dead or dependent in the treatment and control groups at the end of follow up (3–6 months after the stroke: ARR +0.4%, 95% CI −0.9% to +1.7%; RRR 0%, 95% CI −2% to +3%).[23] There was no clear short or long term benefit of anticoagulants in any prespecified subgroups (stroke of presumed cardioembolic origin v others; different anticoagulants). The first subsequent RCT (449 people with acute stroke and atrial fibrillation) found no significant difference between dalteparin (a low molecular weight heparin) versus aspirin for the primary outcome of recurrent ischaemic stroke during the first 14 days (ARI +1.0%, 95% CI −3.6% to +6.2%) or for secondary outcomes, including functional outcome at 3 months.[24] The second RCT randomised 404 people to one of four different doses of certoparin (a low molecular weight heparin) within 12 hours of stroke onset.[25] There was no difference in neurological outcome between the four groups 3 months after treatment. The third RCT (1486 people) compared aspirin versus two different doses of tinzaparin (a low molecular weight heparin) within 48 hours of stroke onset.[26] It found no significant difference among the three groups for achieving functional independence at 6 months (AR for independence 41.5% with tinzaparin 175 anti Xa IU/kg/daily v 42.4% with tinzaparin 100 anti-Xa IU/kg/daily v 42.5% with aspirin 300 mg/daily). **Deep venous thrombosis and pulmonary embolism:** We found three systematic reviews.[23,27,28] The first systematic review (search date 1999) included 10 small heterogeneous RCTs (22 000 people), which assessed anticoagulants in 916 people at high risk of deep venous thrombosis after their stroke.[23] Anticoagulation compared with control reduced the risk of deep vein thrombosis (ARR 29%, 95% CI 24% to 35%; RRR 64%, 95% CI 54% to 71%; NNT 3, 95% CI 2 to 4) and reduced symptomatic pulmonary embolism (ARR 0.3%, 95% CI 0.1% to 0.6%; RRR 38%, 95% CI 16% to 54%; NNT 333, 95% CI 167 to 1000). No RCT performed investigations in all people to rule out silent events. The frequency of reported pulmonary emboli was low and varied among RCTs, so there may have been under ascertainment. Two other systematic reviews (search dates 1999[28] and 2001,[27] same 5 RCTs in each review, 705 people with acute ischaemic stroke) found that low molecular weight heparins or heparinoids versus unfractionated heparin significantly reduced deep venous thrombosis (AR 13% with low molecular weight heparins or heparinoids v 22% with unfractionated heparin; ARR 9%, 95% CI 4.5% to 16%). The number of events was too small to estimate the effects of low molecular weight heparins or heparinoids versus unfractionated heparin on death, intracranial haemorrhage, or functional outcome in survivors.

Harms: One systematic review found that anticoagulation slightly increased symptomatic intracranial haemorrhages within 14 days of starting treatment compared with control (ARI 0.93%, 95% CI 0.68% to 1.18%; RRI 163%, 95% CI 95% to 255%; NNH 108, 95% CI 85 to 147).[23] The large trial of subcutaneous heparin found that this effect was dose dependent (symptomatic intracranial haemorrhage by using medium dose compared with low dose heparin for 14 days; RRI 143%, 95% CI 82% to 204%; NNH 97, 95% CI 68 to 169).[10] The review also found a dose dependent increase in major extracranial haemorrhages after 14 days of treatment with anticoagulants (ARI 0.91%, 95% CI 0.67% to 1.15%; RRI 231%, 95% CI 136% to 365%; NNH 109, 95% CI 87 to 149).[23] The subsequent RCT of dalteparin versus aspirin for people with acute stroke and atrial fibrillation found no difference in adverse events, including symptomatic or asymptomatic intracerebral haemorrhage, progression of symptoms, or early or late death.[24] As in the systematic review,[23] the RCT comparing different doses of certoparin found that intracranial haemorrhage occurred more often in those receiving a higher dose of anticoagulant.[25] However, the overall number of people experiencing haemorrhagic complications in the RCT may have been artificially lowered because the study protocol was changed during the trial period so as to exclude people with early ischaemic changes on computerised tomography scan. The RCT comparing different doses of tinzaparin found that high dose tinzaprin versus aspirin significantly increased symptomatic intracranial haemorrhage (AR 1.5% with high dose tinzaparin v 0.2% with aspirin; OR 7.2, 95% CI 1.1 to 163).[26]

Comment: Alternative treatments to prevent deep venous thrombosis and pulmonary embolism after acute ischaemic stroke include aspirin and compression stockings. The evidence relating to these will be reviewed in future *Clinical Evidence* updates.

OPTION BLOOD PRESSURE REDUCTION

One systematic review found insufficient evidence about the effects of antihypertensives versus placebo, but RCTs have suggested that people treated with antihypertensive agents may have a worse clinical outcome and increased mortality.

Benefits: We found one systematic review (search date 2000, 5 RCTs, 281 people with acute stroke) comparing blood pressure lowering treatment with placebo.[29] Several different antihypertensive agents were used. The trials collected insufficient clinical data to allow an analysis of the relation between changes in blood pressure and clinical outcome.

Harms: Two placebo controlled RCTs have suggested that people treated with antihypertensive agents may have a worse clinical outcome and increased mortality.[30,31] The first RCT (295 people with acute ischaemic stroke) compared nimodipine (a calcium channel antagonist) with placebo.[30] The trial was stopped prematurely because of an excess of unfavourable neurological outcomes in the nimodipine treated group. Exploratory analyses confirmed that this negative correlation was related to reductions in mean arterial blood pressure (CI not provided; $P = 0.02$) and diastolic blood pressure ($P = 0.0005$). The second RCT (302 people with acute ischaemic stroke) assessed β blockers (atenolol or propranolol).[31] There was a non-significant increase in death for people taking β blockers, and no difference in the proportion of people achieving a good outcome. One systematic review (search date 1994, 9 RCTs, 3719 people with acute stroke) compared nimodipine versus placebo; no net benefit was found.[32] A second review (24 RCTs, 6894 people) found a non-significant increase in the risk of death with calcium channel antagonists versus placebo (RRI 8%, 95% CI 1% reduction to 18% increase).[33] Although treatment with calcium channel antagonists in these trials was intended for neuroprotection, blood pressure was lower in the treatment group in several trials.

Comment: Population based studies suggest a direct and continuous association between blood pressure and the risk of recurrent stroke.[34] However, acute blood pressure lowering in acute ischaemic stroke may lead to increased cerebral ischaemia. The systematic review[29] identified several ongoing RCTs. We identified one additional ongoing RCT not included in the review.[35]

OPTION   NEUROPROTECTIVE AGENTS

RCTs found no evidence that compared with placebo, calcium channel antagonists, lubeluzole, γ-aminobutyric acid agonists, tirilazad, glycine antagonists, or N-methyl-D-aspartate antagonists significantly improved clinical outcomes. One systematic review found that lubeluzole versus placebo was associated with a significant increase in the risk of having Q-T prolongation to more than 450 ms on electrocardiography.

Benefits: We found no systematic reviews assessing the general effectiveness of neuroprotective agents in acute ischaemic stroke. **Calcium channel antagonists:** We found two systematic reviews comparing calcium channel antagonists with placebo.[36,37] The first review (search date 1999, 28 RCTs, 7521 people with acute ischaemic stroke) found that calcium channel antagonists did not significantly reduce the risk of poor outcome (including death) at the end of the follow up period compared with placebo (ARI of poor outcome +4.9%, 95% CI −2.5% to +7.3%; RRI +4%, 95% CI −2% to +9%).[36] The second review (search date 1999)[37] includes one additional RCT (454 people)[38] that was stopped prematurely because of publication of the first review.[36] Inclusion of its data does not change the results of the first review. **γ-Aminobutyric acid agonists:** We found one systematic review (search date not stated, 3 RCTs, 1002 people with acute ischaemic stroke), which found no significant difference between piracetam (a γ-aminobutyric acid agonist) and control groups for the number of people dead or dependent at the end of follow up (ARI +0.2%, 95% CI −6.0% to +6.4%; RRI 0%, 95% CI −11% to +9%).[39] We found one RCT (1360 people with acute stroke), which identified no significant effect of clomethiazole (chlormethiazole; a γ-aminobutyric acid agonist) versus placebo on achievement of functional independence (ARR +1.5%, 95% CI –4.0% to +6.6%; RRR +3.0%, 95% CI –7% to +13%).[40] **Lubeluzole:** We found one systematic review (search date 2001, 5 RCTs, 3510 people) that compared lubeluzole (5, 10, or 20 mg daily for 5 days) versus placebo.[41] It found no significant difference with any dose of lubeluzole versus placebo in death or dependency at the end of follow up (after 4–12 wks' follow up, AR 54.6% with lubeluzole v 53.4% with placebo; ARI +1.2%, 95% CI –2.5% to +6.2%). **Glycine antagonists:** We found two RCTs.[42,43] One RCT (1804 conscious people with limb weakness assessed within 6 h of stroke onset) found no significant difference between gavestinel (a glycine antagonist) versus placebo in survival and outcome at 3 months as measured using the Barthel Index (ARR +1.0%, 95% CI –3.5% to +6.0%).[42] The second RCT (1367 people with predefined level of limb weakness and functional independence before stroke) also found no significant difference in survival and outcome at 3 months, measured using the Barthel Index (ARI +1.9%, 95% CI –3.8% to +6.4%).[43] **N-methyl-D-aspartate antagonists:** Two recent RCTs assessing the N-methyl-D-aspartate antagonist (see glossary, p 240) selfotel found no significant difference in the proportion of people with a Barthel Index over 60, but data were limited as the trials were terminated because of adverse outcomes after only 31% of the total planned patient enrolment.[44] **Tirilazad:** We found one systematic review (search date 2001, 6 RCTs, 1757 people) comparing tirilazad (a steroid derivative) versus placebo in people with acute ischaemic stroke.[45] Tirilazad increased death and disability at 3 months' follow up when measured using the expanded Barthel Index (ARI +3.9%, 95% CI –0.8% to +8.6%).[45]

Harms: In the systematic review of calcium channel antagonists, indirect and limited comparisons of intravenous versus oral administration found no significant difference in adverse events (ARI of adverse events, iv v oral, +2.3%, 95% CI –0.9% to +3.7%; RRI +17%, 95% CI –3% to +41%).[36] In the systematic review of piracetam, there was a non-significant increase in death with piracetam versus placebo, which was no longer apparent after correction for imbalance in stroke severity.[39] The systematic review of lubeluzole found that at any dose, lubeluzole was associated with a significant increase in the risk of having a heart conduction disorder (Q-T prolongation to more than 450 ms on electrocardiography) at the end of follow up (AR with lubeluzole 11.9% v 9.74% with control; ARI 2.2%, 95% CI 0.1% to 4.2%; NNH 45, 95% CI 23 to 1000).[41] Lubeluzole did not significantly increase heart rhythm disorders (atrial fibrillation, ventricular tachycardia or fibrillation, torsade de pointes) at the end of the scheduled follow up (OR 1.28, 95% CI 0.97 to 1.69) The trials of selfotel were terminated after enrolling 567 people because of greater early mortality in the selfotel groups.[44] The systematic review of tirilazad found an increased risk of injection site phlebitis compared with placebo (ARI 12.2%, 95% CI 8.7% to 15.7%).[45]

Comment: The effects of the cell membrane precursor citicholine have been assessed in small trials, and a systematic review is in progress.[46] Systematic reviews are being developed for antioxidants and for excitatory amino acid modulators.[47] Several RCTs are ongoing, including one of intravenous magnesium sulphate[48] and another of diazepam (a γ-aminobutyric acid agonist).[49]

QUESTION	What are the effects of surgical treatment for intracerebral haematomas?

OPTION	EVACUATION

We found that the balance between benefits and harms has not been clearly established for the evacuation of supratentorial haematomas. We found no evidence from RCTs on the role of evacuation or ventricular shunting in people with infratentorial haematoma whose consciousness level is declining.

Benefits: **For supratentorial haematomas:** We found three systematic reviews.[50–52] The first review (search date 1998)[50] and second review (search date 1997)[51] both assessed the same four RCTs comparing surgery (craniotomy in 3 trials and endoscopy in 1 trial) versus best medical treatment in 354 people with primary supratentorial intracerebral haemorrhage. The second review also assessed information from case series.[51] Overall, neither review found significant short or long term differences between surgical and medical treatment for death or disability (ARI +3.3%, 95% CI –5.9% to +12.5%; RRI +5%, 95% CI –7% to +19%). The third review (search date 1999)[52] includes several analyses. The first analysis includes results from seven RCTs (530 people), including two RCTs not included in either of the first two systematic reviews. The overall results are similar to those of the first two systematic reviews, with no significant difference in death or disability for surgically treated people (ARI +3.5%, 95% CI –4.4% to +11.4%). A further analysis of results from only recent, post-computerised tomography, well constructed, balanced trials (5 trials, 224 people in total) did not find a significant difference between the two groups (ARR +9.3%, 95% CI –2.6% to +21.2%). **For infratentorial haematomas:** We found no evidence from systematic reviews or RCTs on the role of surgical evacuation or ventricular shunting.[53]

Harms: The two earlier reviews undertook subgroup analyses separating results for craniotomy and endoscopy. They found that for the 254 people randomised to craniotomy rather than best medical treatment, there was increased death and disability (ARI 12%, 95% CI 1.8% to 22%; RRI 17%, 95% CI 2% to 34%; NNH 8, 95% CI 5 to 56).[50,51] For the 100 people randomised to endoscopy rather than best medical practice, there was no significant effect on death and disability (RRR 24%, 95% CI –2% to +44%). The third systematic review did not evaluate these adverse outcomes.[52]

Cardiovascular disorders

Comment: Current practice is based on the consensus that people with infratentorial (cerebellar) haematomas whose consciousness level is declining probably benefit from evacuation of the haematoma. We identified one ongoing multicentre trial comparing a policy of "early surgical evacuation" of haematoma versus "initial conservative treatment" in people with spontaneous intracerebral haemorrhage.[54]

GLOSSARY

Integrated care pathway A model of care that includes definition of therapeutic goals and specification of a timed plan designed to promote multidisciplinary care, improve discharge planning, and reduce the duration of hospital stay.

N-methyl-D-aspartate antagonist Glutamate can bind to N-methyl-D-aspartate receptors on cell surfaces. One hypothesis proposed that glutamate released during a stroke can cause further harm to neurones by stimulating the N-methyl-D-aspartate receptors. N-Methyl-D-aspartate antagonists block these receptors.

REFERENCES

1. Hatano S. Experience from a multicentre stroke register: a preliminary report. *Bull World Health Organ* 1976;54:541–553.
2. Bonita R. Epidemiology of stroke. *Lancet* 1992;339:342–344.
3. Bamford J, Sandercock P, Dennis M, et al. A prospective study of acute cerebrovascular disease in the community: the Oxfordshire community stroke project, 1981–1986. 1. Methodology, demography and incident cases of first ever stroke. *J Neurol Neurosurg Psychiatry* 1988;51:1373–1380.
4. Bamford J, Dennis M, Sandercock P, et al. A prospective study of acute cerebrovascular disease in the community: the Oxfordshire community stroke project, 1981–1986. 2. Incidence, case fatality rates and overall outcome at one year of cerebral infarction, primary intracerebral and subarachnoid haemorrhage. *J Neurol Neurosurg Psychiatry* 1990;53:16–22.
5. Bamford J, Dennis M, Sandercock P, et al. The frequency, causes and timing of death within 30 days of a first stroke: the Oxfordshire community stroke project. *J Neurol Neurosurg Psychiatry* 1990;53:824–829.
6. Wade DT. Functional abilities after stroke: measurement, natural history and prognosis. *J Neurol Neurosurg Psychiatry* 1987;50:177–182.
7. Stroke Unit Trialists' Collaboration. Organised inpatient (stroke unit) care for stroke. In: The Cochrane Library, Issue 1, 2002. Oxford: Update Software. Search date 2001; primary sources Cochrane Stroke Group Specialised Trials Register and hand searches of reference lists of relevant articles and personal contact with colleagues.
8. Wardlaw JM, del Zoppo G, Yamaguchi T. Thrombolysis for acute ischaemic stroke. In: The Cochrane Library, Issue 1, 2002. Oxford: Update Software. Search date 1999; primary sources Cochrane Stroke Group Specialised Register of Controlled Trials, Embase, hand searches of relevant journals and references listed in relevant papers, and personal contact with pharmaceutical companies and principal investigators of trials.
9. CAST (Chinese Acute Stroke Trial) Collaborative Group. Randomised placebo-controlled trial of early aspirin use in 20 000 patients with acute ischaemic stroke. *Lancet* 1997;349:1641–1649.
10. International Stroke Trial Collaborative Group. The international stroke trial (IST): a randomised trial

of aspirin, heparin, both or neither among 19 435 patients with acute ischaemic stroke. *Lancet* 1997;349:1569–1581.
11. Indredavik B, Bakke RPT, Slordahl SA, et al. Stroke unit treatment. 10-year follow-up. *Stroke* 1999;30:1524–1527.
12. Sulch D, Perez I, Melbourn A, Kalra L. Randomized controlled trial of integrated (managed) care pathway for stroke rehabilitation. *Stroke* 2000;31:1929–1934.
13. Indredavik B, Bakke RPT, Slordahl SA, et al. Treatment in a combined acute and rehabilitation stroke unit. Which aspects are most important. *Stroke* 1999;30:917–923.
14. Stegmayr B, Asplund K, Hulter-Asberg K, et al. Stroke units in their natural habitat: can results of randomized trials be reproduced in routine clinical practice? For the risk-stroke collaboration. *Stroke* 1999;30:709–714.
15. Cornu C, Boutitie F, Candelise L, et al. Streptokinase in acute ischemic stroke: an individual patient data meta-analysis: the thrombolysis in acute stroke pooling project. *Stroke* 2000;31:1555–1560.
16. Kwiatkowski T, Libman R, Frankel M, et al. Effects of tissue plasminogen activator for acute ischemic stroke at one year. National Institute of Neurological Disorders and stroke recombinant tissue plasminogen activator stroke study group. *N Engl J Med* 1999;340:1781–1787.
17. Internet Stroke Center: http://www.strokecenter.org/trials (last accessed 5 Sept 2002).
18. Gubitz G, Sandercock P, Counsell C. Antiplatelet therapy for acute ischaemic stroke. In: The Cochrane Library, Issue 1, 2002. Oxford: Update Software. Search date 1999; primary sources Cochrane Stroke Group Specialised Register of Controlled Trials, the Register of the Antiplatelet Trialists' Collaboration, MedStrategy, and personal contact with pharmaceutical companies.
19. Chen Z, Sandercock P, Pan H, et al. Indications for early aspirin use in acute ischemic stroke: a combined analysis of 40 000 randomized patients from the Chinese Acute Stroke Trial and the International Stroke Trial. *Stroke* 2000;31:1240–1249.
20. Antithrombotic Trialists' Collaboration. Collaborative meta-analysis of randomised trials of antiplatelet therapy for prevention of death, myocardial infarction, and stroke in high risk patients. *BMJ* 2002;324:71–86. Search date

1997; primary sources Medline, Embase, Derwent, Scisearch, Biosis, Cochrane Stroke Group Controlled Trials Register, Cochrane Peripheral Vascular Disease Group Controlled Trials Register, hand searches of journals, abstracts and proceedings of meetings, reference lists from relevant articles, and personal contact with colleagues and pharmaceutical companies.

21. Slattery J, Warlow CP, Shorrock CJ, Langman MJS. Risks of gastrointestinal bleeding during secondary prevention of vascular events with aspirin analysis of gastrointestinal bleeding during the UK-TIA trial. *Gut* 1995;37:509–511.

22. Johnson ES, Lanes SF, Wentworth CE, et al. A metaregression analysis of the dose–response effect of aspirin on stroke. *Arch Intern Med* 1999;159:1248–1253.

23. Gubitz G, Counsell C, Sandercock P, et al. Anticoagulants for acute ischaemic stroke. In: The Cochrane Library, Issue 1, 2002. Oxford: Update Software. Search date 1999; primary sources Cochrane Stroke Group Specialised Register of Controlled Trials, trials register held by the Antithrombotic Therapy Trialist's Collaboration, MedStrategy, and personal contact with pharmaceutical companies.

24. Berge E, Abdelnoor M, Nakstad P, et al. Low-molecular weight heparin versus aspirin in people with acute ischaemic stroke and atrial fibrillation: a double-blind randomised study. HAEST Study Group. Heparin in Acute Embolic Stroke Trial. *Lancet* 2000;355:1205–1210.

25. Diener H, Ringelstein E, von Kummer R, et al. Treatment of acute ischemic stroke with the low-molecular-weight heparin certoparin: results of the TOPAS Trial. *Stroke* 2001;32:22–29.

26. Bath P, Lindenstrome E, Bioysen G, et al. Tinzaparin in acute ischaemic stroke (TAIST): a randomised aspirin-controlled trial. *Lancet* 2001;358:702–710.

27. Counsell C, Sandercock P. Low-molecular-weight heparins or heparinoids versus standard unfractionated heparin for acute ischaemic stroke (Cochrane Review). In: The Cochrane Library, Issue 1, 2002. Oxford: Update Software. Search date 2001; primary sources Cochrane Stroke Group Specialised Trials Register, MedStrategy, and personal contact with pharmaceutical companies.

28. Bath P, Iddenden R, Bath F. Low-molecular-weight heparins and heparinoids in acute ischemic stroke: a meta-analysis of randomized controlled trials. *Stroke* 2000;31:1770–1778. Search date 1999; primary sources Cochrane Stroke Group Database of Trials in Acute Stroke, Cochrane Library, and hand searches of reference lists of identified publications.

29. Blood pressure in Acute Stroke Collaboration (BASC). Interventions for deliberately altering blood pressure in acute stroke. In: The Cochrane Library, Issue 1, 2002. Oxford: Update Software. Search date 2000; primary sources Cochrane Stroke Group Specialised Register of Controlled Trials, Cochrane Library (CDSR, CCTR), Medline, Embase, Bids, ISI Science Citation Index, hand searches of reference lists of existing reviews and the ongoing trials section of the journal *Stroke*, and personal contact with research workers in the field and pharmaceutical companies.

30. Wahlgren NG, MacMahon DG, DeKeyser J, et al. Intravenous nimodipine west European stroke trial (INWEST) of nimodipine in the treatment of acute ischaemic stroke. *Cerebrovasc Dis* 1994;4:204–210.

31. Barer DH, Cruickshank JM, Ebrahim SB, et al. Low dose beta blockade in acute stroke (BEST trial): an evaluation. *BMJ* 1988;296:737–741.

32. Mohr JP, Orgogozo JM, Harrison MJG, et al. Meta analysis of oral nimodipine trials in acute ischaemic stroke. *Cerebrovasc Dis* 1994;4:197–203. Search date 1994; primary source Bayer database.

33. Horn J, Orgogozo JM, Limburg M. Review on calcium antagonists in ischaemic stroke; mortality data. *Cerebrovasc Dis* 1998;8(suppl 4).27.

34. Rodgers A, MacMahon S, Gamble G. Blood pressure and risk of stroke patients with cerebrovascular disease. *BMJ* 1996;313:147.

35. Schrader J, Rothemeyer M, Luders S, et al. Hypertension and stroke – rationale behind the ACCESS trial. *Basic Res Cardiol* 1998;93(suppl 2):69–78.

36. Horn J, Limburg M. Calcium antagonists for acute ischemic stroke. In: The Cochrane Library, Issue 1, 2002. Oxford: Update Software. Search date 1999; primary sources Cochrane Stroke Group Specialised Register of Controlled Trials and personal contact with trialists.

37. Horn J, Limburg M. Calcium antagonists for ischemic stroke: a systematic review. *Stroke* 2001;32:570–576. Search date 1999; primary sources Cochrane Collaboration Stroke Group Specialized Register of Controlled Trials, and personal contact with principal investigators and company representatives.

38. Horn J, de Haan R, Vermeulen M, et al. Very Early Nimodipine Use in Stroke (VENUS). A randomized, double-blind, placebo-controlled trail. *Stroke* 2001;32:461–465.

39. Ricci S, Celani MG, Cantisani AT, et al. Piracetam for acute ischaemic stroke (Cochrane Review). In: The Cochrane Library, Issue 1, 2002. Oxford: Update Software. Search date not stated; primary sources Cochrane Stroke Review Group trials register, Medline, Embase, BIDIS ISI, hand searches of relevant journals, and personal contact with the manufacturer.

40. Wahlgren NG, Ranasinha KW, Rosolacci T, et al. Clomethiazole acute stroke study (CLASS): results of a randomised, controlled trial of clomethiazole versus placebo in 1360 acute stroke patients. *Stroke* 1999;30:21–28.

41. Gandolfo C, Sandercock P, Conti M. Lubeluzole for acute ischaemic stroke. In: The Cochrane Library, Issue 1, 2002. Oxford: Update Software. Search date 2001; primary sources Cochrane Stroke Group Specialised Register of Controlled Trials, Cochrane Controlled Trials Register (CENTRAL/CCTR), Medline, Embase, Pascal BioMed, Current Contents, hand searches of all references in relevant papers, and personal contact with Janssen Research Foundation.

42. Lees K, Asplund K, Carolei A, et al. Glycine antagonist (gavestinel) in neuroprotection (GAIN International) in people with acute stroke: a randomised controlled trial. *Lancet* 2000;355:1949–1954.

43. Sacco R, DeRosa J, Haley E Jr, et al. for the GAIN Americas Investigators. Glycine Antagonist in Neuroprotection for Patients with Acute Stroke. GAIN Americas: a randomized controlled trial. *JAMA* 2001;285:1719–1728.

44. Davis S, Lees K, Albers G, et al. for the ASSIST Investigators. Selfotel in acute ischemic stroke. Possible neurotoxic effects of an NMDA antagonist. *Stroke* 2000;31:347–354.

45. The Tirilazad International Steering Committee. Tirilazad for acute ischaemic stroke. In: The Cochrane Library, Issue 1, 2002. Oxford: Update Software. Search date 2001; primary sources Cochrane Stroke Group Specialised Trials Register, Cochrane Controlled Trials Register (CENTRAL/CCTR), the Cochrane Library, hand

Cardiovascular disorders

searches of a publication on the quality of acute stroke RCTs, and personal contact with Pharmacia & Upjohn.

46. Saver JL, Wilterdink J. Choline precursors for acute and subacute ischemic and hemorrhagic stroke (Protocol for a Cochrane Review). In: The Cochrane Library, Issue 1, 2002. Oxford: Update Software.

47. Cochrane Stroke Review Group. Department of Clinical Neurosciences, Western General Hospital, Crewe Road, Edinburgh, UK EH4 2XU. http://www.dcn.ed.ac.uk/csrg (last accessed 5 Sept 2002).

48. Muir KW, Lees KR. IMAGES. Intravenous magnesium efficacy in stroke trial [abstract]. *Cerebrovasc Dis* 1996;6:75P383.

49. Lodder J, van Raak L, Kessels F, Hilton A. Early GABA-ergic activation study in stroke (EGASIS). *Cerebrovasc Dis* 2000;10(suppl 2):80.

50. Prasad K , Shrivastava A. Surgery for primary supratentorial intracerebral haemorrhage. In: The Cochrane Library, Issue 1, 2002. Oxford: Update Software. Search date 1998; primary sources Cochrane Stroke Group Trials Register and hand searches of reference lists of articles identified, three relevant monographs and issues of *Curr Opin Neurol Neurosurg* and *Neurosurg Clin N Am.*

51. Hankey G, Hon C. Surgery for primary intracerebral hemorrhage: is it safe and effective? A systematic review of case series and randomised trials. *Stroke* 1997;28:2126–2132. Search date 1997; primary sources Medline, and hand searches of reference lists of identified articles, published epidemiological studies, and reviews.

52. Fernandes HM, Gregson B, Siddique S, et al. Surgery in intracerebral hemorrhage: the uncertainty continues. *Stroke* 2000;31:2511–2516. Search date 1999; primary sources Ovid databases (unspecified), Medline, and hand searches of the reference lists of identified articles and relevant cited references.

53. Warlow CP, Dennis MS, van Gijn J, et al, eds. Treatment of primary intracerebral haemorrhage. In: *Stroke: a practical guide to management.* Oxford: Blackwell Science, 1996:430–437.

54. Mendelow A. International Surgical Trial in Intracerebral Haemorrhage (ISTICH). *Stroke* 2000;31:2539.

Gord Gubitz

Assistant Professor
Division of Neurology
Dalhousie University
Halifax
Canada

Peter Sandercock

Professor of Neurology
Neurosciences Trials Unit
University of Edinburgh
Edinburgh
UK

Competing interests: GG none declared. PS was the Principal Investigator of the second International Stroke Trial (IST-2). The trial was partly funded by Glaxo-Wellcome. He is also Chairman of the Steering Committee for the third International Stroke Trial (IST3) of thrombolysis in acute stroke. The start-up phase of trial is currently funded by a grant from the Stroke Association. Boehringer Ingelheim have donated trial drug and placebo for the 300 patients to be included in the start-up phase. PS has received honoraria for lectures, single consultations and travel expenses from a variety of pharmaceutical companies including: Boehringer Ingelheim, Sanofi, BNS, MSD, Servier, Glaxo-Wellcome, Lilly, Centocor.

Cardiovascular disorders

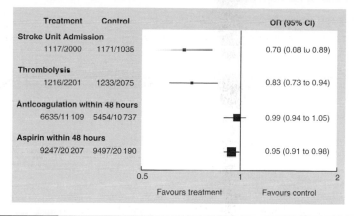

Proportional effects on "death or dependency" at the end of scheduled follow up: results of systematic reviews.[7-10] Data refer only to benefits and not to harms (see text, p 234).

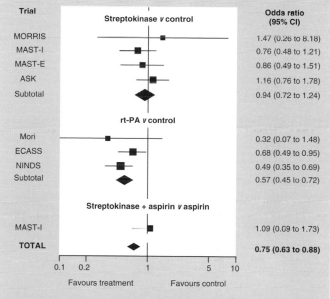

rt-PA, recombinant tissue plasminogen activator

Effect of thrombolysis on death and dependency at end of trial: results of review (see text, p 232). Figure reproduced with permission. Wardlaw JM, Warlow CP, Counsell C. Systematic review of evidence on thrombolytic therapy for acute ischaemic stroke. *Lancet* 1997;350:607–614. © by The Lancet Ltd, 1997.

Search date May 2002

Clinical Evidence writers on stroke prevention

Key Messages

In people with a prior stroke or transient ischaemic attack

■ **Alternative antiplatelet agents to aspirin** Systematic reviews have found no good evidence that any antiplatelet treatment is superior to aspirin for long term secondary prevention of serious vascular events.

■ **Antiplatelet treatment** One systematic review found that antiplatelet treatment reduces the risk of serious vascular events in people with prior stroke or transient ischaemic attack compared with placebo or no antiplatelet treatment.

- **Blood pressure reduction** One systematic review and one subsequent RCT found that antihypertensive treatment reduced stroke among people with a prior stroke or transient ischaemic attack, whether they were hypertensive or not

- **Carotid angioplasty** RCTs found insufficient evidence about the effects of carotid angioplasty versus best "medical treatment".

- **Carotid endarterectomy in people with severe asymptomatic carotid artery stenosis** Systematic reviews in people with no carotid territory transient ischaemic event or minor stroke within the past few months found limited evidence suggesting that carotid endarterectomy versus medical treatment may significantly reduce the risk of perioperative stroke or death or subsequent ipsilateral stroke over 3 years. However, as the risk of death without surgery in asymptomatic people is relatively low, the balance of benefits and harms from surgery remains unclear.

- **Carotid endarterectomy in people with moderate or severe symptomatic carotid artery stenosis** One systematic review in people with a recent carotid territory transient ischaemic event or non-disabling ischaemic stroke has found that carotid endarterectomy versus control treatment significantly reduces the risk of major stroke or death (NNT 15, 95% CI 10 to 31).

- **Cholesterol reduction** One large RCT has found that simvastatin versus placebo reduced major vascular events, including stroke, in people with prior stroke or transient ischaemic attack over about 5 years. RCTs have found no evidence that non-statin treatments versus placebo or no treatment reduced stroke.

- **Different blood pressure lowering regimens** Systematic reviews found no clear evidence of a difference in effectiveness between different antihypertensive drugs. One systematic review found that more intensive treatment reduced stroke and major cardiovascular events, but not mortality, compared with less intensive treatment.

- **High dose versus low dose aspirin (no additional benefit but may increase harms)** One systematic review and one subsequent RCT have found that low dose aspirin (75–150 mg) daily is as effective as higher doses in the prevention of serious vascular events. There was insufficient evidence that doses lower than 75 mg daily are as effective. One systematic review found no association between the dose of aspirin and risk of major extracranial haemorrhage in either direct or indirect comparisons. Another systematic review found no association between the dose of aspirin and risk of gastrointestinal bleeding in an indirect comparison. RCTs directly comparing different doses of aspirin found an increased risk of upper gastrointestinal upset with high (500–1500 mg daily) versus medium (75–325 mg daily) doses. One systematic review of observational studies found an increased risk of gastrointestinal complications with doses of aspirin greater than 300 mg daily. One systematic review found no association between dose of aspirin and risk of intracranial haemorrhage.

- **Oral anticoagulation in people with prior cerebrovascular ischaemia and sinus rhythm** One systematic review in people with prior cerebral ischaemia and in normal sinus rhythm found no significant difference with anticoagulation versus placebo for death or dependency, mortality, or recurrent stroke at about 2 years, but found a significantly increased risk of fatal intracranial haemorrhage (NNH 49, 95% CI 27 to 240). One systematic review has found no significant difference between high intensity (international normalised ratio 3.0–4.5) or low intensity (international normalised ratio 2.5–3.5) anticoagulation versus antiplatelet treatment for preventing recurrent stroke in people with recent cerebral ischaemia of presumed arterial (non-cardiac) origin. High intensity anticoagulation increased the risk of major bleeding compared with antiplatelet treatment.

In people with atrial fibrillation and a prior stroke or transient ischaemic attack

- **Aspirin in people with contraindications to anticoagulants** Systematic reviews have found that aspirin versus placebo reduces the risk of stroke, but found that aspirin is less effective than anticoagulants. These findings support the use of aspirin in people with atrial fibrillation and contraindications to anticoagulants.

- **Oral anticoagulation** Systematic reviews have found that adjusted dose warfarin versus placebo significantly reduces the risk of stroke. Systematic reviews have also found that warfarin versus aspirin significantly reduces the risk of stroke in people with previous stroke or transient ischaemic attack.

In people with atrial fibrillation but no other major risk factors for stroke

- **Aspirin in people with contraindications to anticoagulants** One systematic review has found that aspirin versus placebo significantly reduces the risk of stroke (NNT 45, 95% CI 24 to 333), but another review found no significant difference. These findings support the use of aspirin in people with atrial fibrillation and contraindications to anticoagulants.

- **Oral anticoagulation** One systematic review has found that warfarin versus placebo significantly reduces fatal and non-fatal ischaemic stroke (NNT 25, 95% CI 18 to 42), provided there is a low risk of bleeding and careful monitoring. The people in the review had a mean age of 69 years. One overview in people less than 65 years old has found no significant difference in the annual stroke rate with warfarin versus placebo.

DEFINITION Prevention in this context is the long term management of people with a prior stroke or transient ischaemic attack, and of people at high risk of stroke (see glossary, p 262) for other reasons such as atrial fibrillation. **Stroke:** See definition under stroke management, p 229. **Transient ischaemic attack:** Similar to a mild ischaemic stroke except that symptoms last for less than 24 hours.[1]

INCIDENCE/ PREVALENCE See incidence/prevalence under stroke management, p 229.

AETIOLOGY/ RISK FACTORS See aetiology under stroke management, p 229. Risk factors for stroke include prior stroke or transient ischaemic attack, increasing age, hypertension, diabetes, cigarette smoking, and emboli associated with atrial fibrillation, artificial heart valves, or myocardial infarction. The relation with cholesterol is less clear; an overview of prospective studies among healthy middle aged individuals found no association between total cholesterol and overall stroke risk.[2] However, one review of prospective observational studies in eastern Asian people found that cholesterol was positively associated with ischaemic stroke but negatively associated with haemorrhagic stroke.[3]

PROGNOSIS   People with a history of stroke or transient ischaemic attack are at high risk of all vascular events, such as myocardial infarction, but are at particular risk of subsequent stroke (about 10% in the first year and about 5% each year thereafter); see figure 1, p 268, and figure 1 in secondary prevention of ischaemic cardiac events, p 189.[5,6] People with intermittent atrial fibrillation treated with aspirin should be considered at similar risk of stroke, compared to people with sustained atrial fibrillation treated with aspirin (rate of ischaemic stroke/year: 3.2% with intermittent _v_ 3.3% with sustained).[7]

AIMS   To prevent death or disabling stroke, as well as other serious non fatal outcomes, especially myocardial infarction, with minimal adverse effects from treatment.

OUTCOMES   Dependency; myocardial infarction; stroke; and mortality.

METHODS   _Clinical Evidence_ update search and appraisal May 2002, plus handsearches of vascular, neurology, and general medical journals for options authored by Cathie Sudlow.

QUESTION	What are the effects of interventions in people with prior stroke or transient ischaemic attack?

OPTION	BLOOD PRESSURE REDUCTION VERSUS NO BLOOD PRESSURE REDUCTION

Cathie Sudlow

One systematic review and one subsequent RCT found that antihypertensive treatment reduced stroke in people with a prior stroke or transient ischaemic attack, whether they were hypertensive or not.

Benefits: We found one systematic review[8] and one subsequent RCT[9] of antihypertensive treatment versus placebo, no treatment, or usual care in people with a prior stroke or transient ischaemic attack. The systematic review (9 RCTs, search date not stated, 6753 people with a prior stroke or transient ischaemic attack) found that antihypertensive treatment significantly reduced stroke and major cardiovascular events compared with placebo, no treatment, or usual care over 2–7 years (stroke: RR 0.72, 95% CI 0.61 to 0.85; major cardiovascular events: RR 0.79, 95% CI 0.68 to 0.91).[8] Over 80% of people in the review were included in a single large RCT, the results of which have only been published in preliminary form.[10] The subsequent RCT (6105 people with a prior stroke or transient ischaemic attack with and without hypertension) compared the angiotensin converting enzyme inhibitor perindopril plus indapamide (added at the discretion of the physician) versus placebo.[9] It found that active treatment versus placebo reduced stroke but not deaths after about 4 years (stroke: AR 10% with treatment _v_ 14% with placebo; RR 0.72, 95% CI 0.62 to 0.83; deaths: AR with treatment 10% _v_ 10% with placebo; RR 0.96, 95% CI 0.82 to 1.12). Relative risks were similar in people with and without hypertension.

Stroke prevention

Harms: In people with a history of stroke, reports of an apparently J-shaped relationship between blood pressure and subsequent stroke have led to concerns that blood pressure reduction may increase the risk of recurrent stroke, perhaps because of reduced cerebral perfusion, particularly among people with extracranial carotid or vertebral artery stenosis.[11] However, observational studies found no evidence of a threshold of diastolic blood pressure below which there was no reduction in stroke.[11,12]

Comment: The systematic review found that the effects of blood pressure lowering were similar in people with and without a history of stroke or transient ischaemic attack.[8]

OPTION	DIFFERENT BLOOD PRESSURE LOWERING REGIMENS

Cathie Sudlow

Systematic reviews found no clear evidence of a difference in effectiveness between different antihypertensive drugs. One systematic review found that more intensive treatment reduced stroke and major cardiovascular events, but not mortality, compared with less intensive treatment.

Benefits: We found no RCTs comparing different antihypertensive regimens specifically among people with a prior stroke or transient ischaemic attack. We found three systematic reviews[13-15] and one subsequent RCT[16] that compared effects of different antihypertensive treatments on stroke and other vascular outcomes in people with hypertension. One systematic review (search date 1997, 5 RCTs, about 18 000 people) found no significant difference between diuretics versus β blockers in death, stroke, or coronary artery disease.[13] The second systematic review (search date not stated, 15 RCTs)[14] compared more intensive versus less intensive treatment (3 RCTs, about 20 000 people); angiotensin converting enzyme inhibitors versus diuretics or β blockers (3 RCTs, about 16 000 people); calcium channel antagonists versus diuretics or β blockers (5 RCTs, about 23 000 people); and angiotensin converting enzyme inhibitors versus calcium channel antagonists (2 RCTs, about 5000 people). It found that more intensive treatment (target diastolic blood pressure 75–85 mm Hg) versus less intensive treatment (target diastolic blood pressure 85–105 mm Hg) significantly reduced stroke and major cardiovascular events, but not death (stroke: RR 0.80, 95% CI 0.65 to 0.98; major cardiovascular events: RR 0.85, 95% CI 0.76 to 0.96; death: RR 0.97, 95% CI 0.85 to 1.11). It found no significant difference with angiotensin converting enzyme inhibitors versus diuretics or β blockers in stroke, other vascular outcomes, or death (stroke: RR 1.05, 95% CI 0.92 to 1.19; death: RR 1.03, 95% CI 0.93 to 1.14). Calcium channel antagonists versus diuretics or β blockers reduced stroke (stroke: RR 0.87, 95% CI 0.77 to 0.98), but slightly increased coronary heart disease (RR 0.81, 95% CI 0.68 to 0.97), and had no significant effect on death or other vascular outcomes (death: RR 1.01, 95% CI 0.92 to 1.11). Angiotensin converting enzyme inhibitors versus calcium channel antagonists reduced coronary heart disease, but had no significant effect on stroke or death (coronary heart disease: RR 0.81, 95% CI 0.68 to 0.97; stroke: RR 1.02,

95% CI 0.85 to 1.21; death: RR 1.03, 95% CI 0.91 to 1.18). However, the RCTs included in this comparison were statistically heterogeneous so the results of the analysis should be treated with caution. The third systematic review (search date not stated) found similar results to the second review.[15] It suggested that results for different antihypertensive drugs could be explained by the blood pressure differences between randomised groups. The subsequent RCT (9193 people with hypertension, 728 of whom had a history of cerebrovascular disease) compared an angiotensin II receptor blocker (losartan) with a β blocker (atenolol).[16] It found that losartan versus atenolol significantly reduced the combined outcome of cardiovascular death, myocardial infarction, and stroke after 5 years (AR 14% with atenolol v 12% with losartan; HR 0.85, 95% CI 0.76 to 0.96). Blood pressure reduction was similar in both treatment groups (systolic/diastolic: about 30/17 mm Hg).

Harms: See harms under blood pressure reduction, p 248.

Comment: It has been suggested that both angiotensin converting enzyme inhibitors and angiotensin II receptor blockers produce reductions in vascular outcomes beyond what might be expected from their effects on blood pressure.[16,17]

OPTION   CHOLESTEROL REDUCTION

Cathie Sudlow

One large RCT has found that simvastatin versus placebo reduced major vascular events, including stroke, in people with prior stroke or transient ischaemic attack. RCTs have found no evidence that non-statin treatments versus placebo or no treatment reduced stroke.

Benefits: **Statins:** We found several systematic reviews (about 38 000 people with and without a history of coronary heart disease) that assessed the effects of reducing cholesterol with a statin on coronary heart disease and also reported on stroke as an outcome. The RCTs included did not specifically aim to include people with a prior stroke or transient ischaemic attack (TIA). One systematic review (search date 1995, 14 RCTs)[18] and one additional RCT[19] included all of the relevant results, which are summarised in table 1 (see table 1, p 267). The review found that reducing mean total cholesterol with a statin by 21% over an average of 4 years reduced the relative odds of stroke by 24% (see table 1, p 267). We found one subsequent RCT (20 536 people with coronary heart disease, other occlusive vascular disease, or diabetes, 3280 of whom had a history of cerebrovascular disease and over 4000 of whom had a pretreatment cholesterol of < 5.0 mmol/L) that compared simvastatin 40 mg daily versus placebo[20] (see table 1, p 267). It found that simvastatin versus placebo reduced mean total cholesterol by 24%, reduced stroke, major vascular events (major coronary events, strokes, and coronary or non-coronary revascularisations), and deaths over 5 years (stroke: AR 4% with simvastatin v 6% with placebo; RR 0.75, 95% CI 0.66 to 0.85; major vascular events: AR 20% with simvastatin v 25% with placebo; RR 0.76, 95% CI 0.72 to 0.81; deaths: AR 13% with simvastatin v 15% with placebo; RR 0.87, 95% CI 0.81 to 0.94). The relative risk of major vascular events was similar and separately significant in people with and without a history of coronary artery disease, among those with a history of ischaemic stroke or TIA, peripheral vascular disease, and diabetes, and among those with different pretreatment concentrations of cholesterol and triglycerides. **Non-statin treatments:** We found one overview,[21] one subsequent RCT,[22] and one additional RCT[23] that assessed the outcome of stroke. The overview (11 RCTs) compared reducing cholesterol with a non-statin treatment (fibrate, resin, or diet) versus placebo or no treatment.[21] It found no significant difference with a non-statin treatment versus placebo in the risk of stroke (OR 0.99, 95% CI 0.82 to 1.21). Results for people with previous stroke or TIA were not provided separately. The subsequent RCT (2531 men with coronary heart disease)[22] found no significant difference with gemfibrozil versus placebo in the risk of stroke (AR 5% with gemfibrozil v 6% with placebo; RRR +25%, 95% CI −6% to +47%). Results on people with previous stroke or TIA were not provided separately. The additional RCT (532 men who had a previous stroke or TIA)[23] found no significant difference between clofibrate versus placebo in death after 3.5 years (AR 13% with clofibrate v 19% with placebo; P value not provided).

Harms: It had been suggested that statins may increase haemorrhagic stroke.[3,18] However, the subsequent RCT found that simvastatin did not increase haemorrhagic stroke.[20]

Comment: An RCT comparing atorvastatin versus placebo in 4200 people with minor stroke or TIA is in progress.[24] A planned overview of individual participant data from all RCTs of cholesterol reduction aims to summarise the effects of reducing cholesterol in different groups of people, including those with a prior stroke or TIA.[25]

| OPTION | ANTIPLATELET TREATMENT VERSUS NO ANTIPLATELET TREATMENT |

Cathie Sudlow

One systematic review found that prolonged antiplatelet treatment versus placebo or no antiplatelet treatment reduces the risk of serious vascular events in people with prior stroke or transient ischaemic attack.

Benefits: We found one systematic review (search date 1997, 195 RCTs, about 135 640 people at high risk of vascular disease: previous stroke or transient ischaemic attack [TIA], acute stroke, ischaemic heart disease, heart failure, cardiac valve disease, atrial fibrillation, peripheral arterial disease, diabetes, and haemodialysis) comparing antiplatelet treatment (mostly aspirin) versus placebo or no antiplatelet treatment.[4] It found that in people with prior stroke or TIA (21 RCTs, 18 270 people), antiplatelet treatment reduced serious vascular events (stroke, myocardial infarction, or vascular death) compared with placebo or no antiplatelet treatment after

3 years (AR 18% with antiplatelet v 21% with placebo or no antiplatelet treatment; OR 0.78, 95% CI 0.73 to 0.85). Antiplatelet treatment also reduced the separate outcomes of stroke, myocardial infarction, vascular death, and death (see figure 1, p 268). For every 1000 people with a prior stroke or TIA treated for about 3 years, antiplatelet treatment prevented 25 non-fatal strokes, six non-fatal myocardial infarctions, and 15 deaths.[4]

Harms: The systematic review found that antiplatelet treatment versus no antiplatelet treatment in people with prior stroke or TIA increased major extracranial haemorrhage (haemorrhages requiring hospital admission or blood transfusion), and intracranial haemorrhage (intracranial haemorrhage: AR 0.64% with antiplatelet v 0.56% with no antiplatelet; OR 1.2; CI not provided; major extracranial haemorrhage: AR 0.97% with antiplatelet v 0.47% with no antiplatelet; OR 2.0; CI not provided).[4] We found one systematic review (search date 1999, 24 RCTs) assessing the effects of aspirin on gastrointestinal bleeding.[26] It found that aspirin versus placebo or no aspirin increased gastrointestinal bleeding (OR 1.68, 95% CI 1.51 to 1.88). Another systematic review (search date 1997, 16 RCTs, 55 462 people)[27] found that aspirin increased intracranial haemorrhage by about one event per 1000 people treated for 3 years.

Comment: In people at high risk of vascular disease, including those with a prior ischaemic stroke or TIA, the large absolute reductions in serious vascular events produced by antiplatelet treatment far outweighed any absolute hazards.

OPTION   HIGH DOSE VERSUS LOW DOSE ASPIRIN

Cathie Sudlow

One systematic review and one subsequent RCT have found that low dose aspirin (75–150 mg daily) is as effective as higher doses in the prevention of serious vascular events. There was insufficient evidence that doses lower than 75 mg daily are as effective. One systematic review found no association between the dose of aspirin and risk of major extracranial haemorrhage in either direct or indirect comparisons. Another systematic review found no association between the dose of aspirin and risk of gastrointestinal bleeding in an indirect comparison. RCTs directly comparing different doses of aspirin found an increased risk of upper gastrointestinal upset with high (500–1500 mg daily) versus medium (75–325 mg daily) daily doses. One systematic review of observational studies found an increase in risk of gastrointestinal complications with doses of aspirin greater than 300 mg daily. One systematic review found no association between dose of aspirin and risk of intracranial haemorrhage.

Benefits: We found one systematic review (search date 1997, 7225 people at high risk of vascular disease in RCTs comparing different doses of aspirin; and about 60 000 people at high risk of vascular disease, excluding those with acute stroke, in RCTs comparing different doses of aspirin versus placebo or no aspirin)[4] and one subsequent RCT[28] that compared the effects of higher versus lower dose aspirin on stroke. The systematic review found no significant difference between aspirin 500–1500 mg daily versus 75–325 mg daily in serious vascular events (stroke, myocardial infarction, or vascular death; OR 0.97, 95% CI 0.79 to 1.19).[4] It also found that doses of 75 mg or more did not reduce serious vascular events compared with doses lower than 75 mg (OR 1.08, 95% CI 0.90 to 1.31). However, the comparison lacked power to exclude a clinically important difference. The results in people with prior stroke or transient ischaemic attack were not presented separately. The systematic review also found that different aspirin doses versus placebo or no antiplatelet treatment reduced serious vascular events by similar amounts for the higher daily doses (500–1500 mg daily v placebo or no antiplatelet treatment: OR 0.81, 95% CI 0.75 to 0.87; 160–325 mg daily v placebo or no antiplatelet treatment: OR 0.74, 95% CI 0.69 to 0.80; 75–150 mg daily v placebo or no antiplatelet treatment: OR 0.68, 95% CI 0.59 to 0.79) but by a smaller amount for lower doses (< 75 mg daily v placebo or no antiplatelet treatment: OR 0.87, 95% CI 0.74 to 1.03). See figure 2 in secondary prevention of ischaemic cardiac events, p 189. People with acute stroke were excluded from these analyses. The results in people with prior stroke or transient ischaemic attack were not presented separately. The subsequent RCT (2849 people scheduled for carotid endarterectomy, most of whom had prior stroke or transient ischaemic attack) compared low dose aspirin (81 and 325 mg daily) versus high dose aspirin (650 and 1300 mg daily).[28] It found that high dose versus low dose aspirin increased the combined outcome of stroke, myocardial infarction, and death after 3 months (AR 8.4% with high dose v 6.2% with low dose; RR 1.34, 95% CI 1.03 to 1.75).

Harms: **Extracranial haemorrhage:** The systematic review found that the proportional increase in risk of major extracranial haemorrhage was similar with all daily aspirin doses. In direct comparisons, 75–325 mg aspirin did not increase major extracranial haemorrhage compared with doses lower than 75 mg (AR 2.5% with 75–325 mg daily v 1.8% with < 75 mg daily; P > 0.05).[6] We found one systematic review (search date 1999, 24 RCTs) of the effects of aspirin on gastrointestinal bleeding.[26] Indirect comparisons in a metaregression analysis found no association between dose of aspirin and risk of gastrointestinal bleeds. RCTs directly comparing different daily doses of aspirin have found a trend towards more gastrointestinal haemorrhage and a significant increase in upper gastrointestinal symptoms with high (500–1500 mg) versus medium (75–325 mg) doses (upper gastrointestinal symptoms, OR 1.3, 95% CI 1.1 to 1.5), but no significant difference in these outcomes between 283 mg and 30 mg daily.[28–30] We found one systematic review of observational studies (search date 2001, 5 studies) of the effects of different doses of aspirin on the risk of upper gastrointestinal complications (bleeding, perforation, or upper gastrointestinal event leading to hospital admission or visit to specialist).[31] It found greater risks of upper gastrointestinal complications with doses of aspirin greater than 300 mg daily. **Intracranial haemorrhage:** We found one systematic review (search date 1997, 16 RCTs, 55 462 people) of the effects of aspirin on intracranial haemorrhage.[27] It found no clear variation in risk with the dose of aspirin used. Three RCTs directly compared different daily doses of aspirin and found no significant differences in the risk of intracranial haemorrhage, but lacked power to detect clinically important differences.[28–30]

Comment: None

| OPTION | ALTERNATIVE ANTIPLATELET AGENTS TO ASPIRIN |

Cathie Sudlow

Systematic reviews have found no good evidence that any antiplatelet regimen is superior to aspirin for long term secondary prevention of serious vascular events.

Benefits: **Thienopyridines (clopidogrel and ticlopidine) versus aspirin:** We found two systematic reviews (search dates 1997[4] and 1999[32]) that compared thienopyridines versus aspirin. The first systematic review (4 RCTs, 3791 people at high risk of vascular disease) found no significant difference with ticlopidine versus aspirin in serious vascular events (stroke, myocardial infarction, or vascular death) (AR 21% with ticlopidine v 23% with aspirin; OR presented graphically; P value not provided).[4] It also found that the risk of serious vascular events was similar with clopidogrel versus aspirin (1 RCT; 19 185 people; AR 10% with clopidogrel v 11% with aspirin; OR 0.90, 95% CI 0.82 to 0.99). The second systematic review (4 RCTs)[32] found that ticlopidine or clopidogrel versus aspirin marginally reduced vascular events after about 2 years (OR 0.91, 95% CI 0.84 to 0.98; ARR 1.1%, 95% CI 0.2% to 1.9%). **Dipyridamole plus aspirin:** We found one systematic review (search date 1997, 25 relevant RCTs, 10 404 people comparing dipyridamole plus aspirin versus aspirin alone).[4] It found no significant difference with adding dipyridamole to aspirin in serious vascular events (stroke, myocardial infarction, or vascular death) (AR 11.8% with combination treatment v 12.4% with aspirin alone; OR 0.94, 95% CI 0.83 to 1.06).

Harms: **Thienopyridines (clopidogrel and ticlopidine):** The second systematic review[32] of thienopyridines versus aspirin found that the thienopyridines reduced gastrointestinal haemorrhage and upper gastrointestinal symptoms compared with aspirin (gastrointestinal haemorrhage: OR 0.71, 95% CI: 0.59 to 0.86; indigestion, nausea, or vomiting: OR 0.84, 95% CI: 0.78 to 0.90). However, thienopyridines increased the incidence of skin rash and diarrhoea compared with aspirin (skin rash: clopidogrel v aspirin, OR 1.3, 95% CI 1.2 to 1.5; ticlopidine v aspirin, OR 2.2, 95% CI 1.7 to 2.9; diarrhoea: clopidogrel v aspirin, OR 1.3, 95% CI 1.2 to 1.6; ticlopidine v aspirin, OR 2.3, 95% CI 1.9 to 2.8). Ticlopidine (but not clopidogrel) increased neutropenia compared with aspirin (OR 2.7, 95% CI 1.5 to 4.8). Observational studies have found that ticlopidine is associated with thrombocytopenia and thrombotic thrombocytopenic purpura.[33,34] **Dipyridamole:** One RCT found that combination treatment with dipyridamole plus aspirin was discontinued more frequently for adverse effects than aspirin alone.[35]

Cardiovascular disorders

Comment: One large RCT has assessed effects of adding clopidogrel to aspirin among people with unstable angina (see benefits of antiplatelet treatments in unstable angina, p 285).[36] A further large RCT is currently assessing the effects of alternative antiplatelet regimens among people with acute myocardial infarction.[37] One ongoing RCT is comparing effects of oral anticoagulation, aspirin plus dipyridamole, and aspirin alone among 4500 people with a prior transient ischaemic attack or minor ischaemic stroke.[38]

OPTION	LONG TERM ORAL ANTICOAGULATION IN PEOPLE WITH RECENT CEREBRAL ISCHAEMIA AND IN SINUS RHYTHM

Gord Gubitz and Peter Sandercock

One systematic review has found no significant difference between anticoagulation versus placebo for preventing recurrent stroke after presumed ischaemic stroke in people in normal sinus rhythm. Anticoagulants increased the risk of fatal intracranial and extracranial haemorrhage compared with placebo. One systematic review has found no significant difference between high or low intensity anticoagulation versus antiplatelet treatment for preventing recurrent stroke in people with recent cerebral ischaemia of presumed arterial (non-cardiac) origin. High intensity anticoagulation increased the risk of major bleeding compared with antiplatelet treatment.

Benefits: **Versus placebo:** We found one systematic review (search date not stated, 9 small RCTs, 1214 people in sinus rhythm with previous non-embolic presumed ischaemic stroke or transient ischaemic attack, mean duration 1.8 years).[39] It found no clear benefit of oral anticoagulants (warfarin, dicoumarol, or phenindione) versus placebo on death or dependency (ARR +4%, 95% CI −6% to +14%; RRR +5%, 95% CI −9% to +18%), or on mortality or recurrent stroke. **Versus antiplatelet treatment:** We found one systematic review (search date 1999, 4 RCTs, 1870 people) comparing long term (> 6 months) treatment with oral anticoagulants (warfarin, phenprocoumarin, or acenocoumarol [nicoumalone]) versus antiplatelet treatment in people with a history of transient ischaemic attack or minor stroke of presumed arterial (non-cardiac) origin in the past 6 months.[40] It found no significant difference between high intensity (INR [see glossary, p 262] 3.0–4.5) or low intensity (INR 2.1–3.5) anticoagulation versus antiplatelet treatment for preventing recurrent stroke (low intensity anticoagulation v antiplatelet treatment: ARR +0.2%, 95% CI −4.0% to +4.3%; RR 0.96, 95% CI 0.38 to 2.42; high intensity anticoagulation v antiplatelet treatment: ARR −0.1%, 95% CI −1.7% to +1.5%; RR 1.02, 95% CI 0.49 to 2.13).

Harms: **Versus placebo:** The first review found that anticoagulants increased the risk of fatal intracranial haemorrhage (ARI 2.0%, 95% CI 0.4% to 3.6%; RR 2.51, 95% CI 1.12 to 5.60; NNH 49 people treated with anticoagulants over 1.8 years for 1 additional non-fatal extracranial haemorrhage, 95% CI 27 to 240).[39] The risk of fatal and non-fatal extracranial haemorrhage was also increased by anticoagulants compared with placebo (ARI 5.1%, 95% CI 3.0% to 7.2%; RR 5.86, 95% CI 2.39 to 14.3; NNH 20, 95% CI 14 to 33).

Versus antiplatelet treatment: The review comparing anticoagulants versus antiplatelet treatment found no significant difference in risk of major intracranial or extracranial bleeding with low intensity anticoagulation (INR 2.1–3.6) versus antiplatelet treatment (RR 1.19, 95% CI 0.59 to 2.41).[40] However, high intensity anticoagulation (INR 3.0–4.5) significantly increased the risk of major intracranial or extracranial bleeding (RR 1.08, 95% CI 1.03 to 1.20).

Comment: **Versus placebo:** The trials in the systematic review all had major problems with their methods, including poor monitoring of anticoagulation.[39] All were completed before introducing routine computerised tomography scanning, which means that people with primary haemorrhagic strokes could have been included. The systematic review could not, therefore, provide a reliable and precise overall estimate of the balance of risk and benefit regarding death or dependency. Most people in the trial comparing warfarin and aspirin did have a computerised tomography scan, but an adverse outcome was still seen with anticoagulants. Two further RCTs are in progress: one compares a lower intensity of adjusted dose warfarin (to maintain an INR of 1.4–2.8) with aspirin 325 mg four times daily within 30 days after stroke and treated for at least 2 years,[41] whereas the other assesses warfarin (to maintain an INR of 2.0–3.0) versus aspirin (any dose between 30–325 mg daily) versus aspirin plus dipyridamole (400 mg daily).[42]

OPTION   **CAROTID ENDARTERECTOMY FOR PEOPLE WITH RECENT CAROTID TERRITORY ISCHAEMIA**

Gord Gubitz and Peter Sandercock

One systematic review has found that carotid endarterectomy reduces the risk of major stroke and death in people with a recent carotid territory transient ischaemic attack or non-disabling ischaemic stroke who have moderate or severe symptomatic stenosis of the ipsilateral carotid artery. Evidence from two other systematic reviews suggest a possible benefit in people with asymptomatic but severe stenosis, but the results of a new large scale trial are awaited. One systematic review found no evidence that eversion carotid endarterectomy is more beneficial than conventional carotid endarterectomy.

Benefits: **People with symptomatic stenosis:** We found one systematic review (search date 1999, 3 RCTs, 6143 people with a recent neurological event in the territory of a stenosed ipsilateral carotid artery) comparing carotid surgery versus control treatment;[43] 96% of these data came from two large RCTs.[44,45] People were randomised within 4 and 6 months of the onset of vascular symptoms. The trials used different methods to measure degree of stenosis. The trials included 1247 people with severe stenosis (80–99%[44] and 70–99%[45]), 1259 people with moderate stenosis (70–79%[44] and 50–69%[45]), and 3397 people with mild stenosis (< 70%[44] and < 50%[45]). The degree of benefit from surgery was related to the degree of stenosis. For people with severe stenosis, there was a significant decrease in the subsequent risk of major stroke or death (ARR 6.7%, 95% CI 3.2% to 10.0%; RR 0.52, 95% CI 0.37 to 0.73; NNT 15, 95% CI 10 to 31). People with moderate stenosis also benefited (ARR 4.7%, 95% CI 0.8% to 8.7%; RR 0.73, 95% CI 0.56 to 0.95; NNT 21, 95% CI 11 to 125). People with mild stenosis did not have a significantly reduced risk of stroke (RR 0.80, 95% CI 0.56 to 1.0). In the trial with longer follow up, the annual risk of stroke after 3 years was not significantly different between people who had had surgery and those who had not.[44] In the other trial, people with severe stenosis had a benefit from endarterectomy at 8 years' follow up.[46] **People with asymptomatic stenosis:** We found two systematic reviews (search dates 1998) assessing carotid endarterectomy for asymptomatic carotid stenosis (no carotid territory transient ischaemic attack or minor stroke within the past few months).[47,48] One review included results from five RCTs (2440 people).[47] The other review included results from 2203 people from four of these five RCTs, after excluding the fifth RCT because of weak methods.[48] Both reviews found similar results. Carotid endarterectomy reduced the risk of perioperative stroke, death, or subsequent ipsilateral stroke (for the review of 4 RCTs:[48] AR 4.9% over 3 years in the surgical group v 6.8% in the medical group; ARR 1.9%, 95% CI 0.1% to 3.9%; NNT 52, 95% CI 26 to 1000; for the review of 5 RCTs:[47] 4.7% over 3 years in the surgical group v 7.4% in the medical group; ARR 2.7%, 95% CI 0.8% to 4.6%; NNT 37, 95% CI 22 to 125). Although the risk of perioperative stroke or death from carotid surgery for people with asymptomatic stenosis seems to be lower than in people with symptomatic stenosis, the risk of stroke or death without surgery in asymptomatic people is relatively low and so, for most people, the balance of risk and benefit from surgery remains unclear.[47,48] **Eversion carotid endarterectomy versus conventional carotid endarterectomy:** We found one systematic review (search date 1999, 5 RCTs, 2645 people, 2590 carotid arteries) that compared eversion carotid endarterectomy versus conventional carotid endarterectomy (see glossary, p 262) performed either with primary closure or patch angioplasty.[49] Overall, the review found no significant differences in the rate of perioperative stroke, stroke or death, local complication rate, and rate of neurological events (for stroke or death: AR 1.7% with eversion v 2.6% with conventional, ARR +0.9%, 95% CI −0.3% to +2.1%; for stroke: AR 1.4% with eversion v 1.7% with conventional, ARR +0.3%, 95% CI −0.7% to +1.3%).

Harms:

People with symptomatic stenosis: The systematic review of endarterectomy for symptomatic stenosis found that carotid surgery was associated with a definite risk of recurrent stroke or death.[43] The relative risk of disabling stroke or death within 30 days of randomisation was 2.5 (95% CI 1.6 to 3.8). A second systematic review (search date 1996, 36 studies) identified several risk factors for operative stroke and death from carotid endarterectomy, including female sex, occlusion of the contralateral internal carotid artery, stenosis of the ipsilateral external carotid artery, and systolic blood pressure greater than 180 mm Hg.[50] Endarterectomy is also associated with other postoperative complications, including wound infection (3%), wound haematoma (5%), and lower cranial nerve injury (5–7%). **People with asymptomatic stenosis:** Given the low prevalence of severe carotid stenosis in the general population, there is concern that screening and surgical intervention in asymptomatic people may result in more strokes than it prevents.[51]

Comment: **People with symptomatic stenosis:** The two RCTs contributing most of the data to the systematic review[44,45] used different techniques to measure the degree of carotid stenosis, but conversion charts are available and were used in the systematic review.[43] The trials, as well as observational studies,[5] found that risk of recurrent stroke was highest about the time of the symptomatic event. Subgroup analysis of one RCT included in the review found that, compared to medical treatment, endarterectomy for greater than 70% symptomatic stenosis reduced ipsilateral stroke to a greater extent in older people than younger people (at 2 years, for people > 75 years: ARR of stroke with endarterectomy v medical treatment 28.9%, 95% CI 12.9% to 44.9%; NNT 3, 95% CI 2 to 8, for people aged 65–74 years: ARR 15.1%, 95% CI 7.2% to 23.0%; NNT 7, 95% CI 4 to 14; for people aged < 65 years: ARR 9.7%, 95% CI 1.5% to 17.9%; NNT 10, 95% CI 6 to 67).[52] Among people with 50–69% stenosis, only the older (> 75 years) age group significantly benefited from endarterectomy (ARR for ipsilateral stroke at 2 years 17.3%, 95% CI 6.6% to 28.0%; NNT 6, 95% CI 4 to 15). Participating surgeons were experienced and people with other life threatening comorbidity were excluded. **People with asymptomatic stenosis:** A large scale trial is ongoing.[53]

OPTION	CAROTID AND VERTEBRAL PERCUTANEOUS TRANSLUMINAL ANGIOPLASTY

Gord Gubitz and Peter Sandercock

We found that carotid or vertebral percutaneous transluminal angioplasty has not been adequately assessed in people with a recent carotid or vertebral territory transient ischaemic attack or non-disabling ischaemic stroke who have severe stenosis of the ipsilateral carotid or vertebral artery.

Benefits: We found no systematic review. **Carotid percutaneous transluminal angioplasty:** One RCT (504 people with a recent carotid territory transient ischaemic attack or non-disabling ischaemic stroke with stenosis of the ipsilateral carotid artery) compared "best medical treatment" plus carotid percutaneous transluminal angioplasty (PTA) versus "best medical treatment" plus carotid endarterectomy.[54] The rates of major outcome events within 30 days of first treatment did not differ significantly between endovascular treatment and surgery (AR for disabling stroke or death 6.4% with PTA v 5.9% with surgery; AR for stroke lasting more than 7 days or death 10.0% with PTA v 9.9% with surgery). The trial found no significant difference between treatments for ipsilateral stroke rate up to 3 years after randomisation (adjusted HR 1.04, 95% CI 0.63 to 1.70, P = 0.9). **Vertebral artery; PTA:** The RCT also compared vertebral PTA versus "best medical treatment" in 16 people, but did not provide enough data for reliable estimates of efficacy.[54]

Harms: The RCT found that cranial neuropathy was more common with surgery (22 people [8.7%] undergoing surgery v 0 people after endovascular treatment; P < 0.0001). Major groin or neck haematoma occurred less often after endovascular treatment than after surgery (3 people with endovascular treatment [1.2%] v 17 people with surgery [6.7%]; P < 0.0015).[54]

Stroke prevention

Comment: The RCT comparing endovascular treatment versus surgery had low power, and results lacked precision.[54] Two ongoing RCTs are comparing carotid endarterectomy versus primary stenting in people with recently symptomatic severe carotid stenosis.[55,56]

QUESTION	What are the effects of anticoagulant and antiplatelet treatment in people with atrial fibrillation?

Gord Gubitz, Peter Sandercock, and Gregory YH Lip

Systematic reviews have found that people with atrial fibrillation at high risk of stroke and with no contraindications are likely to benefit from anticoagulation. However, one recent systematic review has questioned the quality of existing RCTs and reviews and suggested that more trials are needed to establish effects of anticoagulation. Antiplatelet agents are less effective than warfarin and are associated with a lower bleeding risk, but are a reasonable alternative if warfarin is contraindicated or if risk of ischaemic stroke is low. The best time to begin anticoagulation after an ischaemic stroke is unclear.

Benefits: Three risk strata have been identified based on evidence derived from one overview of five RCTs[57] and one subsequent RCT.[58] Most reviews have stratified effects of treatment in terms of these risk categories. However, one recent systematic review (search date 1999), which did not stratify for perceived risk, has suggested that RCTs may be too heterogeneous to determine effects of long term oral anticoagulation versus placebo among people with non-rheumatic atrial fibrillation (see comment below).[59] **People with atrial fibrillation at high risk of stroke, adjusted dose warfarin versus placebo:** We found one overview[57] and three systematic reviews[60–62] examining the effect of warfarin in different groups of people with atrial fibrillation at high risk of stroke (see glossary, p 262). The overview (5 RCTs, 2461 elderly people with atrial fibrillation and a variety of stroke risks) compared warfarin versus placebo.[57] It found that anticoagulation reduced the risk of stroke (ARR after a mean of 5 years 4.4%, 95% CI 2.8% to 6.0%; RR 0.32, 95% CI 0.21 to 0.50; NNT 23 over 1 year, 95% CI 17 to 36). The first systematic review (search date not stated) identified two RCTs comparing warfarin with placebo in 1053 people with chronic non-rheumatic atrial fibrillation and a history of prior stroke or transient ischaemic attack (TIA).[60] Most people (98%) came from one double blind RCT (669 people within 3 months of a minor stroke or TIA,[63] which compared anticoagulant (target INR [see glossary, p 262] 2.5–4.0) versus aspirin versus placebo. It found that anticoagulants reduced the risk of recurrent stroke over about 2 years (ARR 13.7%, 95% CI 7.3% to 20.1%; RR 0.39, 95% CI 0.25 to 0.63; NNT 7 over 1 year, 95% CI 5 to 14). The second systematic review (search date 1999, 16 RCTs, 9874 people) included six RCTs (2900 people) of adjusted dose warfarin versus placebo (5 RCTs) or versus control (1 RCT) in high risk people (45% had hypertension, 20% had experienced a previous stroke or TIA).[61] These six RCTs included five trials in people without prior cerebral ischaemia (primary prevention trials) and one RCT in people with prior cerebral ischaemia (secondary prevention trial).[64] Target INR varied among RCTs (2.0–2.6 in primary prevention RCTs and 2.9 in the secondary prevention RCT). The results of this systematic review were similar to the others. The meta-analysis found that adjusted dose warfarin reduced the risk of stroke (5 primary prevention RCTs: ARR 4.0%, 95% CI 2.3% to 5.7%; NNT 25, 95% CI 18 to 43; 1 secondary prevention RCT: ARR 14.5%, 95% CI 7.7% to 21.3%; NNT 7, 95% CI 5 to 13; combined primary and secondary prevention RCTs: ARR 5.5%, 95% CI 3.7% to 7.3%; NNT 18, 95% CI 14 to 27). The third systematic review (search date 1999, 14 RCTs) identified the same warfarin versus placebo trials and found similar results.[62] **Adjusted dose warfarin versus minidose warfarin in people with atrial fibrillation and high risk of stroke:** We found no systematic review or RCTs of low dose warfarin regimens in people with atrial fibrillation and a recent TIA or acute stroke. We found one RCT (1044 people with atrial fibrillation at high risk of stroke), which compared low, fixed dose warfarin (target INR 1.2–1.5) plus aspirin (325 mg daily) with standard adjusted dose warfarin treatment (target INR 2.0–3.0).[58] Adjusted dose warfarin significantly reduced the combined rate of ischaemic stroke or systemic embolism (ARR 6.0%, 95% CI 3.4% to 8.6%; NNT 17, 95% CI 12 to 29), and of disabling or fatal stroke (ARR 3.9%, 95% CI 1.6% to 6.1%; NNT 26, 95% CI 16 to 63). We found two additional RCTs,[65][67] which aimed to assess adjusted dose warfarin versus low dose warfarin and aspirin, but were stopped prematurely when the results of the earlier trial[58] were published. Analyses of the optimal anticoagulation intensity for stroke prevention in atrial fibrillation found that stroke risk was substantially increased at INR levels below 2.[64,68] **Adjusted dose warfarin versus aspirin in people with atrial fibrillation and high risk of stroke:** We found two systematic reviews of warfarin versus different antiplatelet regimens in people at high risk of stroke.[61,69] The first systematic review (search date not stated, 1 RCT)[69] found that in elderly people with atrial fibrillation and a prior history of stroke or TIA, warfarin (target INR 2.5–4.0) reduced the risk of stroke compared to aspirin 300 mg daily (22.6% with aspirin v 8.9% with warfarin; ARR 14%, 95% CI 7% to 20%; RR 0.39, 95% CI 0.24 to 0.64; NNT 7, 95% CI 5 to 14).[69] The second systematic review (search date 1999, 16 RCTs, 9874 people) included five RCTs (4 primary prevention and 1 secondary prevention RCTs, 2837 people) of adjusted dose warfarin versus aspirin in high risk people (45% had hypertension, 20% had experienced a previous stroke or TIA).[61] Target INR varied among RCTs (2.0–4.5 in primary prevention RCTs, 2.5–4.0 in the secondary prevention RCT). Adjusted dose warfarin versus aspirin reduced the overall risk of stroke (ARR 2.9%, 95% CI 0.9% to 4.8%; NNT 34, 95% CI 21 to 111). The effect varied widely among the five RCTs, none of which were blinded. **Adjusted dose warfarin versus other antiplatelet treatment in people with atrial fibrillation and high risk of stroke:** One systematic review (search date 1999) compared adjusted dose warfarin versus other antiplatelet agents such as indobufen.[61] One RCT included in the review (916 people within 15 days of stroke onset) compared warfarin (INR 2.0–3.5) with indobufen.[70] It found no significant difference in the rate of recurrent stroke between the two groups (5% for indobufen v 4% for warfarin; ARR +1.0%, 95% CI −1.7% to +3.7%). **Adjusted warfarin versus any antiplatelet agents in people with atrial**

fibrillation and high risk of stroke: We found one systematic review (search date 1999, 6 RCTs, 3298 people) of aspirin or indobufen versus warfarin.[59] It found that warfarin reduced stroke more than antiplatelet agents (ARR 1.8%, 95% CI 0.4% to 3.2%; NNT 56, 95% CI 31 to 250). **Aspirin versus placebo in people with atrial fibrillation and high risk of stroke:** We found one systematic review (search date 1999, 5 RCTs, 2769 people with atrial fibrillation and prior stroke or TIA).[62] Aspirin reduced the risk of stroke, although the confidence interval included the possibility of no benefit (ARR +1.8%, 95% CI −0.4% to +4.0%). **In people with atrial fibrillation at moderate risk of stroke:** See glossary, p 263. We found no RCT that considered this group specifically. **Anticoagulants in people with atrial fibrillation at low risk of stroke:** See glossary, p 263. We found one systematic review[71] and one overview[57] comparing warfarin versus placebo in people with atrial fibrillation and a variety of stroke risks. Both reviews included the same five RCTs. The overview (2461 people) found that, for people younger than 65 years with atrial fibrillation (but no history of hypertension, stroke, TIA, or diabetes), the annual stroke rate was the same with warfarin or placebo (1% a year).[57] The systematic review (search date 1999, 2313 people, mean age 69 years, 20% aged > 75 years; 45% had hypertension, 15% diabetes, and 15% a prior history of myocardial infarction) found that warfarin (INR 2.0–2.6) versus placebo reduced fatal and non-fatal ischaemic stroke (ARR 4.0%, 95% CI 2.4% to 5.6%; NNT 25, 95% CI 18 to 42), reduced all ischaemic strokes or intracranial haemorrhage (ARR 4.5%, 95% CI 2.8% to 6.2%; NNT 22, 95% CI 16 to 36), and reduced the combined outcome of disabling or fatal ischaemic stroke or intracranial haemorrhage (ARR 1.8%, 95% CI 0.5% to 3.1%; NNT 56, 95% CI 32 to 200).[71] **Antiplatelet treatment in people with atrial fibrillation and low risk of stroke:** We found two systematic reviews.[61,72] The first (search date 1999, 2 RCTs, 1680 people with either paroxysmal or sustained non-valvular atrial fibrillation confirmed by electrocardiogram but without previous stroke or TIA, 30% aged > 75 years) compared aspirin with placebo.[72] In primary prevention, aspirin did not significantly reduce ischaemic stroke (OR 0.71, 95% CI 0.46 to 1.10; ARR +1.6%, 95% CI −0.5% to +3.7%), all stroke (OR 0.70, 95% CI 0.45 to 1.08; ARR +1.8%; 95% CI −0.5% to +3.9%), all disabling or fatal stroke (OR 0.88, 95% CI 0.48 to 1.58; ARR +0.4%, 95% CI −1.2% to +2.0%), or the composite end point of stroke, myocardial infarction, or vascular death (OR 0.76, 95% CI 0.54 to 1.05; ARR +2.3%, 95% CI −0.4% to +5.0%). The second systematic review (search date 1999)[61] included three RCTs of primary prevention. The average rate of stroke among people taking placebo was 5.2%. Meta-analysis of the three RCTs found that antiplatelet treatment versus placebo reduced the risk of stroke (ARR 2.2%, 95% CI 0.3% to 4.1%; NNT 45, 95% CI 24 to 333).

Harms: The major risk of anticoagulants and antiplatelet agents was haemorrhage. In the overview assessing elderly people with variable risk factors for stroke, the absolute risk of major bleeding was 1% for placebo, 1% for aspirin, and 1.3% for warfarin.[57] Another systematic review[61] found the absolute risk of intracranial haemorrhage increased from 0.1% a year with control to 0.3% a year with warfarin, but the difference was not significant. The absolute risks were three times higher in people who had bled previously. Both bleeding and haemorrhagic stroke were more common in people aged over 75 years. The risk of death after a major bleed was 13–33%, and risk of subsequent morbidity in those who survived a major bleed was 15%. The risk of bleeding was associated with an INR greater than 3, fluctuating INRs, and uncontrolled hypertension. In a systematic review (search date not stated, 2 RCTs) major extracranial bleeding was more frequent with anticoagulation treatment than placebo (ARI 4.9%, 95% CI 1.6% to 8.2%; RR 6.2, 95% CI 1.4 to 27.1; NNH 20, 95% CI 12 to 63).[60] The studies were too small to define the rate of intracranial haemorrhage (none occurred). In a systematic review (search date not stated) comparing anticoagulants and antiplatelet treatment, major extracranial bleeding was more frequent with anticoagulation (ARI 4.9%, 95% CI 1.6% to 8.2%; RR 6.4, 95% CI 1.5 to 28.1; NNH 20, 95% CI 12 to 63).[69] The studies were too small to define the rate of intracranial haemorrhage (in 1 RCT, none of the people on anticoagulant and 1 person on aspirin had an intracranial bleed). In the systematic review of oral anticoagulants versus placebo in low risk people,[71] the number of intracranial haemorrhages was small with a non-significant increase in the treatment group (5 in the treatment group and 2 in the control group). Likewise, in the systematic review assessing antiplatelet treatment in low risk people with atrial fibrillation,[72] too few haemorrhages occurred to characterise the effects of aspirin. One more recent systematic review found no evidence that warfarin significantly increased the risk of major haemorrhage compared with placebo among people with no prior TIA or stroke (5 RCTs, 2415 people; ARI for major haemorrhage warfarin v placebo +0.8%, 95% CI −1.3% to +2.9%).[62] However, if people with prior stroke or TIA were included, warfarin significantly increased major haemorrhage (6 RCTs, ARI warfarin v placebo 1.3%, 95% CI 0.4% to 2.2%; NNH 77, 95% CI 45 to 250). The systematic review found no evidence of a difference in major haemorrhage between warfarin and aspirin; warfarin and any antiplatelet agent; warfarin and low dose warfarin plus aspirin; and low molecular weight heparin and placebo; however, the review may have lacked power to detect a clinically important difference.[62]

Comment: One recent systematic review (search date 1999, 5 RCTs, 3298 people) has found results that conflict with those of previous reviews.[59] The review questions the methods and highlights the heterogeneity of RCTs of oral anticoagulation in people with non-rheumatic atrial fibrillation. People in the RCTs were highly selected (< 10%, range 3–40% of eligible people were randomised); many were excluded after assessments for the absence of contraindications and physicians' refusal to enter them into the study. Many of the studies were not double blinded and in some studies there was poor agreement between raters for "soft" neurological end points. The frequent monitoring of warfarin treatment under trial conditions and motivation of people/investigators was probably more than that seen in usual clinical practice. The review has suggested that considerable uncertainty remains about benefits of long term anticoagulation in people with non-rheumatic atrial fibrillation. The review has different inclusion and exclusion criteria than previously published reviews and includes a trial not included in previous reviews.[58] Unlike previous reviews, the recent systematic review did not stratify people for perceived stroke risk and identified no significant difference between anticoagulant versus placebo with either a fixed effects model or a random effects model, which was employed to account for heterogeneity of underlying trials (fixed effects: OR 0.74, 95% CI 0.39 to 1.40 for stroke deaths; OR 0.86, 95% CI 0.16 to 1.17 for vascular deaths; random effects: OR 0.79, 95% CI 0.61 to 1.02 for combined fatal and non-fatal events).[59] The publication of this review has led to debate and uncertainty about clinical effectiveness of long term anticoagulation in people with non-rheumatic atrial fibrillation. Decisions to treat should be informed by considering trade-offs between benefits and harms, and each person's treatment preferences.[73-78] We found net benefit of anticoagulation for people in atrial fibrillation who have had a TIA or stroke, or who are over 75 years of age and at a high risk of stroke. We found less clear cut evidence for those aged 65–75 years at high risk, and for those with moderate risk (i.e. > 65 years and not in a high risk group or < 65 years with clinical risk factors), or for those at low risk (< 65 years with no other risk factors). The benefits of warfarin in the RCTs may not translate into effectiveness in clinical practice.[59,79,80] In the RCTs, most strokes in people randomised to warfarin occurred while they were not in fact taking warfarin, or were significantly underanticoagulated at the time of the event. A recent systematic review[81] (search date not stated, 410 people) identified three trials comparing the outcomes of people treated with anticoagulants in the community to the pooled results of the RCTs. The authors confirmed that people who undergo anticoagulation for atrial fibrillation in actual clinical practice are generally older and have more comorbid conditions than people enrolled in RCTs. However, both groups had similar rates of stroke and major bleeding. This risk of minor bleeding was higher in the community group, and it was suggested that these people may require more intensive monitoring in routine practice. **Timing of anticoagulation:** The best time to start anticoagulation after an ischaemic stroke is unclear, but aspirin reduces the risk of recurrent stroke in such people with or without atrial fibrillation, suggesting that it is reasonable to use aspirin until it is considered safe to start oral anticoagulants.[82]

GLOSSARY

Conventional carotid endarterectomy This is more commonly employed and involves a longitudinal arteriotomy of the carotid artery.

Eversion carotid endarterectomy This involves a transverse arteriotomy and reimplantation of the carotid artery.

International normalised ratio (INR) A value derived from a standardised laboratory test that measures the effect of an anticoagulant like warfarin. The laboratory materials used in the test are calibrated against internationally accepted standard reference preparations, so that variability between laboratories and different reagents is minimised. Normal blood has an INR of 1. Therapeutic anticoagulation often aims to achieve an INR value of 2.0–3.5.

People at high risk of stroke People of any age with a previous transient ischaemic attack or stroke or a history of rheumatic vascular disease, coronary artery disease, congestive heart failure, and impaired left ventricular function or

Cardiovascular disorders

echocardiography; and people aged 75 years and over with hypertension, diabetes, or both.

People at moderate risk of stroke People aged over 65 years who are not in the high risk group; and people aged under 65 years with clinical risk factors, including diabetes, hypertension, peripheral arterial disease, and ischaemic heart disease. **People at low risk of stroke** All other people aged less than 65 years with no history of stroke, transient ischaemic attack, embolism, hypertension, diabetes, or other clinical risk factors.

REFERENCES

1. Hankey GJ, Warlow CP. *Transient ischaemic attacks of the brain and eye.* London: WB Saunders, 1994.

2. Prospective Studies Collaboration. Cholesterol, diastolic blood pressure, and stroke: 13 000 strokes in 450 000 people in 45 prospective cohorts. *Lancet* 1995;346:1647–1653.

3. Eastern Stroke and Coronary Heart Disease Collaborative Research Group. Blood pressure, cholesterol, and stroke in eastern Asia. *Lancet* 1998;352:1801–1807.

4. Antithrombotic Trialists' Collaboration. Collaborative meta-analysis of randomised trials of antiplatelet therapy for prevention of death, myocardial infarction, and stroke in high risk patients. *BMJ* 2002;324:71–86. Corrections: *BMJ* 2002;324:141. Search date 1997; primary sources Medline, Embase, Derwent, SciSearch, Biosis, searching the trials registers of the Cochrane Stroke and Peripheral Vascular Disease Groups trials registers, and hand searches of selected journals, proceedings of meetings, reference lists of trials and review articles, and personal contact with colleagues and representatives of pharmaceutical companies.

5. Warlow CP, Dennis MS, Van Gijn J, et al. Predicting recurrent stroke and other serious vascular events. In: *Stroke. A practical guide to management.* Oxford: Blackwell Science, 1996:545–552.

6. Antiplatelet Trialists' Collaboration. Collaborative overview of randomised trials of antiplatelet therapy — I: prevention of death, myocardial infarction, and stroke by prolonged antiplatelet therapy in various categories of patients. *BMJ* 1994;308:81–106. Search date 1990; primary sources Medline, Current Contents, hand searches of journals, reference lists, and conference proceedings, and contact with authors of trials and manufacturers.

7. Hart RG, Pearce LA, Rothbart RM, et al. Stroke with intermittent atrial fibrillation: incidence and predictors during aspirin therapy. Stroke Prevention in Atrial Fibrillation Investigators. *J Am Coll Cardiol* 2000;35:183–187.

8. The INDANA Project Collaborators. Effect of antihypertensive treatment in patients having already suffered from stroke. *Stroke* 1997;28:2557–2562. Search date not stated; primary sources electronic medical databases; survey of specialised and general medical journals and congress proceedings and consultanting experts.

9. PROGRESS Collaborative Group. Randomised trial of a perindopril-based blood-pressure-lowering regimen among 6105 individuals with previous stroke or transient ischaemic attack. *Lancet* 2001;358:1033–1041.

10. PATS Collaborating Group. Post-stroke antihypertensive treatment study: a preliminary result. *Chinese Med J* 1995;108:710–717.

11. Rodgers A, MacMahon S, Gamble G, et al, for the United Kingdom Transient Ischaemic Attack Collaborative Group. Blood pressure and risk of stroke in patients with cerebrovascular disease. *BMJ* 1996;313:147.

12. Neal B, Clark T, MacMahon S, et al, on behalf of the Antithrombotic Trialists' Collaboration. Blood pressure and the risk of recurrent vascular disease. *Am J Hypertension* 1998;11:25A–26A.

13. Wright JM, Lee C-H, Chambers GK. Systematic review of antihypertensive therapies: does the evidence assist in choosing a first line drug? *Can Med Assoc J* 1999;161:25–32. Search date 1997; primary sources Medline, Cochrane Library (Issue 2, 1998), and references from previous meta-analyses published between 1980 and 1997.

14. Blood Pressure Lowering Treatment Trialists' Collaboration. Effects of ACE inhibitors, calcium antagonists, and other blood-pressure-lowering drugs: results of prospectively designed overviews of randomised trials. *Lancet* 2000;356:1955–1964. Search date not stated; primary sources result from a collaboration of trialists providing a limited data set for inclusion in the overview analyses.

15. Staessen JA, Wang J-G, Thijs L. Cardiovascular protection and blood pressure reduction: a meta-analysis. *Lancet* 2001;358:1305–1315. Search date not stated; primary sources Medline and hand searches of reference lists of previous overviews.

16. Dahlöf B, Devereux RB, Kjeldsen SE, et al, for the LIFE study group. Cardiovascular morbidity and mortality in the Losartan Intervention for Endpoint reduction in hypertension study (LIFE): a randomised trial against atenolol. *Lancet* 2002;359:995–1003.

17. Sleight P, Yusuf S, Pogue J, et al, for the Heart Outcomes Prevention Evaluation (HOPE) study investigators. Blood-pressure reduction and cardiovascular risk in HOPE study. *Lancet* 2001;358:2130–2131.

18. Hebert PR, Gaziano JM, Chan KS, et al. Cholesterol lowering with statin drugs, risk of stroke, and total mortality: an overview of randomized trials. *JAMA* 1997;278:313–321. Search date 1995; primary sources electronic databases, reference lists, authors of trials and funding agencies. Cholesterol and Current Events (CARE) data added in 1996.

19. The Long-term Intervention with Pravastatin in Ischaemic Disease (LIPID) study group. Prevention of cardiovascular events and death with pravastatin in patients with coronary heart disease and a broad range of initial cholesterol levels. *N Engl J Med* 1998;339:1349–1357.

20. Heart Protection Study Collaborative Group. MRC/BHF Heart Protection Study of cholesterol lowering with simvastatin in 20 536 high-risk individuals: a randomised placebo-controlled trial. *Lancet* 2002;360:7–22.

21. Hebert PR, Gaziano M, Hennekens CH. An overview of trials of cholesterol lowering and risk of stroke. *Arch Intern Med* 1995;155:50–55.

22. Rubins HB, Robins SJ, Collins D, et al. Gemfibrozil for the secondary prevention of coronary heart disease in men with low levels of high-density lipoprotein cholesterol. *N Engl J Med* 1999;341:410–418.

23. Anonymous. The treatment of cerebrovascular disease with clofibrate. Final report of the Veterans' Administration Cooperative Study of Atherosclerosis, neurology section. *Stroke* 1973;4:684–693.

24. Welch KMA. Stroke Prevention by Aggressive Reduction in Cholesterol Levels (SPARCL). *Stroke* 2000;31:2541.

25. Cholesterol Treatment Trialists' Collaboration. Protocol for a prospective collaborative overview of all current and planned randomized trials of cholesterol treatment regimens. *Am J Cardiol* 1995;75:1130–1134.

26. Derry S, Loke YK. Risk of gastrointestinal haemorrhage with long term use of aspirin: meta-analysis. *BMJ* 2000;321:1183–1187. Search date 1999; primary sources Medline, Embase, and hand searches of reference lists from previous review papers and retrieved trials.

27. He J, Whelton PK, Vu B, et al. Aspirin and risk of hemorrhagic stroke. A meta-analysis of randomised controlled trials. *JAMA* 1998;280:1930–1935. Search date 1997; primary sources Medline and hand searches of reference lists of relevant articles.

28. The Dutch TIA Study Group. A comparison of two doses of aspirin (30 mg vs 283 mg a day) in patients after a transient ischaemic attack or minor ischaemic stroke. *N Engl J Med* 1991;325:1261–1266.

29. Farrell B, Godwin J, Richards S, et al. The United Kingdom transient ischaemic attack (UK-TIA) aspirin trial: final results. *J Neurol Neurosurg Psychiatry* 1991;54:1044–1054.

30. Taylor DW, Barnett HJM, Haynes RB, et al, for the ASA and Carotid Endarterectomy (ACE) Trial Collaborators. Low-dose and high-dose acetylsalicylic acid for patients undergoing carotid endarterectomy: a randomised controlled trial. *Lancet* 1999;353:2179–2184.

31. Garc a Rodr guez LA, Hernández-D az S, de Abajo FJ. Association between aspirin and upper gastrointestinal complications. Systematic review of epidemioligic studies. *Br J Clin Pharmacol* 2001;52;563–571. Search date 2001; primary sources Medline and hand searches of reference lists of reviews.

32. Hankey GJ, Sudlow CLM, Dunbabin DW. Thienopyridine derivatives (ticlopidine, clopidogrel) versus aspirin for preventing stroke and other serious vascular events in high vascular risk patients. In: The Cochrane Library, Issue 3, 2001. Oxford: Update Software. Search date 1999; primary sources Cochrane Stroke Group Trials Register, Antithrombotic Trialists' Collaboration database, and personal contact with the Sanofi pharmaceutical company.

33. Moloney BA. An analysis of the side effects of ticlopidine. In: Hass WK, Easton JD, eds. *Ticlopidine, platelets and vascular disease.* New York: Springer, 1993:117–139.

34. Bennett CL, Davidson CJ, Raisch DW, et al. Thrombotic thrombocytopenic purpura associated with ticlopidine in the setting of coronary artery stents and stroke prevention. *Arch Int Med* 1999;159:2524–2528.

35. Diener HC, Cunha L, Forbes C, et al. European secondary prevention study 2: dipyridamole and acetylsalicylic acid in the secondary prevention of stroke. *J Neurol Sci* 1996;143:1–13.

36. The Clopidogrel in Unstable Angina to Prevent Recurrent Events (CURE) Trial Investigators. Effects of clopidogrel in addition to aspirin in patients with acute coronary syndromes without ST-segment elevation. *N Engl J Med* 2001;345:494–502.

37. Second Chinese Cardiac Study (CCS-2) Collaborative Group. Rationale, design and organisation of the Second Chinese Cardiac Study (CCS-2): a randomised trial of clopidogrel plus aspirin, and of metoprolol, among patients with suspected acute myocardial infarction. *J Cardiovasc Risk* 2000;7:435–441.

38. De Schryver ELLM, on behalf of the European/Australian Stroke Prevention in Reversible Ischaemia Trial (ESPRIT) Group. Design of ESPRIT: an international randomized trial for secondary prevention after non-disabling cerebral ischaemia of arterial origin. *Cerebrovasc Dis* 2000;10:147–150.

39. Liu M, Counsell C, Sandercock P. Anticoagulants for preventing recurrence following ischaemic stroke or transient ischaemic attack. In: The Cochrane Library, Issue 3, 2001. Oxford: Update Software. Search date not stated; primary sources Cochrane Stroke Group Trials Register, and contact with companies marketing anticoagulant agents.

40. Algra A, De Schryver ELLM, van Gijn J, et al. Oral anticoagulants versus antiplatelet therapy for preventing further vascular events after transient ischaemic attack or minor stroke of presumed arterial origin (Cochrane Review). In: The Cochrane Library, Issue 2, 2002. Oxford: Update Software.

41. Mohr J, for the WARSS Group. Design considerations for the warfarin-antiplatelet recurrent stroke study. *Cerebrovasc Dis* 1995;5:156–157.

42. De Schryvfer E, for the ESPRIT Study Group. ESPRIT: mild anticoagulation, acetylsalicylic acid plus dipyridamole or acetylsalicylic acid alone after cerebral ischaemia of arterial origin [abstract]. *Cerebrovasc Dis* 1998;8(suppl 4):83.

43. Cina C, Clase C, Haynes R. Carotid endarterectomy for symptomatic stenosis. In: The Cochrane Library, Issue 3, 2001. Oxford: Update Software. Search date 1999; primary sources Cochrane Stroke Group Specialised Register of Trials, Medline, Embase, Healthstar, Serline, Cochrane Controlled Trials Register, DARE, and Best Evidence.

44. European Carotid Surgery Trialists' Collaborative Group. Randomised trial of endarterectomy for recently symptomatic carotid stenosis: final results of the MRC European carotid surgery trial. *Lancet* 1998;351:1379–1387.

45. North American Symptomatic Carotid Endarterectomy Trial Collaborators. Beneficial effect of carotid endarterectomy in symptomatic patients with high-grade carotid stenosis. *N Engl J Med* 1991;325:445–453.

46. Barnett HJ, Taylor DW, Eliasziw M, et al. Benefit of carotid endarterectomy in patients with symptomatic moderate or severe stenosis. North American symptomatic carotid endarterectomy trial collaborators. *N Engl J Med* 1998;339:1415–1425.

47. Benavente O, Moher D, Pham B. Carotid endarterectomy for asymptomatic carotid stenosis: a meta-analysis. *BMJ* 1998;317:1477–1480. Search date 1997; primary sources Medline, Cochrane Controlled Trials Register, Ottawa Stroke Trials Register, Current Contents, and hand searches.

48. Chambers BR, You RX, Donnan GA. Carotid endarterectomy for asymptomatic carotid stenosis. In: The Cochrane Library, Issue 3, 2001. Oxford: Update Software. Search date 1998; primary sources Cochrane Stroke Group Trials Register,

Medline, Current Contents, hand searches of reference lists, and contact with researchers in the field.

49. Cao PG, De Rango P, Zannetti S, et al. Eversion versus conventional carotid endarterectomy for preventing stroke. In: The Cochrane Library, Issue 4, 2001. Oxford: Update Software. Search date 1999; primary sources Medline, Cochrane Stroke Group Trials Register, hand searches of surgical journals and conference proceedings, and contact with experts.

50. Rothwell P, Slattery J, Warlow C. Clinical and angiographic predictors of stroke and death from carotid endarterectomy: systematic review. BMJ 1997;315:1571–1577. Search date 1996; primary sources Medline, Cochrane Collaboration Stroke database, and hand searches of reference lists.

51. Whitty C, Sudlow C, Warlow C. Investigating individual subjects and screening populations for asymptomatic carotid stenosis can be harmful. J Neurol Neurosurg Psychiatry 1998;64:619 623.

52. Alamowitch S, Eliasziw, M, Algra A, et al, for the North American Symptomatic Carotid Endarterectomy Trial (NASCET) Group. Risk, causes, and prevention of ischaemic stroke in elderly patients with symptomatic internal-carotid-artery stenosis. Lancet 2001;357:1154–1160.

53. Halliday A, Thomas D, Manssfield A. The asymptomatic carotid surgery trial (ACST). Rationale and design. Eur J Vascular Surg 1994;8:703–710.

54. CAVATAS Investigators. Endovascular versus surgical treatment in patients with carotid stenosis in the Carotid and Vertebral Artery Transluminal Angioplasty Study (CAVATAS): a randomised trial. Lancet 2001;357;1729–1737.

55. Brown M. The International Carotid Stenting Study [abstract]. Stroke 2000;31:2812.

56. Al-Mubarek N, Roubin G, Hobson R, et al. Credentialing of Stent Operators for the Carotid Revascularization Endarterectomy vs Stenting Trial (CREST) [abstract]. Stroke 2000;31:292.

57. Atrial Fibrillation Investigators. Risk factors for stroke and efficacy of antithrombotic therapy in atrial fibrillation. Arch Intern Med 1994;154:1449–1457.

58. Stroke Prevention in Atrial Fibrillation Investigators. Adjusted-dose warfarin versus low-intensity, fixed-dose warfarin plus aspirin for high risk patients with atrial fibrillation: stroke prevention in atrial fibrillation III randomised clinical trial. Lancet 1996;348:633–638.

59. Taylor F, Cohen H, Ebrahim S. Systematic review of long term anticoagulation or antiplatelet treatment in patients with non-rheumatic atrial fibrillation. BMJ 2001;322:321–326. Search date 1999; primary sources Cochrane Central database, Embase, Medline, Cinahl, Sigle, hand searches of reference lists, and personal contact with experts.

60. Koudstaal P. Anticoagulants for preventing stroke in patients with non-rheumatic atrial fibrillation and a history of stroke or transient ischemic attacks. In: The Cochrane Library, Issue 2, 2002. Oxford: Update Software. Search date not stated; primary source Cochrane Stroke Group Trials Register and contact with trialists.

61. Hart R, Benavente O, McBride R, et al. Antithrombotic therapy to prevent stroke in patients with atrial fibrillation: a meta-analysis. Ann Intern Med 1999;131:492–501. Search date 1999; primary sources Medline, Cochrane Database, and Antithrombotic Trialists' Collaboration database.

62. Segal JB, McNamara RL, Miller MR, et al. Anticoagulants or antiplatelet therapy for non-rheumatic atrial fibrillation and flutter. In: The Cochrane Library, Issue 2, 2002. Oxford: Update Software. Search date 1999; primary sources Medline, Embase, Cochrane Heart Group Trials Register, hand searches of selected journals and conference proceedings, and contact with experts.

63. European Atrial Fibrillation Trial Study Group. Secondary prevention in non rheumatic atrial fibrillation after transient ischaemic attack or minor stroke. Lancet 1993;342:1255.

64. The European Atrial Fibrillation Trial Study Group. Optimal oral anticoagulant therapy in patients with non-rheumatic atrial fibrillation and recent cerebral ischemia. N Engl J Med 1995;333:5–10.

65. Pengo V, Zasso Z, Barbero F, et al. Effectiveness of fixed minidose warfarin in the prevention of thromboembolism and vascular death in nonrheumatic atrial fibrillation. Am J Cardiol 1998;82:433 437.

66. Gullov A, Koefoed B, Petersen P, et al. Fixed minidose warfarin and aspirin alone and in combination vs adjusted-dose warfarin for stroke prevention in atrial fibrillation. Second Copenhagen Atrial Fibrillation, Aspirin, and Anticoagulation Study. Arch Intern Med 1998;158:1513–1521.

67. Hellemons B, Langenberg M, Lodder J, et al. Primary prevention of arterial thrombo-embolism in non-rheumatic atrial fibrillation in primary care: randomised controlled trial comparing two intensities of coumarin with aspirin. BMJ 1999;319:958–964.

68. Hylek EM, Skates SJ, Sheehan MA, et al. An analysis of the lowest effective intensity of prophylactic anticoagulation for patients with non-rheumatic atrial fibrillation. N Engl J Med 1996;335:540–546.

69. Koudstaal P. Anticoagulants versus antiplatelet therapy for preventing stroke in patients with non-rheumatic atrial fibrillation and a history of stroke or transient ischemic attacks. In: The Cochrane Library, Issue 2, 2002. Oxford: Update Software. Search date not stated; primary sources Cochrane Stroke Group Trials Register and contact with trialists.

70. Morocutti C, Amabile G, Fattapposta F, et al, for the SIFA Investigators. Indobufen versus warfarin in the secondary prevention of major vascular events in non-rheumatic atrial fibrillation. Stroke 1997;28:1015–1021.

71. Benavente O, Hart R, Koudstaal P, et al. Oral anticoagulants for preventing stroke in patients with non-valvular atrial fibrillation and no previous history of stroke or transient ischemic attacks. In: The Cochrane Library, Issue 2, 2002. Oxford: Update Software. Search date 1999; primary sources Cochrane Stroke Group Specialised Register of Trials, Medline, Antithrombotic Trialists' Collaboration database, and hand searches of reference lists of relevant articles.

72. Benavente O, Hart R, Koudstaal P, et al. Antiplatelet therapy for preventing stroke in patients with non-valvular atrial fibrillation and no previous history of stroke or transient ischemic attacks. In: The Cochrane Library, Issue 2, 2002. Oxford: Update Software. Search date 1999; primary sources Medline, Cochrane Specialised Register of Trials, and hand searches of reference lists of relevant articles.

73. Lip G. Thromboprophylaxis for atrial fibrillation. Lancet 1999;353:4–6.

74. Ezekowitz M, Levine J. Preventing stroke in patients with atrial fibrillation. JAMA 1999;281:1830–1835.

75. Hart R, Sherman D, Easton D, et al. Prevention of stroke in patients with non-valvular atrial fibrillation. Neurology 1998;51:674–681.

76. Feinberg W. Anticoagulation for prevention of stroke. *Neurology* 1998;51(suppl 3):20–22.
77. Albers G. Choice of antithrombotic therapy for stroke prevention in atrial fibrillation. Warfarin, aspirin, or both? *Arch Intern Med* 1998;158:1487–1491.
78. Nademanee K, Kosar E. Long-term antithrombotic treatment for atrial fibrillation. *Am J Cardiol* 1998;82:37N–42N.
79. Green CJ, Hadorn DC, Bassett K, et al. Anticoagulation in chronic non-valvular atrial fibrillation: a critical appraisal and meta-analysis. *Can J Cardiol* 1997;13:811–815.
80. Blakely J. Anticoagulation in chronic non-valvular atrial fibrillation: appraisal of two meta-analyses. *Can J Cardiol* 1998;14:945–948.
81. Evans A, Kalra L. Are the results of randomized controlled trials on anticoagulation in patients with atrial fibrillation generalizable to clinical practice? *Arch Intern Med* 2001;161:1443–1447. Search date not stated; primary sources Medline, Cochrane Library, and hand searches of reference lists of relevant retrieved articles.
82. Chen ZM, Sandercock P, Pan HC, et al. Indications for early aspirin use in acute ischemic stroke: a combined analysis of 40 000 randomized patients from the Chinese acute stroke trial and the international stroke trial. On behalf of the CAST and IST collaborative groups. *Stroke* 2000;31:1240–1249.

Cathie Sudlow
Wellcome Clinician Scientist
Department of Clinical Neurosciences
University of Edinburgh
Edinburgh, UK

Gord Gubitz
Assistant Professor
Division of Neurology
Dalhousie University
Halifax, Canada

Peter Sandercock
Professor in Neurology
Neurosciences Trials Unit
University of Edinburgh
Edinburgh, UK

Gregory Lip
Consultant Cardiologist and Professor of Cardiovascular Medicine
City Hospital
Birmingham, UK

Competing interests: PS was the Principal Investigator of the second International Stroke Trial (IST-2). The trial was partly funded by Glaxo-Wellcome. He is also Chairman of the Steering Committee for the third International Stroke Trial (IST3) of thrombolysis in acute stroke. The start-up phase of trial is currently funded by a grant from the Stroke Association. Boehringer Ingelheim have donated trial drug and placebo for the 300 patients to be included in the start-up phase. PS has received honoraria for lectures, single consultations and travel expenses from a variety of pharmaceutical companies including: Boehringer Ingelheim, Sanofi, BNS, MSD, Servier, Glaxo-Wellcome, Lilly, Centocor. GG and GL none declared. CS on one occasion received fee from Sanofi-Synthelabo for giving a talk at a GP meeting.

TABLE 1 Effects of cholesterol reduction with a statin on risk of stroke: results of systematic review[18] and RCTs (see text, p 249),[19,20]

| | Number of | | Mean pretreatment cholesterol (mmol/L) | Average follow up duration (years) | Mean reduction in cholesterol* (%) | Summary OR (95% CI) for active treatment v control | |
	People	Strokes				Fatal or non-fatal stroke	Fatal stroke
1997 overview (14 RCTs)[18] + LIPID trial[19]	38 000	827	6.3	4	21	0.76† (0.66 to 0.87)	0.99† (0.67 to 1.45)
Heart Protection Study[20]	20 000	1029	5.9	5	24	0.75 (0.66 to 0.85)	0.81 (0.52 to 1.1)
All trials	58 000	1856	6.2	4.4	23	0.75 (0.67 to 0.83)	0.86 (0.39 to 1.1)

*Weighted by trial size; †the findings of other published overviews were consistent with the results shown here.

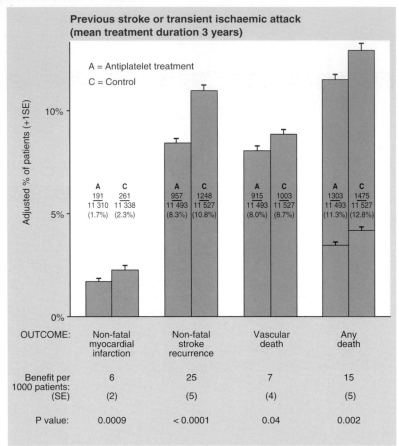

Previous stroke or transient ischaemic attack (mean treatment duration 3 years)

A = Antiplatelet treatment
C = Control

Adjusted % of patients (+1SE)

	A	C	A	C	A	C	A	C
	191	261	957	1248	915	1003	1303	1475
	11 310	11 338	11 493	11 527	11 493	11 527	11 493	11 527
	(1.7%)	(2.3%)	(8.3%)	(10.8%)	(8.0%)	(8.7%)	(11.3%)	(12.8%)

OUTCOME:	Non-fatal myocardial infarction	Non-fatal stroke recurrence	Vascular death	Any death
Benefit per 1000 patients: (SE)	6 (2)	25 (5)	7 (4)	15 (5)
P value:	0.0009	< 0.0001	0.04	0.002

FIGURE 1 Absolute effects of antiplatelet treatment on various outcomes in 21 trials in people with a prior (presumed ischaemic) stroke or transient ischaemic attack. The columns show the absolute risks over 3 years for each outcome. The error bars represent standard deviations. In the "any death" column, non-vascular deaths are represented by lower horizontal lines (see text, p 250). Adapted with permission.[4]

Key Messages

Proximal deep vein thrombosis

- **Oral anticoagulants** One RCT found that combined acenocoumarol plus intravenous unfractionated heparin versus acenocoumarol alone for initial treatment reduced recurrence of proximal deep vein thrombosis within 6 months. Systematic reviews have found that longer versus shorter duration of anticoagulation is associated with significantly fewer deep vein thrombosis recurrences or thromboembolic complications. One non-systematic review found limited evidence that longer versus shorter duration of warfarin treatment was associated with a significantly increased risk of major haemorrhage, but another non-systematic review found no significantly increased risk. The absolute risk of recurrent venous thromboembolism decreases with time, but the relative risk reduction with treatment remains constant. Harms of treatment, including major haemorrhage, continue during prolonged treatment. Individual people have different risk profiles. It is likely that the optimal duration of anticoagulation will vary between people.

- **Unfractionated and low molecular weight heparin** One systematic review has found no significant difference with long term low molecular weight heparin versus oral anticoagulation in recurrent thromboembolism, major haemorrhage, or mortality. Systematic reviews have found that low molecular weight heparin is at least as effective as unfractionated heparin in reducing the incidence of recurrent thromboembolic disease, and have found that short term low molecular weight heparin versus unfractionated heparin is associated with a significantly decreased risk of major haemorrhage.

Isolated calf vein thrombosis

- **Warfarin plus heparin** One RCT found that warfarin plus intravenous unfractionated heparin versus heparin alone (international normalised ratio 2.5–4.2) reduced the rate of proximal extension. One unblinded RCT found no significant difference in recurrent thromboembolism with 6 versus 12 weeks of anticoagulation.

Pulmonary embolism

- **Oral anticoagulants** We found no direct evidence about the optimum intensity and duration of anticoagulation in people with pulmonary embolism. The best available evidence requires extrapolation of results from studies of people with proximal deep vein thrombosis.
- **Thrombolysis** One systematic review in people with pulmonary embolism has found no significant difference in mortality with thrombolysis plus heparin versus heparin alone, and has found that thrombolysis may increase the incidence of intracranial haemorrhage. One small RCT identified by the review found limited evidence that thrombolysis may reduce mortality in people with shock due to massive pulmonary embolism.
- **Unfractionated and low molecular weight heparin** One small RCT found that heparin plus warfarin versus no anticoagulation significantly reduced mortality at 1 year in people with pulmonary embolism (NNT 4, 95% CI 2 to 16). One RCT in people with symptomatic pulmonary embolism who did not receive thrombolysis or embolectomy found no significant difference with low molecular weight heparin versus unfractionated heparin in mortality or new episodes of thromboembolism. Another RCT in people with proximal deep vein thrombosis without clinical signs or symptoms of pulmonary embolism but with high probability lung scan findings found that fixed dose low molecular weight heparin versus intravenous heparin significantly reduced the proportion of people with new episodes of venous thromboembolism.

Computerised decision support of oral anticoagulation

- We found no RCTs of computerised decision support versus usual management of oral anticoagulation that used clinically important outcomes (major haemorrhage or death).
- One systematic review and three subsequent RCTs have found that computerised decision support in oral anticoagulation significantly increases time spent in the target international normalised ratio range. Another subsequent RCT found no significant difference with computerised decision support versus standard manual support in the time spent in the target international normalised ratio range. A subsequent RCT of initiation of warfarin found no significant difference with computerised decision support versus usual care in the time taken to reach therapeutic levels of anticoagulation.

DEFINITION **Venous thromboembolism** is any thromboembolic event occurring within the venous system, including deep vein thrombosis and pulmonary embolism. **Deep vein thrombosis** is a radiologically confirmed partial or total thrombotic occlusion of the deep venous system of the legs sufficient to produce symptoms of pain or swelling. **Proximal deep vein thrombosis** affects the veins above the knee (popliteal, superficial femoral, common femoral, and iliac veins). **Isolated calf vein thrombosis** is confined to the deep veins of the calf and does not affect the veins above the knee. **Pulmonary embolism** is radiologically confirmed partial or total thromboembolic occlusion of pulmonary arteries, sufficient to cause symptoms of breathlessness, chest pain, or both. **Post-thrombotic syndrome** is oedema, ulceration, and impaired viability of the subcutaneous tissues of the leg occurring after deep vein thrombosis. **Recurrence** refers to symptomatic deterioration due to a further (radiologically confirmed) thrombosis, after a previously confirmed thromboembolic event, where there had been an initial partial or total symptomatic improvement. **Extension** refers to a radiologically confirmed new, constant, symptomatic intraluminal filling defect extending from an existing thrombosis.

INCIDENCE/ PREVALENCE We found no reliable study of the incidence/prevalence of deep vein thrombosis or pulmonary embolism in the UK. A prospective Scandinavian study found an annual incidence of 1.6–1.8/1000 people in the general population.[1,2] One postmortem study estimated that 600 000 people develop pulmonary embolism each year in the USA, of whom 60 000 die as a result.[3]

AETIOLOGY/ RISK FACTORS Risk factors for deep vein thrombosis include immobility, surgery (particularly orthopaedic), malignancy, smoking, pregnancy, older age, and inherited or acquired prothrombotic clotting disorders.[4] Evidence for these factors is mainly observational. The oral contraceptive pill is associated with increased risk of death due to venous thromboembolism (ARI with any combined oral contraception: 1–3/ million women a year).[5] The principal cause of pulmonary embolism is a deep vein thrombosis.[4]

PROGNOSIS The annual recurrence rate of symptomatic calf vein thrombosis in people without recent surgery is over 25%.[6,7] Proximal extension develops in 40–50% of people with symptomatic calf vein thrombosis.[8] Proximal deep vein thrombosis may cause fatal or non-fatal pulmonary embolism, recurrent venous thrombosis, and the post thrombotic syndrome. One observational study published in 1946 found 20% mortality from pulmonary emboli in people in hospital with untreated deep vein thrombosis.[9] One non-systematic review of observational studies found that, in people after recent surgery who have an asymptomatic calf vein deep vein thrombosis, the rate of fatal pulmonary embolism was 13–15%.[10] The incidence of other complications without treatment is not known. The risk of recurrent venous thrombosis and complications is increased by thrombotic risk factors.[11]

AIMS To reduce acute symptoms of deep vein thrombosis and to prevent morbidity and mortality associated with thrombus extension, the post-thrombotic syndrome, and pulmonary embolisation; to reduce recurrence; to minimise any adverse effects of treatment.

Thromboembolism

OUTCOMES	Rates of symptomatic recurrence, post-thrombotic syndrome, symptomatic pulmonary embolism, and death. Proxy outcomes include radiological evidence of clot extension or pulmonary embolism.
METHODS	*Clinical Evidence* update search and appraisal March 2002. Observational studies were used for estimating incidence, prevalence, and adverse event rates. RCTs were included only if participants and outcomes were objectively defined, and if the trial provided dose ranges (with adjusted dosing schedules for oral anticoagulation and unfractionated heparin) and independent, blinded outcome assessment.

QUESTION **What are the effects of treatments for proximal deep vein thrombosis?**

OPTION **ANTICOAGULATION**

Warfarin versus placebo: we found no RCTs. Acenocoumarol plus intravenous unfractionated heparin versus acenocoumarol alone for initial treatment: one RCT found reduced recurrence of proximal deep vein thrombosis. Longer versus shorter duration of anticoagulation: systematic reviews have found significantly fewer deep vein thrombosis recurrences with longer anticoagulation. One non-systematic review found limited evidence of significantly increased major haemorrhage, but another non-systematic review found no significant increase. Low molecular weight heparin versus unfractionated heparin: systematic reviews have found that low molecular weight heparin is at least as effective as unfractionated heparin in reducing the incidence of recurrent thromboembolic disease, and have found that short term low molecular weight heparin versus unfractionated heparin is associated with a significantly decreased risk of major haemorrhage. Long term low molecular weight heparin versus oral anticoagulation: one systematic review has found no significant difference with long term low molecular weight heparin versus oral anticoagulation in recurrent thromboembolism, major haemorrhage, or mortality. Heparin treatment at home versus in hospital: one systematic review has found limited evidence of no significant difference in recurrence of thromboembolism.

Benefits: **Warfarin versus placebo:** We found no systematic review and no RCTs. **Acenocoumarol plus intravenous unfractionated heparin versus acenocoumarol alone for initial treatment:** We found no systematic review. One RCT (120 people with proximal deep vein thrombosis) found that combined intravenous unfractionated heparin plus acenocoumarol versus acenocoumarol alone reduced recurrence at interim analysis at 6 months; although the difference did not quite reach significance and, as a result, the trial was stopped (12/60 [20%] with warfarin alone *v* 4/60 [7%] with combined treatment; P = 0.058).[12] **Longer versus shorter duration of anticoagulation:** We found two systematic reviews[13,14] and two subsequent open label RCTs.[15,16] The first systematic review (search date 2000, 4 RCTs, 1500 people) included two RCTs of people with a first episode of venous thromboembolism, one RCT in people with a second episode of venous thromboembolism, and one RCT in people with acute proximal deep vein thrombosis.[13] The periods of treatment compared were different in all four RCTs: 4 weeks versus 3 months, 6 weeks versus 6 months, 3 months versus 27 months, and 6 months versus 4 years. In all RCTs, anticoagulant doses were adjusted to achieve an international normalised ratio (see glossary, p 282) of 2.0–3.0. The review found that prolonged versus shorter treatment significantly reduced thromboembolic complications (AR 7/758 [0.9%] in the long arm v 91/742 [12.3%] in the short arm; RR 0.08, 95% CI 0.04 to 0.16; NNT 9, 95% CI 8 to 12). However, it found no significant reduction in mortality with prolonged versus shorter treatment (AR 37/758 [4.9%] in the long arm v 50/742 [6.7%] in the short arm; RR 0.72, 95% CI 0.48 to 1.08).[13] The second systematic review (search date not stated, 7 RCTs, 2304 people) included three of the same RCTs as the first systematic review plus four RCTs that had been excluded from the first systematic review on methodological grounds (either because of problems with blinding of outcomes or lack of an objective test to confirm thromboembolism).[14] There was wide variation in the duration of short term (3–12 wks) and longer term (12 wks to 2 years) RCTs. This review also found that longer versus shorter duration of anticoagulation reduced the risk of recurrent thromboembolism (74/1156 [6.4%] events per person with longer duration v 127/1148 [11.1%] with shorter duration; RR 0.60, 95% CI 0.45 to 0.79; NNT 22, 95% CI 15 to 43). The first subsequent RCT (736 people, including 539 with proximal deep vein thrombosis and/or pulmonary embolism; open label) comparing fluindione for 3 months versus 6 months found no significant difference in the risk of recurrent thromboembolism, although the confidence interval was wide (AR 21/270 [7.8%] with 3 months treatment v 23/269 [8.6%] with 6 months; ARR +0.8%, 95% CI −3.9% to +5.4%; RR 0.93, 95% CI 0.53 to 1.65).[15] The second subsequent RCT (267 people with a first episode of symptomatic proximal deep vein thrombosis; open label) compared warfarin or acenocoumarol treatment for 3 months versus 12 months.[16] It found no significant difference in recurrence of venous thromboembolism over a mean of 3 years (21/134 [15.7%] with 12 months v 21/133 [15.8%] with 3 months treatment; RR 0.99, 95% CI 0.57 to 1.73). Mean time to recurrence was shorter with 3 months versus 12 months treatment (11.2 months with 3 months v 16 months with 12 months; no further data provided).[16] **Intensity of anticoagulation:** We found one RCT (96 people with a first episode of idiopathic venous thromboembolism) comparing international normalised ratio targets of 2.0–3.0 versus 3.0–4.5 for 12 weeks' treatment with warfarin after an initial course of intravenous heparin. It found similar recurrence rates at 10 months for both international normalised ratio target ranges (1/47 [2.1%] with lower range v 1/49 [2.0%] with higher range; P > 0.05), but found significantly fewer haemorrhagic events with the lower target range (2/47 [4.3%] v 11/49 [22.4%]; ARR 18%, 95% CI 5% to 32%; RR 0.19, 95% CI 0.04 to 0.81; NNT 6, 95% CI 4 to 23).[17] **Abrupt versus gradual discontinuation of warfarin:** One RCT (41 people with deep vein thrombosis who had received intravenous heparin for 3–5 days followed by warfarin for 3–6 months) compared abrupt withdrawal of warfarin versus an additional month of warfarin at a fixed low dose of 1.25 mg daily.[18]

It found no difference in recurrence (3 people with abrupt withdrawal v 1 person with gradual withdrawal). **Low molecular weight heparin (LMWH) versus unfractionated heparin in people with proximal deep vein thrombosis:** We found two systematic reviews[19,20] and one subsequent unblinded RCT[21] in people with symptomatic proximal deep vein thrombosis. The first systematic review (search date 1993, 16 RCTs, 2045 people) found that LMWH (see glossary, p 282) versus unfractionated heparin significantly reduced thrombus extension (ARs not provided; OR 0.45, 95% CI 0.25 to 0.81).[19] The second systematic review (search date 1994, 10 RCTs, 1424 people) found that LMWH versus unfractionated heparin significantly reduced symptomatic thromboembolic complications (ARs not provided; RR 0.47, 95% CI 0.27 to 0.82) and mortality (RR 0.53, 95% CI 0.31 to 0.90).[20] The subsequent unblinded RCT (961 people) compared LMWH twice daily for 1 week versus LMWH once daily for 4 weeks versus intravenous unfractionated heparin.[21] It found that both LMWH regimens versus unfractionated heparin significantly increased thrombus regression at 21 days (167/312 [53.5%] with once daily LMWH v 129/321 [40.2%] with unfractionated heparin; RR 1.29, 97.5% CI 1.08 to 1.53; 175/328 [53.4%] with twice daily LMWH v 129/321 [40.2%] with unfractionated heparin; RR 1.28, 97.5% CI 1.08 to 1.52). It found that twice daily LMWH versus unfractionated heparin significantly reduced recurrent thromboembolism at 90 days (7/388 [1.8%] with twice daily LMWH v 24/375 [6.4%] with unfractionated heparin; RR 0.28, 97.5% CI 0.11 to 0.74), but found no significant difference with once daily LMWH versus unfractionated heparin in recurrent thromboembolism (13/374 [3.5%] with once daily LMWH v 24/375 [6.4%] with unfractionated heparin; RR 0.55, 97.5% CI 0.24 to 1.16). **LMWH versus unfractionated heparin in people with symptomatic venous thromboembolism:** We found six systematic reviews[22–27] and two subsequent RCTs[28,29] of LMWH versus unfractionated heparin in people with symptomatic venous thromboembolism located at sites other than just the proximal calf. The first systematic review (search date 1999, 14 RCTs, 4754 people) included five RCTs (blinded and unblinded, 1636 people) of proximal deep vein thrombosis.[22] It found that LMWH versus unfractionated heparin significantly reduced thrombotic complications (AR 39/814 [4.8%] with LMWH v 64/822 [7.8%] with unfractionated heparin; OR 0.60, 95% CI 0.40 to 0.89). Overall mortality was also reduced (AR 44/814 [5.4%] with LMWH v 68/822 [8.3%] with unfractionated heparin; OR 0.64, 95% CI 0.43 to 0.93). Eight of the 14 RCTs in the systematic review included people with symptomatic deep vein thrombosis of the leg without symptoms of pulmonary embolism, and these accounted for about 75% of all participants. Analysis of the seven RCTs that concealed treatment allocation found no difference in recurrent venous thromboembolism during initial treatment (AR 34/1569 [2.2%] with LMWH v 43/1595 [2.7%] with unfractionated heparin; OR 0.80, 95% CI 0.51 to 1.26), in recurrent venous thromboembolism at the end of 1–6 months' follow up (AR 75/1671 [4.5%] with LMWH v 92/1693 [5.4%] with unfractionated heparin; OR 0.82, 95% CI 0.60 to 1.12), in overall mortality (AR 123/1671 [7.4%] with LMWH v 150/1694 [8.9%] with unfractionated heparin; OR 0.82,

95% CI 0.64 to 1.05), or in major haemorrhage (see glossary, p 282).[22] The second systematic review (search date 1999, 21 blinded and unblinded RCTs, 4472 people) included nine RCTs excluded from the first systematic review on methodological grounds (dose of unfractionated heparin not adjusted, adjustment of dose of LMWH, and intravenous administration of LMWH).[26] Results for people with proximal deep vein thrombosis alone were not analysed separately. It found that LMWH versus unfractionated heparin significantly improved clot regression (OR 0.73, 95% CI 0.59 to 0.90), reduced the incidence of haemorrhage (OR 0.65, 95% CI 0.43 to 0.98; P = 0.04 7), and reduced mortality (OR 0.68, 95% CI 0.50 to 0.91; P = 0.01). It found no significant difference in recurrent thromboembolism (OR 0.78, 95% CI 0.59 to 1.04; P = 0.10). The third systematic review (search date not stated, 16 unblinded and blinded RCTs, 6042 people) included 14 RCTs from the first systematic review and two RCTs published after the search date of the first review.[27] It found that LMWH versus unfractionated heparin significantly reduced recurrent venous thromboembolism (ARs not provided; OR 0.66, 95% CI 0.51 to 0.86). The other three systematic reviews (search dates 1996,[23] 1999,[24] and not stated[25]), which included many of the same trials, found no significant difference in recurrent venous thromboembolism or pulmonary embolism with unfractionated heparin versus LMWH, and found a significant difference in favour of LMWH for total mortality over 3 months. The first subsequent RCT (294 people with acute proximal deep vein thrombosis, unblinded) compared intravenous unfractionated heparin in hospital versus LMWH twice daily given mainly at home (outpatients) or alternatively in hospital versus subcutaneous heparin calcium given at home. It found no significant difference in recurrent deep vein thrombosis (6/98 [6%] with unfractionated heparin v 6/97 [6%] with LMWH v 7/99 [7%] with subcutaneous heparin calcium).[28] See systematic anticoagulation under stroke management, p 229. The second subsequent RCT (900 people with symptomatic lower extremity deep vein thrombosis, including 287 with pulmonary embolism) compared unfractionated heparin versus enoxaparin once or twice daily. It found no significant difference in recurrent thromboembolism at 3 months (12/290 [4.1%] with unfractionated heparin v 22/610 [3.6%] with enoxaparin; ARR +0.5%, 95% CI −2% to +3%).[29] **Once daily versus twice daily LMWH:** We found one systematic review (search date 1999, 5 RCTs, 1522 people with symptomatic proximal deep vein thrombosis) comparing once versus twice daily LMWH for 5–10 days.[30] It found that once versus twice daily LMWH reduced the proportion of people with symptomatic or asymptomatic venous thromboembolism at 10 days or 3 months, but the difference was not significant (symptomatic venous thromboembolism at 10 days: 5 RCTs, OR 0.82, 95% CI 0.26 to 2.49; at 3 months: 3 RCTs, OR 0.85, 95% CI 0.48 to 1.49). **Long term LMWH versus oral anticoagulation:** We found one systematic review (search date 2001, 7 RCTs, 1137 people with proximal deep vein thrombosis treated initially with LMWH or unfractionated heparin for 5–10 days) comparing long term oral anticoagulation versus long term LMWH.[31] It found no significant difference with

LMWH versus oral anticoagulation in recurrent symptomatic thromboembolism (27/568 [4.8%] v 38/569 [6.7%]; OR 0.70, 95% CI 0.42 to 1.16) or mortality (21/568 [4.0%] v 14/569 [2.5%]; OR 1.51, 95% CI 0.77 to 2.97).[31] **Home versus hospital treatment with short term heparin:** We found one systematic review (search date 2000, 3 RCTs, 1104 people).[32] Two of the RCTs in the systematic review compared LMWH at home versus unfractionated heparin in hospital, the other RCT compared LMWH both at home and in hospital. The RCTs had methodological problems, including high exclusion rates and partial hospital treatment in the home treatment arms. The systematic review found no significant difference between treatments in recurrence of thromboembolism, minor bleeding, major haemorrhage, or mortality.[32]

Harms:　**Warfarin:** Two non-systematic reviews of RCTs and cohort studies found annual bleeding rates of 0–5% (fatal bleeding) and 2–8% (major bleeds).[33,34] Rates depended on how bleeding was defined and the intensity of anticoagulation. **Acenocoumarol plus intravenous unfractionated heparin versus acenocoumarol alone for initial treatment:** In the RCT comparing acenocoumarol plus heparin versus acenocoumarol alone: one person in the combined treatment group committed suicide at 6 months. There were two cancer related deaths, confirmed by postmortem examination, in the group treated with warfarin alone; one in week 11 and the other in week 12.[12] **Longer versus shorter duration of anticoagulation:** No individual study in either review comparing length of anticoagulation found a significant increase in bleeding complications during prolonged versus shorter treatment for venous thromboembolism.[13,14] Both reviews included studies with different periods of treatment and the populations studied had different types of venous thromboembolism (see benefits above). The first review found that prolonged versus shorter anticoagulation significantly increased the risk of major haemorrhage (19/758 [2.5%] with prolonged anticoagulation v 4/742 [0.5%] with shorter anticoagulation; OR 3.75, 95% CI 1.63 to 8.62).[13] The second review found a greater risk of major haemorrhage with prolonged versus shorter anticoagulation, but the difference was not significant (10/917 [1.1%] with prolonged treatment v 6/906 [0.7%] with shorter treatment; RR 1.43, 95% CI 0.51 to 4.01).[14] **LMWH versus unfractionated heparin:** One systematic review (3306 people treated for at least 5 days) found no significant difference with LMWH versus unfractionated heparin in the risk of thrombocytopenia (RR 0.85, 95% CI 0.45 to 1.62).[23] Another systematic review in people with venous thromboembolism found no significant difference with LMWH versus unfractionated heparin in the risk of major haemorrhage (AR 27/1791 [1.5%] v 39/1827 [2.1%]; OR 0.71, 95% CI 0.43 to 1.15).[22] In this systematic review, pooling of blinded and unblinded RCTs found that the risk of major haemorrhage was 1–2% for up to 10 days' treatment with either LMWH or unfractionated heparin. Analysis of the five RCTs in the review of people with proximal thrombosis (blinded and unblinded, 1636 people) found that short term LMWH versus unfractionated heparin significantly reduced major haemorrhage (8/814 [1.0%] v 19/822 [2.3%]; OR 0.44, 95% CI 0.21 to 0.95).[22] Three other systematic reviews, covering many of the same trials, found similar significant reductions in major haemorrhage.[23–25] A fifth systematic review (4472 people) found no significant difference

with twice daily LMWH versus unfractionated heparin in major haemorrhage (OR 0.79, 95% CI 0.47 to 1.32), but found that once daily
LMWH versus unfractionated heparin significantly reduced major
haemorrhage (OR 0.07, 95% CI 0.01 to 0.54).[26] A sixth systematic
review (6055 people) found that LMWH versus unfractionated heparin
significantly reduced the frequency of major haemorrhage (OR 0.56,
95% CI 0.38 to 0.83).[27] One of the systematic reviews in people with
deep vein thrombosis found that unfractionated heparin versus LMWH
was associated with higher rates of clinically important bleeding (ARs
not provided; unfractionated heparin v LMWH RR 2.48, 95% CI 1.27 to
6.67) and death.[20] **Long term LMWH versus anticoagulation:** One
systematic review found that long term anticoagulation versus long
term LMWH significantly reduced major haemorrhage (7 RCTs; 5/568
[0.9%] v 14/569 [2.5%]; OR 0.38, 95% CI 0.15 to 0.94) but, when
only high quality RCTs were included, it found no significant difference
in major haemorrhage with long term LMWH versus anticoagulation (3
RCTs; 4/236 [1.7%] v 5/241 [2.1%]; OR 0.80, 95% CI 0.21 to
3.00).[31]

Comment: **Studies assessing harm:** These varied in regard to diagnostic criteria,
definitions of adverse events, and intensity of anticoagulation, making
interpretation difficult. **Duration of warfarin treatment:** The absolute
risk of recurrent venous thromboembolism decreases with time,
whereas the relative risk reduction with treatment remains constant.
Observed recurrence of venous thromboembolism is therefore
dependent on length of follow up. Harms of treatment, including major
haemorrhage, continue during prolonged treatment. Individual people
have different risk profiles and it is likely that the optimal duration of
anticoagulation will vary between people.

QUESTION   **What are the effects of treatment for isolated calf vein
thrombosis?**

OPTION   **ANTICOAGULATION**

One RCT found that warfarin plus intravenous unfractionated heparin versus
heparin alone (international normalised ratio 2.5–4.2) reduced rates of
proximal extension. One unblinded RCT found no significant difference in
recurrent thromboembolism with 6 versus 12 weeks of anticoagulation.

Benefits: **Warfarin versus placebo:** We found no systematic review and no
RCTs. **Warfarin plus heparin versus warfarin alone:** We found no
systematic review. We found one RCT that compared intravenous
unfractionated heparin (international normalised ratio [see glossary, p 282] 2.5–4.2) for at least 5 days with or without 3 months
of warfarin. It found that heparin plus warfarin reduced proximal
extension of clot at 1 year compared with heparin alone (1/23 [4%]
people with heparin plus warfarin v 9/28 [32%] people with heparin
alone; ARR 28%, 95% CI 9% to 47%).[6] **Duration of
anticoagulation:** We found one unblinded RCT (736 people,
including 197 with isolated calf vein thrombosis) comparing
6 weeks versus 12 weeks of anticoagulation, which found no significant difference in recurrence of venous thromboembolism (AR 2/
105 [1.9%] with 6 wks treatment v 3/92 [3.3%] with 12 wks;
RR 0.58, 95% CI 0.10 to 3.36).[15]

Thromboembolism

Harms: See harms of anticoagulation under treatments for proximal deep vein thrombosis, p 276. **Duration of anticoagulation:** One RCT (197 people) found no significant difference in rate of haemorrhage with 6 weeks versus 12 weeks of anticoagulation (AR 13/105 [12.4%] with 6 wks treatment v 19/92 [20.6%] with 12 wks; RR 0.59, 95% CI 0.31 to 1.26).[15]

Comment: Many reported cases of isolated calf vein thrombosis are asymptomatic but detected radiologically for research purposes. We found limited evidence on the clinical significance of asymptomatic calf vein thrombosis. Similarly, studies into the incidence of pulmonary embolism associated with isolated calf vein thrombosis detected asymptomatic embolism by ventilation–perfusion scanning, and it is not clear what the clinical significance of these findings are.

QUESTION	What are the effects of treatments for pulmonary embolism?

OPTION	ANTICOAGULATION

We found no direct evidence in people with pulmonary embolism about the optimum intensity and duration of anticoagulation. Evidence for intensity and duration of treatment has been extrapolated from studies in people with proximal deep vein thrombosis and any venous thromboembolism. One small RCT found that heparin plus warfarin versus no anticoagulation significantly reduced mortality in people with pulmonary embolism. One RCT in people with symptomatic pulmonary embolism who did not receive thrombolysis or embolectomy found no significant difference with low molecular weight heparin versus unfractionated heparin in mortality or new episodes of thromboembolism. Another RCT in people with proximal deep vein thrombosis without clinical signs or symptoms of pulmonary embolism but with high probability lung scan findings found that low molecular weight heparin versus intravenous heparin significantly reduced the proportion of people with new episodes of venous thromboembolism.

Benefits: We found no RCTs of heparin versus placebo, warfarin versus placebo, or heparin plus warfarin versus heparin alone or versus warfarin alone. **Heparin plus warfarin versus no anticoagulation:** We found no systematic review. We found one RCT (published 1960; 35 people with pulmonary embolism) comparing heparin plus warfarin versus no anticoagulation.[35] It found that anticoagulation significantly reduced mortality at 1 year (0/16 deaths [0%] with anticoagulation v 5/19 deaths [26%] with no anticoagulation; NNT 4, 95% CI 2 to 16). **Duration and intensity of anticoagulation:** We found no direct evidence in people with pulmonary embolism. Evidence for intensity and duration of treatment has been extrapolated from studies in people with proximal deep vein thrombosis and any venous thromboembolism. These trials found that bleeding rates were increased by higher international normalised ratio (see glossary, p 282) target ranges (international normalised ratio 3.0–4.5), but recurrence rates were not significantly different compared with a lower range (international normalised ratio 2.0–3.0), and that longer courses of anticoagulation reduced recurrence compared with shorter courses (see benefits of anticoagulation under treatments for proximal deep vein thrombosis, p 272). **Low molecular weight heparin (LMWH) versus**

unfractionated heparin: We found no systematic review. We found two RCTs.[36,37] The first RCT (612 people with symptomatic pulmonary embolism who did not receive thrombolysis or embolectomy) found no significant difference with LMWH (see glossary, p 282) (tinzaparin) versus intravenous heparin in mortality (AR 12/304 [3.9%] with tinzaparin v 14/308 [4.5%] with heparin; P = 0.7) or recurrent thromboembolism (5/304 [1.6%] with tinzaparin v 6/308 [1.9%] with heparin; P = 0.8).[36] The second RCT (200 people with proximal deep vein thrombosis without clinical signs or symptoms of pulmonary embolism but with high probability lung scan findings) found that fixed dose LMWH given once daily versus dose adjusted intravenous heparin significantly reduced the proportion of people with new episodes of venous thromboembolism (AR 0/97 [0%] with LMWH v 7/103 [6.8%] with iv heparin; P = 0.01).[37]

Harms: The first RCT comparing LMWH versus unfractionated heparin found no significant difference in the rate of major haemorrhage (see glossary, p 282) (3/304 [1.0%] with LMWH v 5/308 [1.6%] with unfractionated heparin; P = 0.5).[36] The second RCT also found no significant difference in the risk of major haemorrhage (1/97 [1%] with LMWH v 2/103 [2%] with iv heparin; P = 0.6).[37] See harms of anticoagulation under treatments for proximal deep vein thrombosis, p 276.

Comment: In the two RCTs,[36,37] the incidence of major haemorrhage was low and the number of people was too small to detect a clinically important difference.

OPTION   THROMBOLYSIS

One systematic review in people with pulmonary embolism has found no significant difference in mortality with thrombolysis plus heparin versus heparin alone, and has found that thrombolysis may increase the incidence of intracranial haemorrhage. One small RCT identified by the review found limited evidence that thrombolysis may reduce mortality in people with shock due to massive pulmonary embolism.

Benefits: We found one systematic review,[38] and one large non-randomised trial (see comment below).[39] **Versus heparin:** The systematic review (search date 1998) identified nine RCTs comparing various thrombolytic agents versus heparin.[38] The review did not perform a meta-analysis. The largest RCT (160 people with angiographically documented pulmonary embolism) identified by the review compared a 12 hour infusion of urokinase followed by heparin versus heparin alone. It found no significant difference between treatments in mortality (7/78 [9%] v 6/82 [7%]; RR 1.23, 95% CI 0.43 to 3.49) or recurrent pulmonary embolism at 12 months (15/78 [19%] v 12/82 [15%]; RR 1.31, 95% CI 0.66 to 2.63). Seven short term RCTs identified by the review compared urokinase, streptokinase, or recombinant tissue-type plasminogen activator followed by heparin versus heparin alone, where heparin was adjusted to maintain a therapeutic partial thromboplastin time. They found no significant difference in mortality or recurrent embolism at 24 hours to 30 days. One small RCT identified by the review (8 people with shock related to pulmonary embolism) comparing bolus streptokinase versus heparin found limited evidence that streptokinase reduced mortality (0/4 [0%] with streptokinase *v* 4/4 [100%] with heparin). However, these results should be interpreted with caution as people receiving heparin alone had a much longer delay between onset of symptoms and initiation of treatment than people receiving streptokinase.[38] **Versus each other:** The systematic review identified six RCTs (491 people) comparing different thrombolytic agents versus each other.[38] It found no significant difference in mortality or recurrent pulmonary embolism with different thrombolytics.

Harms: One systematic review (search date not stated) assessing haemorrhagic complications of anticoagulation identified the same 16 RCTs.[40] It found no difference in the proportion of people who had major bleeding events with thrombolysis versus thrombolytics plus heparin or versus heparin alone (thrombolytics 0–48% *v* thrombolytics plus heparin 0–45% *v* heparin alone 0–27%).[40] It also found no difference between different thrombolytic agents in the proportion of people who had major bleeding events (9–14%). It found that intravenous thrombolytics versus heparin increased the proportion of people who had an intracranial haemorrhage (896 people; 1.2% with thrombolytics [half of which were fatal] *v* 0% with heparin alone).[40]

Comment: **Versus heparin:** One additional, non-randomised trial (719 people), which excluded people with shock, found limited evidence that thrombolytics versus heparin reduced overall mortality (8/169 [5%] *v* 61/550 [11%]; RR 0.43, 95% CI 0.21 to 0.87) and recurrent pulmonary embolism over 30 days (13/169 [8%] *v* 103/550 [19%]; RR 0.25, 95% CI 0.13 to 0.51).[39] However, these results should be interpreted with caution as people receiving heparin were older and more likely to have underlying cardiac or pulmonary disease than those receiving thrombolytics.

QUESTION **What are the effects of computerised decision support on oral anticoagulation management?**

We found no RCTs of computerised decision support versus usual management of oral anticoagulation that used clinically important outcomes (major haemorrhage or death). One systematic review and three subsequent RCTs have found that computerised decision support in oral anticoagulation significantly increases time spent in the target international normalised ratio range. Another subsequent RCT found no significant difference with computerised decision support versus standard manual support in the time spent in the target international normalised ratio range. A subsequent RCT of initiation of warfarin found no significant difference with computerised decision support versus usual care in the time taken to reach therapeutic levels of anticoagulation. Most RCTs were small and brief.

Benefits: **Clinical outcomes:** We found no systematic review and no RCTs. **Laboratory outcomes:** We found three systematic reviews[41–43] and five subsequent RCTs.[44–48] The first review (search date 1997, 9 RCTs, 1336 people) included eight RCTs using warfarin and one using heparin.[41] The computer systems advised the doses for initiation of anticoagulation (2 RCTs) and for maintenance of anticoagulation (6 RCTs). Follow up was short (15 days to 12 months). Indications for treatment included cardiac diseases and venous thrombosis. The outcome reported by 7/9 RCTs (693 people) in the systematic review was the proportion of days within the target range of anticoagulation. The review found that computerised decision support (see glossary, p 282) versus usual care increased the time that the international normalised ratio (see glossary, p 282) was in the target range (OR 1.29, 95% CI 1.12 to 1.49). One included trial (small and with the largest effect) introduced significant heterogeneity between the trials and therefore was excluded (OR for remaining RCTs 1.25, 95% CI 1.08 to 1.45). The other two systematic reviews (search dates 1998[42] and 1996[43]) included computer support for determining the dose for a wider range of drugs and included seven[42] and four[43] RCTs of the nine found by the first systematic review.[41] These reviews did not provide a discrete analysis of the RCTs of computer support of oral anticoagulation. The first subsequent RCT (122 people on warfarin after hip replacement) compared usual care versus computerised decision support.[44] Only initiation of warfarin was studied. It found no significant difference in the time taken to reach therapeutic levels of anticoagulation (4.7 days with usual care v 2.8 days with computerised decision support). The second subsequent RCT compared a computerised decision support dosing system versus physician adjusted dosing in five hospitals.[45] People who were taking warfarin for at least 6 days were selected (285 people) and followed for at least 3 months (results from 254 people [89%] were analysed). People managed by computerised decision support spent significantly more time with their international normalised ratio in the target range than people managed conventionally (63% with computerised decision support v 53% with conventional management; P < 0.05). The third subsequent RCT (244 people) compared a package of care that included computerised decision support versus traditional hospital outpatient management. The intervention was based in primary care: a practice nurse clinic that included near patient international normalised ratio testing and computerised decision support. It found significantly more time spent in the target range after 12 months with packaged care versus traditional outpatient management (69% v 57%; P < 0.001), but no difference in the proportion of tests in range (61% with intervention v 51% with control) or in the point prevalence of tests in range (71% v 62%).[46] The fourth subsequent RCT (101 people receiving oral anticoagulation after heart valve replacement) compared a computerised decision support system versus standard manual monitoring of international normalised ratio over 315 days.[47] It found no significant difference in the proportion of international normalised ratios in the target range or time spent in the target range (no further data and no mean follow up time provided). It found that people had significantly fewer dose changes with computerised versus standard manual monitoring (31% with computerised v 47% with manual; P = 0.02). The fifth subsequent RCT (335 people receiving initiation, 916 people receiving maintenance anticoagulation treatment for a variety of indications) compared a computerised decision support system for both dosing and appointment scheduling versus standard manual monitoring by "expert physicians".[48] It found that significantly more people managed by computerised decision support versus standard monitoring achieved a stable international

Cardiovascular disorders

Thromboembolism

normalised ratio in the first month (39% with computerised decision support v 27% with standard monitoring; P < 0.01) and spent more time with their international normalised ratio in the target range (71% with computerised decision support v 68% with standard monitoring; P < 0.001).

Harms: **Major haemorrhage:** See glossary, p 282. One systematic review (search date 1997, 9 RCTs, 1336 people) found major haemorrhages in 14/700 (2%) people with computerised decision support versus 25/636 (4%) in the control group.[41] Most of the events occurred in one study making meta-analysis inappropriate. One RCT found no significant difference in overall mortality or serious adverse events with computerised decision support versus usual care.[46]

Comment: We found only limited evidence (from small trials with short follow up of proxy outcomes) on the use of computerised decision support in oral anticoagulation management. Computerised decision support for oral anticoagulation seems to be at least as effective as human performance in terms of time spent in the target international normalised ratio range. It is not clear if this will translate to improved clinical outcomes. Larger and longer trials that measure clinical outcomes (particularly harms) are needed.

GLOSSARY

Computerised decision support system A computer program that provides advice on the significance and implications of clinical findings or laboratory results.
International normalised ratio (INR) A value derived from a standardised laboratory test that measures the effect of an anticoagulant. The laboratory materials used in the test are calibrated against internationally accepted standard reference preparations, so that variability between laboratories and different reagents is minimised. Normal blood has an international normalised ratio of 1. Therapeutic anticoagulation often aims to achieve an international normalised ratio value of 2.0–3.5.
Low molecular weight heparins (LMWH) are made from heparin using chemical or enzymatic methods. The various formulations of LMWH differ in mean molecular weight, composition, and anticoagulant activity. As a group, LMWHs have distinct properties and it is not yet clear that one LMWH will behave exactly like another. Some subcutaneously administered LMWHs do not require monitoring.
Major haemorrhage Exact definitions vary between studies but usually a major haemorrhage is one involving intracranial, retroperitoneal, joint, or muscle bleeding leading directly to death or requiring admission to hospital to stop the bleeding or provide a blood transfusion. All other haemorrhages are classified as minor.

REFERENCES

1. Nordstrom M, Linblad B, Bergqvist D, et al. A prospective study of the incidence of deep-vein thrombosis within a defined urban population. *Arch Intern Med* 1992;326:155–160.

2. Hansson PO, Werlin L, Tibblin G, et al. Deep vein thrombosis and pulmonary embolism in the general population. *Arch Intern Med* 1997;157:1665–1670.

3. Rubinstein I, Murray D, Hoffstein V. Fatal pulmonary emboli in hospitalised patients: an autopsy study. *Arch Intern Med* 1988;148:1425–1426.

4. Hirsh J, Hoak J. Management of deep vein thrombosis and pulmonary embolism. *Circulation* 1996;93:2212–2245.

5. Farley TMM, Meirik O, Chang CL, et al. Effects of different progestogens in low oestrogen oral

contraceptives on venous thromboembolic disease. *Lancet* 1995;346:1582–1588.

6. Lagerstedt C, Olsson C, Fagher B, et al. Need for long term anticoagulant treatment in symptomatic calf vein thrombosis. *Lancet* 1985;334:515–518.

7. Lohr J, Kerr T, Lutter K, et al. Lower extremity calf thrombosis: to treat or not to treat? *J Vasc Surg* 1991;14:618–623.

8. Kakkar VV, Howe CT, Flanc C, et al. Natural history of postoperative deep vein thrombosis. *Lancet* 1969;ii:230–232.

9. Zilliacus H. On the specific treatment of thrombosis and pulmonary embolism with anticoagulants, with a particular reference to the post thrombotic sequelae. *Acta Med Scand* 1946;170:1–221.

10. Giannoukas AD, Labropoulos N, Burke P, et al. Calf deep vein thrombosis: a review of the literature. *Eur J Vasc Endovasc Surg* 1995;10:398–404.

11. Lensing AWA, Prandoni P, Prins MH, et al. Deep-vein thrombosis. *Lancet* 1999;353:479–485.

12. Brandjes DPM, Heijboer H, Buller HR, et al. Acenocoumarol and heparin compared with acenocoumarol alone in the initial treatment of proximal-vein thrombosis. *N Engl J Med* 1992;327:1485–1489.

13. Hutten BA, Prins MH. Duration of treatment with vitamin K antagonists in symptomatic venous thromboembolism. In: The Cochrane Library, Issue 1, 2002. Oxford: Update Software. Search date 2000; primary sources Medline, Embase, hand searching relevant journals, and personal contacts.

14. Pinede L, Duhaut P, Cucherat M, et al. Comparison of long versus short duration of anticoagulant therapy after a first episode of venous thromboembolism: a meta-analysis of randomized, controlled trials. *J Intern Med* 2000;247:553–562. Search date not stated; primary sources Medline, Embase, Cochrane Controlled Trials Register, and hand searched reference lists.

15. Pinede L, Ninet J, Duhaut P, et al. Comparison of 3 and 6 months of oral anticoagulant therapy after a first episode of proximal deep vein thrombosis or pulmonary embolism and comparison of 6 and 12 weeks of therapy after isolated calf deep vein thrombosis. *Circulation* 2001;103:2453–2460.

16. Agnelli G, Prandoni P, Santamaria MG, et al. Three months versus one year of oral anticoagulant therapy for idiopathic deep venous thrombosis. Warfarin Optimal Duration Italian Trial Investigators. *N Engl J Med* 2001;345:165–169.

17. Hull R, Hirsh J, Jay RM, et al. Different intensities of oral anticoagulant therapy in the treatment of proximal vein thrombosis. *N Engl J Med* 1982;307:1676–1681.

18. Ascani A, Iorio A, Agnelli G. Withdrawal of warfarin after deep vein thrombosis: effects of a low fixed dose on rebound thrombin generation. *Blood Coagul Fibrinolysis* 1999;10:291–295.

19. Leisorovicz A, Simonneau G, Decousous H, et al. Comparison of efficacy and safety of low molecular weight heparins and unfractionated heparin in initial treatment of deep venous thrombosis: a meta-analysis. *BMJ* 1994;309:299–304. Search date 1993; primary sources Medline and hand searched references.

20. Lensing AWA, Prins MH, Davidson BL, et al. Treatment of deep venous thrombosis with low-molecular weight heparins. *Arch Intern Med* 1995;155:601–607. Search date 1994; primary sources Medline, manual search, and hand searched references.

21. Breddin HK, Hach-Wunderle V, Nakov R, et al. Effects of a low-molecular-weight heparin on thrombus regression and recurrent thromboembolism in patients with deep-vein thrombosis. *N Engl J Med* 2001;344:626–631.

22. Van den Belt AGM, Prins MH, Lensing AWA, et al. Fixed dose subcutaneous low molecular weight heparins versus adjusted dose unfractionated heparin for venous thromboembolism. In: The Cochrane Library, Issue 1, 2002. Oxford: Update Software. Search date 1999; primary sources Medline, Embase, LILACS, contact with researchers and pharmaceutical companies, and hand searched references.

23. Dolovich LR, Ginsberg JS, Douketis JD, et al. A meta-analysis comparing low-molecular-weight heparins with unfractionated heparin in the treatment of venous thromboembolism. *Arch Intern Med* 2000;160:181–188. Search date 1996; primary sources Medline, HEALTH, The Cochrane Library, and hand searched references.

24. Bijsterveld NR, Hettiaraohchi R, Peters R, et al. Low-molecular weight heparins in venous and arterial thrombotic disease. *Thromb Haemost* 1999;82(suppl 1):139–147. Search date 1999; primary sources Medline, Embase, principal study investigators, and hand searched references.

25. Rohan JK, Hettiarachchi RJ, Prins MH, et al. Low molecular weight heparin versus unfractionated heparin in the initial treatment of venous thromboembolism. *Curr Opin Pulmon Med* 1998;4:220–225. Search date not stated; primary sources Medline, Current Contents, and Embase.

26. Rocha E, Martinez-Gonzalez MA, Montes R, et al. Do the low molecular weight heparins improve efficacy and safety of the treatment of deep venous thrombosis? A meta-analysis. *Haematologica* 2000;85:935–942. Search date 1999; primary sources Medline, Excerpta Medica, and conference abstracts.

27. Van der Heijden JF, Prins MH, Buller HR. For the initial treatment of venous thromboembolism: are all low-molecular weight heparin compounds the same? *Thromb Res* 2000;10:V121–V130. Search date not stated; primary sources Medline, Embase, and Current Contents.

28. Belcaro G, Nicolaides AN, Cesarone MR, et al. Comparison of low-molecular-weight heparin, administered primarily at home, with unfractionated heparin, administered in hospital, and subcutaneous heparin, administered at home for deep-vein thrombosis. *Angiology* 1999;50:781–787.

29. Merli G, Spiro TE, Olsson CG, et al. Subcutaneous enoxaparin once or twice daily compared with intravenous unfractionated heparin for treatment of venous thromboembolic disease. *Ann Intern Med* 2001;134:191–202.

30. Couturaud F, Julian JA, Kearon C. Low molecular weight heparin administered once versus twice daily in patients with venous thromboembolism: a meta-analysis. *Thromb Haemost* 2001;86:980–984. Search date 1999; primary sources Medline, the Cochrane Library, hand searches of reference lists, and personal files of local experts.

31. Van Der Heijden JF, Hutten BA, Buller HR, et al. Vitamin K antagonists or low-molecular-weight heparin for the long term treatment of symptomatic venous thromboembolism. In: The Cochrane Library, Issue 1, 2002. Oxford: Update Software. Search date 2001; primary sources Medline, Embase, Current Contents, hand searching relevant journals, and personal contacts.

32. Schraibman IG, Milne AA, Royle EM. Home versus in-patient treatment for deep vein thrombosis. In: The Cochrane Library, Issue 1, 2002. Oxford: Update Software. Search date 2000; primary sources Medline, Embase, Cochrane Controlled Trials Register, and hand searching of relevant journals.

33. Landefeld CS, Beyth RJ. Anticoagulant related bleeding: clinical epidemiology, prediction, and prevention. *Am J Med* 1993;95:315–328.

34. Levine MN, Hirsh J, Landefeld CS, Raskob G. Haemorrhagic complications of anticoagulant treatment. *Chest* 1992;102(suppl):352–363.

35. Barrit DW, Jordan SC. Anticoagulant drugs in the treatment of pulmonary embolism: a controlled trial. *Lancet* 1960;i:1309–1312.

36. Simonneau G, Sors H, Charbonnier B, et al. A comparison of low-molecular weight heparin with

Cardiovascular disorders

unfractionated heparin for acute pulmonary embolism. *N Engl J Med* 1997;337:663–669.

37. Hull RD, Raskob GE, Brant RF, et al. Low-molecular-weight heparin vs heparin in the treatment of patients with pulmonary embolism. American–Canadian Thrombosis Study Group. *Arch Intern Med* 2000;160:229–236.

38. Arcasoy SM, Kreit JW. Thrombolytic therapy for pulmonary embolism. A comprehensive review of current evidence. *Chest* 1999;115:1695–1707. Search date 1998; primary sources Medline and hand searches of reference lists of retrieved articles.

39. Konstantinides S, Geibel A, Olschewski M, et al. Association between thrombolytic treatment and the prognosis of haemodynamically stable patients with major pulmonary embolism: results of a multicentre registry. *Circulation* 1997;96:882–888.

40. Levine MN, Goldhaber SZ, Gore JM, et al. Haemorrhagic complications of thrombolytic therapy in the treatment of myocardial infarction and venous thromboembolism. *Chest* 1995;108:291S–301S. Search date not stated; primary sources not stated.

41. Chatellier G, Colombet I, Degoulet P. An overview of the effect of computer-assisted management of anticoagulant therapy on the quality of anticoagulation. *Int J Med Informatics* 1998;49:311–320. Search date 1997; primary source Medline.

42. Hunt DL, Haynes RB, Hanna SE, et al. Effects of computer-based clinical decision support systems on physician performance and patient outcomes: a systematic review. *JAMA* 1998;280:1339–1346. Search date 1998;

primary sources Medline, Embase, Inspec, SciSearch, Cochrane Library, hand searching of reference lists, and personal contact with authors.

43. Walton RT, Dovey S, Harvey E, et al. Computerised advice on drug dosage to improve prescribing practice. Search date 1996; primary sources The Cochrane Effective Practice and Organisation of Care Group specialised register, Medline, Embase, and hand searches of the journal *Therapeutic Drug Monitoring*, reference lists of articles, and contact with experts in the field.

44. Motykie GD, Mokhtee D, Zebala LP, et al. The use of a Bayseian Forecasting Model in the management of warfarin therapy after total hip arthroplasty. *J Arthroplasty* 1999;14:988–993.

45. Poller L, Shiach CR, MacCallum PK, et al. Multicentre randomised study of computerised anticoagulant dosage. European Concerted Action on Anticoagulation. *Lancet* 1998;352:1505–1509.

46. Fitzmaurice DA, Hobbs FDR, Murray ET, et al. Oral anticoagulation management in primary care with the use of computerized decision support and near-patient testing. Randomized Controlled Trial. *Arch Intern Med* 2000;160:2343–2348.

47. Ageno W, Turpie AG. A randomized comparison of a computer-based dosing program with a manual system to monitor oral anticoagulant therapy. *Thromb Res* 1998;91:237–240.

48. Manotti C, Moia M, Palareti G, et al. Effect of computer-aided management on the quality of treatment in anticoagulated patients: a prospective, randomized, multicenter trial of APROAT (Automated PRogram for Oral Anticoagulant Treatment). *Haematologica* 2001;86:1060–1070.

David Fitzmaurice
Senior Lecturer

FD Richard Hobbs
Professor

Richard McManus
Clinical Research Fellow

Department of Primary Care and General Practice
The Medical School University of Birmingham, Birmingham, UK

Competing interests: RM none declared. FDRH is a member of the European Society of Cardiology (ESC) Working Party on Heart Failure, Treasurer of the British Society for Heart Failure, and Chair of the British Primary Care Cardiovascular Society (PCCS). He has received travel sponsorship and honoraria from several multinational biotechnology and pharmaceutical companies with cardiovascular products for plenary talks and attendance at major cardiology scientific congresses and conferences. DF has received reimbursement for attendance at scientific meetings from Leo Laboratories who make tinzaparin, a low molecular weight heparin. The Department of Primary Care and General Practice at the University of Birmingham, where the authors work, has a computerised decision support programme that is commercially available.

INTERVENTIONS

Key Messages

- **Adenosine diphosphate inhibitors** One RCT found that clopidogrel versus placebo reduced death, myocardial infarction, and stroke after 9 months. Clopidogrel increased the risk of major bleeding, but not haemorrhagic strokes. Another RCT found that ticlopidine versus conventional treatment reduced vascular deaths and non-fatal myocardial infarction after 6 months (NNT 16, 95% CI 9 to 62), but was associated with neutropenia.

- **Aspirin** One systematic review has found that aspirin versus placebo significantly reduces the risk of death, myocardial infarction, and stroke at 6 months (NNT 20, 95% CI 15 to 34).

- **Calcium channel blockers** One systematic review has found that calcium channel blockers versus placebo or versus standard treatment did not reduce death or myocardial infarction.

- **Direct thrombin inhibitors** One systematic review has found that direct thrombin inhibitors versus heparin reduces death and myocardial infarction after 30 days.

- **Intravenous glycoprotein IIb/IIIa inhibitors** One systematic review has found that intravenous glycoprotein IIb/IIIa inhibitors reduce death or myocardial infarction compared with placebo, but increase the risk of major bleeding complications.

- **Low molecular weight heparins** One systematic review has found that low molecular weight heparin reduced death or myocardial infarction in people taking aspirin, and did not increase bleeding complications in the first 7 days after onset of symptoms. It also found that longer term treatment with low molecular weight heparin versus placebo did not reduce death or myocardial infarction, and increased major bleeding. One systematic review found that low molecular weight heparin versus unfrationated heparin did not reduce death or myocardial infarction.

- **Oral glycoprotein IIb/IIIa inhibitors** One systematic review found that oral glycoprotein IIb/IIIa inhibitors did not reduce mortality, myocardial infarction, or recurrent ischaemia but increased bleeding events.

- **Routine early invasive treatment** Two RCTs found that that early invasive treatment reduced death and myocardial infarction, but two RCTs found that early invasive treatment did not reduce death and myocardial infarction.

- **Unfractionated heparin added to aspirin** Two systematic reviews have found that adding unfractionated heparin to aspirin in people with unstable angina reduces death or myocardial infarction with no significant increase in major bleeding after 1 week of treatment. One systematic review found that adding unfractionated heparin to aspirin does not reduce death or myocardial infarction after 12 weeks.

- **Warfarin** Five RCTs found no significant difference in myocardial infarction or death with the addition of warfarin to standard treatment. One RCT found that warfarin was associated with an increase in major bleeding.

- **β Blockers; nitrates** We found insufficient evidence of the effects of these interventions.

DEFINITION Unstable angina is distinguished from stable angina, acute myocardial infarction, and non-cardiac pain by the pattern of symptoms (characteristic pain present at rest or on lower levels of activity), the severity of symptoms (recently increasing intensity, frequency, or duration), and the absence of persistent ST segment elevation on a resting electrocardiogram. Unstable angina includes a variety of different clinical patterns: angina at rest of up to 1 week's duration; angina increasing in severity to moderate or severe pain; non-Q wave myocardial infarction; and post-myocardial infarction angina continuing for longer than 24 hours.

INCIDENCE/ PREVALENCE In industrialised countries, the annual incidence of unstable angina is about 6/10 000 people in the general population.

AETIOLOGY/ RISK FACTORS Risk factors are the same as for other manifestations of ischaemic heart disease: older age, previous atheromatous cardiovascular disease, diabetes mellitus, smoking cigarettes, hypertension, hypercholesterolaemia, male sex, and a family history of ischaemic heart disease. Unstable angina can also occur in association with other disorders of the circulation, including heart valve disease, arrhythmia, and cardiomyopathy.

PROGNOSIS In people taking aspirin, the incidence of serious adverse outcomes (such as death, acute myocardial infarction, or refractory angina requiring emergency revascularisation) is 5–10% within the first 7 days and about 15% at 30 days. Between 5% and 14% of people with unstable angina die in the year after diagnosis, with about half of these deaths occurring within 4 weeks of diagnosis. No single factor identifies people at higher risk of an adverse event. Risk factors include severity of presentation (e.g. duration of pain, rapidity of progression, evidence of heart failure), medical history (e.g. previous unstable angina, acute myocardial infarction, left ventricular dysfunction), other clinical parameters (e.g. age, diabetes), electrocardiogram changes (e.g. severity of ST segment depression, deep T wave inversion, transient ST segment elevation), biochemical parameters (e.g. troponin concentration), and change in clinical status (e.g. recurrent chest pain, silent ischaemia, haemodynamic instability).

AIMS

To relieve pain and ischaemia; to prevent death and myocardial infarction; to identify people at high risk who require revascularisation; to facilitate early hospital discharge in people at low and medium risk; to modify risk factors; to prevent death, myocardial infarction, and recurrent ischaemia after discharge from hospital, with minimum adverse effects.

OUTCOMES

Rate of death or myocardial infarction (often measured at 2, 7, and 30 days, and 6 months after randomisation); and adverse effects of treatment. Some RCTs include rates of refractory ischaemia or readmission for unstable angina.

METHODS

Clinical Evidence update search and appraisal April 2002.

QUESTION What are the effects of antiplatelet treatments?

OPTION ASPIRIN

One systematic review has found that aspirin alone versus placebo reduces the risk of death, myocardial infarction, and stroke in people with unstable angina. The evidence suggests no added cardiovascular benefit, and possible added harm, from doses of aspirin over 325 mg daily.

Benefits:

One systematic review (search date 1990, 145 RCTs, 100 000 people) compared antiplatelet treatment versus placebo.[1] Seven of these trials included a total of 4000 people with unstable angina. The review found that antiplatelet treatment (mostly medium dose aspirin, 75–325 mg daily) reduced the combined outcome of vascular death, myocardial infarction, or stroke at 6 months (AR 14% with placebo v 9% with antiplatelet treatment; RR 0.65, 95% CI 0.51 to 0.79; NNT 20, 95% CI 15 to 34). This means that 20 people would need to be treated with aspirin rather than placebo to prevent one additional event in 6 months. Individual trials within the systematic review showed consistent benefit from daily aspirin in terms of reduced deaths and myocardial infarction.

Harms:

The review found that people taking doses of aspirin of 75–1200 mg daily had no significant adverse events, including gastrointestinal intolerance or bleeding.[1] However, the sum of the evidence suggests no added cardiovascular benefit, and greater incidence of gastrointestinal effects, for aspirin doses greater than 325 mg daily. Some people are allergic to aspirin.

Unstable angina

Comment: The systematic review covered a wide range of people with different morbidities and levels of risk. Its results should be generalisable to routine practice.[1] People with unstable angina who are allergic or who do not respond to aspirin will need alternative antiplatelet treatment.

OPTION   ADENOSINE DIPHOSPHATE INHIBITORS

Two RCTs found that clopidogrel or ticlopidine reduced death and myocardial infarction compared with placebo or conventional treatment alone. One RCT found that clopidogrel increased major bleeding, but not haemorrhagic strokes after 6–9 months. The other RCT found that ticlopidine was associated with neutropenia. These drugs may be an alternative in people who are intolerant of or allergic to aspirin.

Benefits: We found no systematic review. We found two RCTs comparing adenosine diphosphate inhibitors versus placebo or conventional treatment.[2,3] The first RCT (12 562 people) compared clopidogrel (300 mg orally within 24 h of onset of symptoms followed by 75 mg daily) versus placebo.[2] It found that clopidogrel significantly reduced the combined outcome of death, myocardial infarction, and stroke after 9 months (AR 9% with clopidogrel v 11% with placebo; OR 0.8, 95% CI 0.7 to 0.9; NNT 50; CI not provided). The second RCT (652 people)[3] found that ticlopidine versus conventional treatment significantly reduced the combined outcome of vascular deaths and myocardial infarction after 6 months (RR 0.5, 95% CI 0.2 to 0.9; NNT 16, 95% CI 9 to 62).

Harms: In the first RCT, clopidogrel versus placebo increased major bleeding complications, but not haemorrhagic strokes (major bleeding 3.7% with clopidogrel v 2.7% with placebo, OR 1.4, 95% CI 1.1 to 1.7; haemorrhagic stroke 0.1% with clopidogrel v 0.1% with placebo, P value and OR not provided).[2] Reversible neutropenia has been reported in 1–2% of people taking ticlopidine.

Comment: Clopidogrel and ticlopidine are also associated with other adverse effects including diarrhoea and rash.

OPTION   INTRAVENOUS GLYCOPROTEIN IIB/IIIA PLATELET RECEPTOR INHIBITORS

One systematic review found that intravenous glycoprotein IIb/IIIa inhibitors versus placebo reduced death or myocardial infarction, but increased the risk of major bleeding complications.

Benefits: We found one systematic review (search date 2001, 8 RCTs, 30 006 people) comparing intravenous glycoprotein IIb/IIIa inhibitors with placebo.[4] It found that intravenous glycoprotein IIb/IIIa inhibitors significantly reduced the combined outcome of death and myocardial infarction at 30 days and 6 months (at 30 days: 8 RCTs; AR 10.8% with inhibitors v 11.8% with placebo; OR 0.91, 95% CI 0.85 to 0.98; at 6 months: 4 RCTs, AR 13.3% with inhibitors v 14.6% with placebo; OR 0.88, 95% CI 0.81 to 0.95).[4]

Harms: The systematic review found that intravenous glycoprotein IIb/IIIa inhibitors versus placebo increased major bleeding complications at 30 days (AR 3.7% with inhibitors v 3.6% with placebo; OR 1.27, 95% CI 1.22 to 1.44).[4]

Comment: A small trial of adding a glycoprotein IIb/IIIa inhibitor to standard treatment suggests that a "dose ceiling" may exist beyond which escalation of dose results in higher bleeding complications with no increase in efficacy.[5]

ORAL GLYCOPROTEIN IIB/IIIA PLATELET RECEPTOR INHIBITORS

One systematic review found that oral glycoprotein IIb/IIIa inhibitors did not reduce the combined outcome of death, myocardial infarction, and recurrent ischaemia, but increased bleeding events.

Benefits: We found one systematic review (search date not stated, 4 RCTs, 26 462 people) comparing combinations of oral glycoprotein IIb/IIIa inhibitors, aspirin, and placebo.[5] Three of the RCTs were reported as abstracts only. The systematic review found that oral glycoprotein IIb/IIIa inhibitors versus aspirin did not reduce the combined outcome of death, myocardial infarction, and severe ischaemia after 90 days (results from fully reported RCT: AR 10.1% with sibrafiban v 9.8% with aspirin; difference not statistically significant; OR and P value not provided).

Harms: The fully reported RCT in the systematic review found that sibrafiban increased major bleeding versus aspirin (AR 27% with low dose sibrafiban v 19% with aspirin; OR and P value not provided). One RCT in the systematic review comparing sibrafiban plus aspirin versus placebo plus aspirin was stopped early because of the findings of the fully reported RCT. A further RCT in the systematic review comparing orbofiban plus aspirin versus placebo plus aspirin was stopped early because orbofiban plus aspirin increased mortality compared with placebo plus aspirin at 30 days (quantitative data not provided). One RCT in the systematic review comparing different doses of lefradafiban plus aspirin versus placebo plus aspirin stopped recruiting to the high dose lefradafiban plus aspirin group because of increased bleeding (AR 11% with high dose lefradafiban v 3% with low and medium dose lefradafiban v 1% with placebo; P value not provided).

Comment: None.

What are the effects of antithrombin treatments?

UNFRACTIONATED HEPARIN

Two systematic reviews found that adding unfractionated heparin to aspirin in people with unstable angina reduced death or myocardial infarction after 1 week. One systematic review found that adding unfractionated heparin to aspirin did not reduce death or myocardial infarction after 12 weeks.

Benefits: **Added to aspirin:** We found two systematic reviews (search dates 1995[6] and not stated[7]). Both included the same six RCTs in 1353 people with unstable angina who were treated with either unfractionated heparin plus aspirin or aspirin alone for 2–7 days. The most recent review found that unfractionated heparin plus aspirin versus aspirin alone reduced the risk of death or myocardial infarction after

7 days (AR 8% with unfractionated heparin plus aspirin v 10% with aspirin alone; OR 0.67, 95% CI 0.45 to 0.99).[7] The older systematic review found that heparin plus aspirin versus aspirin did not reduce death or myocardial infarction after 12 weeks (AR 12% with unfractionated heparin plus aspirin v 14% with aspirin; RR 0.82, 95% CI 0.56 to 1.20).[6] **Versus low molecular weight heparin:** See benefits of low molecular weight heparin, p 290.

Harms: The older systematic review found that heparin plus aspirin did not significantly increase major bleeding compared with aspirin alone (AR 1.5% with unfractionated heparin plus aspirin v 0.4% with aspirin; RR 1.89, 95% CI 0.66 to 5.38).[6]

Comment: None.

OPTION   **LOW MOLECULAR WEIGHT HEPARINS**

One systematic review has found that low molecular weight heparin versus placebo or no treatment reduced death or myocardial infarction in people taking aspirin and did not increase bleeding complications in the first 7 days after an episode of unstable angina. It also found that longer term treatment with low molecular weight heparin versus placebo did not reduce death or myocardial infarction. One systematic review found no significant difference between low molecular weight heparin versus unfractionated heparin in death or myocardial infarction. Long term low molecular weight heparin increased major bleeding compared with placebo, but not compared with unfractionated heparin.

Benefits: **Versus placebo or no heparin treatment:** We found one systematic review (search date not stated, 7 RCTs) comparing low molecular weight heparin (LMWH) versus placebo or no heparin treatment.[7] The systematic review found two RCTs (1639 people already taking aspirin) comparing LMWH versus no heparin or placebo for up to 7 days. It found that LMWH reduced death or myocardial infarction compared with no heparin or placebo during treatment (OR 0.34, 95% CI 0.20 to 0.58). The systematic review found five RCTs (12 099 people) comparing longer term LMWH (up to 90 days) versus placebo. It found that LMWH did not reduce death or myocardial infarction after 90 days compared with placebo (OR 0.98, 95% CI 0.81 to 1.17). **Versus unfractionated heparin:** We found one systematic review (search date not stated, 5 RCTs, 12 171 people) comparing an equal duration (maximum 8 days) of LMWH versus unfractionated heparin.[7] It found that LMWH did not significantly reduce the combined outcome of death or myocardial infarction compared with unfractionated heparin (OR 0.88, 95% CI 0.69 to 1.12).

Harms: The systematic review found no significant difference between LMWH versus unfractionated heparin in the frequency of major bleeds (OR 1.00, 95% CI 0.64 to 1.57)[7] (see harms of unfractionated heparin, p 290). Long term LMWH versus placebo significantly increased the risk of major bleeding (OR 2.26, 95% CI 1.63 to 3.14): equivalent to an excess of 12 bleeds for every 1000 people treated.[7]

Comment: LMWH may be more attractive than unfractionated heparin for routine short term use because coagulation monitoring is not required and it can be self administered after discharge.

OPTION   DIRECT THROMBIN INHIBITORS

One systematic review has found that direct thrombin inhibitors versus heparin reduce death and myocardial infarction.

Benefits: We found one systematic review (search date not stated, 11 RCTs, 35 070 people) comparing 7 days' treatment with direct thrombin inhibitors (hirudin, argatroban, bivalirudin, efegatran, inogatran) versus heparin.[8] It found that direct thrombin inhibitors reduced death or myocardial infarction compared with heparin after 30 days (AR 7.4% with direct thrombin inhibitors v 8.2% with heparin; RR 0.91, 95% CI 0.84 to 0.99).[8]

Harms: The systematic review found that, compared with heparin, direct thrombin inhibitors reduced the risk of major bleeding during treatment (major bleeding; AR 1.9% with direct thrombin inhibitors v 2.3% with heparin; OR 0.75, 95% CI 0.65 to 0.87), and found no significant difference between the risk of stroke at 30 days (stroke; AR 0.6% with direct thrombin inhibitors v 0.6% with heparin; OR 1.01, 95% CI 0.78 to 1.31).[8]

Comment: None.

OPTION   WARFARIN

Five RCTs found no significant difference in myocardial infarction or death with the addition of warfarin to standard treatment. One RCT found that warfarin was associated with an increase in major bleeding.

Benefits: We found no systematic review. We found five RCTs comparing warfarin versus no warfarin in addition to usual treatment.[9–12] Two of the RCTs were reported in the same journal article.[10] The first RCT (214 people) compared warfarin plus aspirin versus aspirin alone.[9] It found that warfarin (target international normalised ratio [see glossary, p 294] 2.0–2.5) plus aspirin reduced the combined outcome of recurrent angina, myocardial infarction, or death after 12 weeks (AR 13% with warfarin plus aspirin v 25% with aspirin; P = 0.06). The second RCT (309 people) compared warfarin (fixed dose 3 mg daily) plus aspirin versus aspirin alone.[10] It found no significant difference between warfarin plus aspirin versus aspirin alone in the combined outcome of refractory angina, myocardial infarction, and death after 6 months (AR 7% with warfarin plus aspirin v 4% with aspirin alone; RR 1.66, 95% CI 0.62 to 4.44). The third RCT (197 people) compared warfarin (target international normalised ratio 2.0–2.5) plus aspirin versus aspirin alone.[10] It found no significant difference with adding warfarin to aspirin in the combined outcome of refractory angina, myocardial infarction, and death after 6 months (AR 5% with warfarin plus aspirin v 12% with aspirin alone; RR 0.42, 95% CI 0.15 to 1.15). The fourth RCT (3712 people) compared adding warfarin (target international normalised ratio 2.0–2.5) to standard treatment versus no warfarin.[11] It found no significant difference with adding warfarin in the combined outcome of death, myocardial infarction, and stroke after 5 months (8% with warfarin v 8% with no warfarin; RR 0.90, 95% CI 0.72 to 1.14). The fifth RCT (135 people with prior coronary artery bypass grafts) compared warfarin plus aspirin, warfarin plus placebo, and aspirin plus placebo.[12] It found no significant difference between treatments in the combined outcome of death, myocardial infarction, and hospital admission for unstable angina after 1 year (AR 11% with warfarin plus aspirin v 14% with warfarin plus placebo v 12% with aspirin plus placebo; P = 0.76).

Harms: In the fourth RCT, warfarin versus standard treatment alone increased major bleeding (AR 2.7% v 1.3%; RR 1.99, 95% CI 1.23 to 3.22; NNH 71; CI not provided).[11]

Comment: None.

QUESTION What are the effects of anti-ischaemic treatments?

OPTION NITRATES, β BLOCKERS, AND CALCIUM CHANNEL BLOCKERS

We found insufficient evidence on the effects of nitrates and β blockers on mortality or myocardial infarction. One systematic review found no significant difference between calcium channel blockers versus placebo or standard treatment on mortality or myocardial infarction. Short acting dihydropyridine calcium channel blockers may increase mortality.

Benefits: We found no systematic review. **Nitrates:** We found one RCT (162 people) comparing intravenous glyceryl trinitrate versus placebo for 48 hours.[13] It found that glyceryl trinitrate significantly reduced the proportion of people with more than two episodes of chest pain and one new episode lasting more than 20 minutes (18% with glyceryl trinitrate v 36% with placebo; RR 0.50, 95% CI 0.25 to 0.90) and the proportion of people needing more than two additional sublingual glyceryl trinitrate tablets (16% with glyceryl trinitrate v 31% with placebo; RR 0.52, 95% CI 0.26 to 0.97). We found one RCT (200 people within 6 months of percutaneous transluminal coronary angioplasty) comparing intravenous glyceryl trinitrate alone, heparin alone, glyceryl trinitrate plus heparin, and placebo.[14] It found that recurrent angina occurred significantly less frequently in people treated with glyceryl trinitrate alone and glyceryl trinitrate plus heparin compared with placebo, but there was no benefit from heparin alone or additional benefit from combination treatment (P < 0.003 for glyceryl trinitrate alone and for glyceryl trinitrate plus heparin v placebo; CI not provided). **β Blockers:** We found two RCTs.[15,16] The first RCT (338 people with rest angina not receiving a β blocker) compared nifedipine, metoprolol, both, or neither versus placebo.[15] It found that metoprolol versus nifedipine significantly reduced the combined outcome of recurrent angina and myocardial infarction within 48 hours (28% with metoprolol v 47% with nifedipine; RR 0.66, 95% CI 0.43 to 0.98). The second RCT (81 people with unstable angina on "optimal doses" of nitrates and nifedipine) compared propranolol (≥ 160 mg daily) versus placebo.[16] It found no significant difference in death, myocardial infarction, and requirement for coronary artery bypass grafting or percutaneous coronary interventions at 30 days (38% with propranolol v 46% with placebo; RR 0.83, 95% CI 0.44 to 1.30). People taking propranolol had a lower cumulative probability of experiencing recurrent rest angina over the first 4 days of the trial. The mean number of clinical episodes of angina, duration of angina, glyceryl trinitrate requirement, and ischaemic ST changes by continuous electrocardiogram monitoring was also lower. **Calcium channel blockers:** We found one systematic review (search date not stated, 6 RCTs, 1109 people) comparing calcium channel blockers versus control treatment (3 RCTs used propranolol as a control and 3 used placebo).[17] The duration of the RCTs ranged from 48 hours (4 RCTs) to 4 months (2 RCTs). The review found no significant difference between calcium channel blockers versus control in rates of myocardial infarction or death.

Harms: Hypotension is a potential adverse effect of nitrates. Both older and more recent large RCTs in people with other ischaemic conditions showed that nitrates were safe and well tolerated when used judiciously in clinically appropriate doses. Potential adverse effects of β blockers include bradycardia, exacerbation of reactive airways disease, and hypoglycaemia in diabetics. Observational studies have reported increased mortality with short acting calcium channel blockers (such as nifedipine) in people with coronary heart disease.[18,19]

Comment: We found no good evidence that anti-ischaemic drugs (nitrates, β blockers, calcium channel blockers) prevent death or myocardial infarction. Consensus suggests that until further data are available, intravenous nitrates remain the preferred treatment together with heparin and aspirin in unstable angina.

QUESTION What are the effects of invasive treatments?

OPTION EARLY ROUTINE CARDIAC CATHETERISATION AND REVASCULARISATION

Four RCTs found conflicting evidence on the effects of early invasive treatment versus conservative treatment.

Benefits: We found no systematic review. We found four RCTs comparing early routine angiography and revascularisation if appropriate versus medical treatment alone.[20–23] The first RCT (2457 people) compared invasive treatment within the first 7 days versus non-invasive treatment plus planned coronary angiography.[20] Invasive treatment significantly reduced the combined outcome of death and myocardial infarction compared with non-invasive treatment after 6 months (AR 9% with invasive treatment v 12% with non-invasive treatment; RR 0.78, 95% CI 0.62 to 0.98; NNT 38; CI not provided). The second RCT (2220 people) compared cardiac catheterisation at 4–48 hours and revascularisation (if appropriate) after a cardiovascular event versus standard treatment.[21] It found that cardiac catheterisation reduced the combined outcome of death, myocardial infarction, and readmission for unstable angina after 6 months (AR 16% with catheterisation v 19% with standard treatment; OR 0.78, 95% CI 0.62 to 0.97; NNT 34; CI not provided). The third RCT (1473 people) compared early cardiac catheterisation at 18–48 hours versus standard treatment.[22] Early

Unstable angina

cardiac catheterisation did not reduce death or myocardial infarction but did reduce hospital admissions after 1 year (death or myocardial infarction: 11% with cardiac catheterisation v 12% with standard treatment, P = 0.42; hospital admissions: 26% with cardiac catheterisation v 33% with standard treatment; P < 0.005; NNT 14; CI not provided). The fourth RCT (920 people) compared invasive with conservative treatment.[23] Invasive treatment did not reduce the combined outcome of death or myocardial infarction compared with conservative treatment after 12–44 months (RR 0.87, 95% CI 0.68 to 1.10).

Harms: The first RCT found that early invasive treatment increased major bleeding but not stroke compared with non-invasive treatment (major bleeds: AR 1.6% with invasive treatment v 0.7% with non-invasive treatment; NNH 111; CI not provided).[22] The second RCT found that cardiac catheterisation increased bleeding compared with standard treatment (6% with cardiac catheterisation v 3% with standard treatment; P < 0.01: NNH 34; CI not provided).[23] The third RCT found that early cardiac catheterisation did not increase complication rates (death, myocardial infarction, emergency coronary artery bypass grafting, abrupt vessel closure, haemorrhage, serious hypotension) compared with conservative treatment (AR 14% with cardiac catheterisation v 13% with conservative treatment; P = 0.38; NNH 100; CI not provided).[24]

Comment: All trials have reported only short term and medium term follow up, so we cannot exclude a long term difference in effect between early invasive and early non-invasive strategies. There may be subgroups of people who benefit particularly from either invasive or conservative treatment. Advances in catheterisation and revascularisation technology and periprocedural management may reduce the early risks of invasive treatment in the future.

GLOSSARY

International normalised ratio (INR) A value derived from a standardised laboratory test that measures the effect of an anticoagulant. The laboratory materials used in the test are calibrated against internationally accepted standard reference preparations, so that variability between laboratories and different reagents is minimised. Normal blood has an international normalised ratio of 1. Therapeutic anticoagulation often aims to achieve an international normalised ratio value of 2.0–3.5.

REFERENCES

1. Antiplatelet Trialists' Collaboration. Collaborative overview of randomised trials of antiplatelet therapy. I: Prevention of death, myocardial infarction, and stroke by prolonged antiplatelet therapy in various categories of patients. *BMJ* 1994;308:81–106. Search date 1990; primary sources Medline and Current Contents.
2. Yusuf S, Zhao F, Mehta S, et al. The Clopidogrel in Unstable Angina to Prevent Recurrent Events (CURE) trial. *N Engl J Med* 2001;345:494–502.
3. Balsano F, Rizzon P, Violi F, et al, and the Studio della Ticlopidina nell'Angina Instabile Group. Antiplatelet treatment with ticlopidine in unstable angina: a controlled multicentre clinical trial. *Circulation* 1990;82:17–26.
4. Bosch X, Marrugat J. Platelet glycoprotein IIb/IIIa blockers for percutaneous coronary revascularization, and unstable angina and non-ST-segment elevation myocardial infarction

(Cochrane Review). In: The Cochrane Library, Issue 2, 2002. Oxford: Update Software. Search date 2001; primary sources Cochrane Library, Medline, Embase, reference lists of articles, medical internet sites, and hand searches of abstracts from cardiology congresses.
5. McDonagh MS, Bachmann LM, Golder S, et al. A rapid and systematic review of the clinical effectiveness and cost-effectiveness of glycoprotein IIb/IIIa antagonists in the medical management of unstable angina. *Health Technol Assess* 2000;4:1–95. Search date not stated; primary sources Cochrane Library, Embase, Medline, National Research Register, and various Internet and online resources.
6. Oler A, Whooley MA, Oler J, et al. Adding heparin to aspirin reduces the incidence of myocardial infarction and death in patients with unstable angina: a meta-analysis. *JAMA*

1996;276:811–815. Search date 1995; primary sources Medline, hand search of reference lists, and consultation with experts.

7. Eikelboom JW, Anand SS, Malmberg K, et al. Unfractionated heparin and low molecular weight heparin in acute coronary syndrome without ST elevation: a meta-analysis. *Lancet* 2000;355:1936–1942. Search date not stated; primary sources Medline and Embase, reference lists of published papers, and experts canvassed for unpublished trials, and personal data.

8. The Direct Thrombin Inhibitor Trialists' Collaborative Group. Direct thrombin inhibitors in acute coronary syndromes: principal results of a meta-analysis based on individual patients' data. *Lancet* 2002;359:294–302. Search date not stated; primary sources Medline, Embase, Cochrane Library, and conference abstracts and proceedings.

9. Cohen M, Adams PC, Parry G, et al. Combination antithrombotic therapy in unstable rest angina and non-Q-wave infarction in nonprior aspirin users. Primary endpoints analysis from the ATACS trial. Antithrombotic Therapy in Acute Coronary Syndromes Research Group. *Circulation* 1994;89:81–88.

10. Anand SS, Yusuf S, Pogue J, et al. Long-term oral anticoagulant therapy in patients with unstable angina or suspected non-Q-wave myocardial infarction: organization to assess strategies for ischaemic syndromes (OASIS) pilot study results. *Circulation* 1998;98:1064–1070.

11. OASIS Investigators. Effects of long-term, moderate-intensity oral anticoagulation in addition to aspirin in unstable angina. *J Am Coll Cardiol* 2001;37:475–484.

12. Hunyh T, Theroux P, Bogaty P, et al. Aspirin, warfarin, or the combination for secondary prevention of coronary events in patients with acute coronary syndromes and prior coronary artery bypass surgery. *Circulation* 2001;103:3069–3074.

13. Karlberg KE, Saldeen T, Wallin R, et al. Intravenous nitroglycerine reduces ischaemia in unstable angina pectoris: a double-blind placebo-controlled study. *J Intern Med* 1998;243:25–31.

14. Douchet S, Malekianpour M, Theroux P, et al. Randomized trial comparing intravenous nitroglycerin and heparin for treatment of unstable angina secondary or restenosis after coronary artery angioplasty. *Circulation* 2000;101:955–961.

15. HINT Research Group. Early treatment of unstable angina in the coronary care unit: a randomized, double blind, placebo controlled comparison of

recurrent ischaemia in patients treated with nifedipine or metoprolol or both. *Br Heart J* 1986;56:400–413.

16. Gottlieb SO, Weisfeldt ML, Ouyang P, et al. Effect of the addition of propranolol to therapy with nifedipine for unstable angina pectoris: a randomized, double-blind, placebo-controlled trial. *Circulation* 1986;73:331–337.

17. Held PH, Yusuf S, Furberg CD. Calcium channel blockers in acute myocardial infarction and unstable angina: an overview. *BMJ* 1989;299:1187–1192. Search date not stated; primary sources not specified in detail.

18. Furberg CD, Psaty BM, Meyer JV. Nifedipine: dose-related increase in mortality in patients with coronary heart disease. *Circulation* 1995;92:1326–1331. Search date and primary sources not stated.

19. WHO-ISH subcommittee of the liaison committee of the World Health Organization and the International Society of Hypertension: effects of calcium antagonists on the risks of coronary heart disease, cancer and bleeding. *J Hypertens* 1997;15:105–115.

20. FRISC II Investigators. Invasive compared with non-invasive treatment in unstable coronary-artery disease: FRISC II prospective randomised multicentre study. Fragmin and Fast Revascularisation during Instability in Coronary artery disease Investigators. *Lancet* 1999;354(9180):694–695.

21. Cannon CP, Weintraub WS, Demopoulos LA, et al. Treat Angina with Aggrastat and Determine Cost of Therapy with an Invasive or Conservative Strategy (TACTICS). *New Engl J Med* 2001;344:1879–1887.

22. The TIMI IIIB Investigators. Effects of tissue plasminogen activator and a comparison of early invasive and conservative strategies in unstable angina and non-Q-wave myocardial infarction. Results of the TIMI IIIB trial. *Circulation* 1994;89:1545–1556.

23. Anderson V, Cannon CP, Stone PH, et al, for the TIMI IIIB Investigators. One-year results of the thrombolysis in myocardial infarction (TIMI) IIIB clinical trial: a randomized comparison of tissue-type plasminogen activator versus placebo and early invasive versus early conservative strategies in unstable angina and non-Q wave myocardial infarction. *J Am Coll Cardiol* 1995;26:1643–1650.

24. Boden WE, O'Rourke RA, Crawford MH, et al, for the VANQWISH Trial Investigators. Outcomes in patients with acute non-Q-wave myocardial infarction randomly assigned to an invasive as compared with a conservative management strategy. *N Engl J Med* 1998;338:1785–1792.

Madhu Natarajan
Division of Cardiology
McMaster University
Hamilton
Canada

Competing interests: None declared.

Cardiovascular disorders

E Andrea Nelson, Nicky Cullum, and June Jones

INTERVENTIONS

Key Messages

Treatment

- **Compression** One systematic review has found that compression versus no compression significantly increases the proportion of venous leg ulcers healed.
- **Cultured allogenic bilayer skin replacement** One RCT found that cultured allogenic bilayer skin replacement versus a non-adherent dressing significantly increased the proportion of ulcers healed after 6 months (NNT 7, 95% CI 4 to 41).
- **Flavonoids** Two RCTs have found that flavonoids versus placebo or versus standard care significantly increase the proportion of ulcers healed.

- **Hydrocolloid (occlusive) dressings versus simple low adherent dressings in the presence of compression** One systematic review found that, in the presence of compression, hydrocolloid dressings did not heal more venous leg ulcers than simple, low adherent dressings.

- **Pentoxifylline** One systematic review has found that oral pentoxifylline versus placebo significantly increases the proportion of ulcers healed at 6 months (NNT 6, 95% CI 4 to 14).

- **Peri-ulcer injection of granulocyte–macrophage colony stimulating factor (GM-CSF)** One RCT found that peri-ulcer injection of GM-CSF versus placebo significantly increased the proportion of ulcers healed after 13 weeks' treatment (NNT 2, 95 % CI 1 to 7).

- **Sulodexide** One RCT found limited evidence that sulodexide plus compression versus compression alone significantly increased the proportion of ulcers healed after 60 days' treatment.

- **Systemic mesoglycan** One RCT found that systemic mesoglycan plus compression versus compression alone significantly increased the proportion of ulcers healed after 24 weeks' treatment.

- **Topically applied autologous platelet lysate** One RCT found no difference after 9 months in time to healing of ulcers with topically applied autologous platelet lysate versus placebo.

- **Antimicrobial agents; aspirin; debriding agents; foam, film, or alginate (semi-occlusive) dressings versus simple dressings in the presence of compression; intermittent pneumatic compression; low level laser treatment; oral zinc; skin grafting; thromboxane u_2 antagonists; topical calcitonin gene related peptide plus vasoactive intestinal polypeptide; topical mesoglycan; topical negative pressure; therapeutic ultrasound; vein surgery** We found insufficient evidence about the effects of these interventions on ulcer healing.

Preventing recurrence

- **Compression** One RCT found that compression stockings versus no stockings significantly reduced the risk of ulcer recurrence after 6 months (NNT 2, 95% CI 2 to 5).

- **Rutoside; stanozolol; vein surgery** We found insufficient evidence about the effects of these interventions on ulcer recurrence.

DEFINITION Definitions of leg ulcers vary, but the following is widely used: loss of skin on the leg or foot that takes more than 6 weeks to heal. Some definitions exclude ulcers confined to the foot, whereas others include ulcers on the whole of the lower limb. This review deals with ulcers of venous origin in people without concurrent diabetes mellitus, arterial insufficiency, or rheumatoid arthritis.

INCIDENCE/ PREVALENCE Between 1.5 and 3/1000 people have active leg ulcers. Prevalence increases with age to about 20/1000 in people aged over 80 years.[1]

AETIOLOGY/ RISK FACTORS Leg ulceration is strongly associated with venous disease. However, about a fifth of people with leg ulceration have arterial disease, either alone or in combination with venous problems, which may require specialist referral.[1] Venous ulcers (also known as varicose or stasis ulcers) are caused by venous reflux or obstruction, both of which lead to poor venous return and venous hypertension.

Venous leg ulcers

PROGNOSIS People with leg ulcers have a poorer quality of life than age matched controls because of pain, odour, and reduced mobility.[2] In the UK, audits have found wide variation in the types of care (hospital inpatient care, hospital clinics, outpatient clinics, home visits), in the treatments used (topical agents, dressings, bandages, stockings), in healing rates, and in recurrence rates (26–69% in 1 year).[3,4]

AIMS To promote healing; to reduce recurrence; to improve quality of life, with minimal adverse effects.

OUTCOMES Ulcer area; number of ulcers healed; number of ulcer free limbs; recurrence rates; number of new ulcer episodes; number of ulcer free weeks or months; number of people who are ulcer free; frequency of dressing/bandage changes; quality of life; adverse effects of treatment.

METHODS *Clinical Evidence* search and appraisal February 2002. We included RCTs with clinically important and objective outcomes: proportion of wounds healed, healing rates, incidence of new or recurring wounds, infection, and quality of life.

QUESTION What are the effects of treatments?

OPTION COMPRESSION

One systematic review has found that compression (elastomeric multilayer high compression bandages, Unna's boot, high compression hosiery, or short stretch bandages) heals venous leg ulcers more effectively than no compression. RCTs found insufficient evidence to compare different methods of compression. Meta-analysis of four RCTs found no significant difference in the proportion of people whose ulcers healed with 12–26 weeks of high compression versus non-high compression bandages. Small RCTs found insufficient evidence of the effects of multilayer high compression versus short stretch bandages. One systematic review found a significant increase in the proportion of ulcers healed with multilayer compression versus single layer bandages.

Benefits: **Compression versus no compression:** We found one systematic review (search date 2000, 6 RCTs, 260 people) comparing compression versus no compression.[5] It found that compression (e.g. elastomeric multilayer high compression bandages, short stretch bandages, double layer bandages, compression hosiery, or Unna's boot — see glossary, p 308) healed venous leg ulcers more effectively than no compression (e.g. dressing alone). The RCTs were heterogeneous, using different forms of compression in different settings and populations. The results were not pooled. The results of individual RCTs consistently favoured compression. **Elastomeric versus non-elastomeric multilayer compression:** The systematic review[5] identified three RCTs (273 people), and we found one subsequent RCT (112 people)[6] comparing elastomeric multilayer high compression bandages versus non-elastomeric multilayer compression. Meta-analysis of all four RCTs (Nelson EA, Cullum N, Jones J, personal communication, 2002) found no significant difference in the proportion of people whose ulcers healed with

12–26 weeks of high compression versus non-high compression bandages (RR 1.30, 95% CI 0.94 to 1.82). **Multilayer high compression versus short stretch bandages:** The systematic review[5] identified four small RCTs (167 people), and we identified one subsequent RCT (112 people).[7] Meta-analysis of all five RCTs (Nelson EA, Cullum N, Jones J, personal communication, 2002) found no significant difference in healing rates between multilayer high compression and short stretch bandages (RR for healing 0%, 95% CI 0.81 to 1.24). The lack of power in these small studies means that a clinically important difference cannot be excluded. **Multilayer high compression versus single layer bandage:** The systematic review identified four RCTs (280 people) comparing multilayer high compression versus a single layer of bandage.[5] It found a significant increase in the proportion of ulcers healed with multilayer compression versus single layer bandages (82/139 [59%] v 59/141 [42%]; RR 1.41, 95% CI 1.12 to 1.77; NNT for variable periods of treatment 6, 95% CI 4 to 18) (see table 1, p 310).

Harms:
High levels of compression applied to limbs with insufficient arterial supply, or inexpert application of bandages, can lead to tissue damage and, at worst, amputation.[12] Complication rates were rarely reported in RCTs. One observational study (194 people) found that four layer compression bandaging for several months was associated with toe ulceration in 12 (6%) people.[13]

Comment:
People found to be suitable for high compression are those with clinical signs of venous disease (ulcer in the gaiter region, from the upper margin of the malleolus to the bulge of the gastrocnemius; staining of the skin around an ulcer; or eczema), no concurrent diabetes mellitus or rheumatoid arthritis, and adequate arterial supply to the foot as determined by ankle/brachial pressure index. The precise ankle/brachial pressure index below which compression is contraindicated is often quoted as 0.8; however, many RCTs used the higher cut off of 0.9.[5] Effectiveness is likely to be influenced by the ability of those applying the bandage to generate safe levels of compression. Bandages may be applied by the person with the leg ulcer, their carer, nurse, or doctor. We found no comparisons of healing rates between specialist and non-specialist application of compression. Training improves bandaging technique among nurses.[14] Bandages containing elastomeric fibres can be applied weekly as they maintain their tension over time. Bandages made of wool or cotton, or both, such as short stretch bandages, may need to be reapplied more frequently as they do not maintain their tension.

| OPTION | INTERMITTENT PNEUMATIC COMPRESSION |

One small RCT found no significant difference in the proportion of people with healed ulcers over 2–3 months with intermittent pneumatic compression versus compression bandages, but it may have been too small to exclude a clinically important difference. One RCT found improved healing at 3 months with intermittent pneumatic compression plus compression bandaging versus compression bandaging alone, but two RCTs found no significant difference in healing at 6 months.

Venous leg ulcers

Benefits: **Intermittent pneumatic compression versus compression bandaging:** We found one systematic review (search date 2001), which identified one small RCT (16 people).[15] It found no difference in the proportion of people with healed ulcers over 2–3 months with intermittent pneumatic compression (see glossary, p 307) versus compression (0/10 v 0/6), but the RCT may have been too small to exclude a clinically important difference.[15] **Intermittent pneumatic compression plus compression bandaging versus compression bandaging alone:** We found one systematic review (search date 2001), which identified three small RCTs (115 people).[15] The systematic review could not perform a meta-analysis because of clinical and methodological heterogeneity between the trials. The first RCT (45 people) found that intermittent pneumatic compression plus graduated compression stockings versus graduated compression stockings alone significantly increased the proportion of people with healed ulcers at 3 months (10/21 [48%] v 1/24 [4%]; RR 11.4, 95% CI 1.6 to 82). The second RCT (53 people) comparing intermittent pneumatic compression plus elastic stockings versus Unna's boot (see glossary, p 308) found no significant difference in the proportion of people healed at 6 months (20/28 [71%] v 15/20 [75%]; RR 0.95, 95% CI 0.67 to 1.34). The third RCT (22 people) found no significant difference in healing at 6 months with intermittent pneumatic compression plus Unna's boot versus Unna's boot alone (12/12 [100%] v 8/10 [80%]; RR 1.25, 95% CI 0.92 to 1.70).[15]

Harms: The RCTs identified by the review gave no information on adverse effects.[15]

Comment: Availability may vary widely between healthcare settings. Treatment can be delivered in the home, in outpatient clinics, or in the hospital ward. Clinical RCTs have evaluated the use of intermittent pneumatic pressure for 1 hour twice weekly and 3–4 hours daily. Treatment requires resting for 1–4 hours daily, which may reduce quality of life.

OPTION **DRESSINGS AND TOPICAL AGENTS**

One systematic review found insufficient evidence on the effects of semi-occlusive dressings (foam, film, or alginate) versus simple dressings, in the presence of compression. The review found that, in the presence of compression, hydrocolloid dressings did not heal more venous leg ulcers than simple, low adherent dressings. The review found insufficient evidence from small, heterogeneous RCTs about the effects of topical agents, such as growth factors, versus inert comparators. One small RCT found no significant difference in the proportion of people with healed ulcers after 12 weeks' treatment with calcitonin gene related peptide plus vasoactive intestinal polypeptide versus placebo. One RCT found that cultured allogenic bilayer skin replacement versus simple dressings significantly increased complete ulcer healing over 6 months. One RCT found no difference after 9 months in time to healing with topical autologous platelet lysate versus placebo. Another systematic review found insufficient evidence on the effects of topical negative

pressure. **A third systematic review found insufficient evidence on the effects of antimicrobial agents versus placebo or standard care. A fourth systematic review found insufficient evidence on the effects of debriding agents versus traditional dressings.**

Benefits: **Foam, film, or alginate (semi-occlusive) dressings compared with simple dressings, in the presence of compression:** We found one systematic review (search date 1997, 5 RCTs) comparing semi-occlusive dressings (foam, film, alginates) versus simple dressings (such as paraffin-tulle or knitted viscose dressings).[16] Two comparisons of foam dressings versus simple dressings; two of film dressings versus simple dressings, and one comparing an alginate versus a simple dressing found no evidence of benefit. However, the RCTs were too small (10–132 people, median 60) to detect anything but a very large difference in effectiveness. **Hydrocolloid (occlusive) dressings compared with simple low adherent dressings, in the presence of compression:** We found one systematic review (search date 1997), which identified nine RCTs comparing hydrocolloid dressings versus simple dressings in the presence of compression.[16] A pooled analysis of seven RCTs (714 people) found no evidence of benefit. **Comparisons between occlusive or semi-occlusive dressings:** The same systematic review identified 12 small RCTs comparing different occlusive or semi-occlusive dressings.[16] It found no significant difference in healing rates between dressings, or insufficient data were provided to calculate their significance. We found one subsequent RCT comparing hydrocolloid versus hydrocellular dressings, which found no difference in healing rates.[17] **Topical agents (e.g. growth factors) versus inert comparators:** The same systematic review identified 16 RCTs comparing topical agents (such as growth factors, cell suspensions, oxygen free-radical scavengers) versus either placebo or standard care in the treatment of venous leg ulcers.[16] It found insufficient evidence to recommend any topical agent. The studies were small (9–233 people, median 45) and heterogeneous; therefore, results could not be pooled. We found four subsequent RCTs, which are described below.[10,18–20] **Cultured allogenic bilayer skin replacement versus non-adherent dressing:** The first subsequent RCT (293 people) comparing a cultured allogenic bilayer skin replacement (see glossary, p 307), which contained both epidermal and dermal components versus a non-adherent dressing, found a significantly greater proportion of ulcers healed completely in 6 months with the skin replacement (92/146 [63%] v 63/129 [49%]; RR 1.29, 95% CI 1.04 to 1.60; NNT for 6 months' treatment 7, 95% CI 4 to 41) (see table 1, p 310).[10] **Topical calcitonin gene related peptide plus vasoactive intestinal polypeptide versus placebo:** The second subsequent RCT (66 people) of calcitonin (salcatonin) gene related peptide plus vasoactive intestinal polypeptide administered by iontophoresis (see glossary, p 307) versus placebo iontophoresis found no significant difference in the proportion of people with healed ulcers after 12 weeks' treatment (11/33 [37%] v 6/33 [28%]; RR 1.83, 95% CI 0.77 to 4.38), but may have been too small to exclude a clinically important difference.[18] **Topical mesoglycan:** The third subsequent RCT (40 people) of topically applied mesoglycan, a profibrinolytic agent, found no evidence of benefit.[19] **Topically applied autologous platelet lysate:** The fourth subsequent RCT (86 people) found no difference after 9 months in time to healing with topical autologous platelet lysate versus placebo.[20] **Topical negative pressure:** We found one systematic review (search date 2000, 2 small RCTs, 34 people).[21] One of the RCTs included some people with venous leg ulcers. It found no clear evidence of benefit of topical negative pressure (see glossary, p 308), but the RCTs may have been too small to exclude a clinically important difference in outcomes. **Antimicrobial agents versus placebo or standard care:** We found one systematic review (search date 1997, 14 RCTs) comparing antimicrobial agents versus either placebo agents or standard care.[22] The RCTs were small (25–153 people, median 56), of poor quality, and no firm conclusions could be drawn. **Debriding agents:** We found one systematic review (search date 1997) comparing debriding agents versus traditional agents.[23] The review did not perform a meta-analysis specifically in people with venous leg ulcers.[23] Six RCTs (277 people) identified by the review compared dextranomer polysaccharide bead dressings versus traditional dressings, but only two RCTs reported complete ulcer healing. Data pooling of these RCTs (137 ulcers) found no significant difference in the proportion of ulcers completely healed over 3 weeks (RR 2.15, 95% CI 0.34 to 13.3), but the size of the trials meant that a clinically important difference cannot be excluded (Nelson EA, Cullum N, Jones J, personal communication, 2002). Seven RCTs (451 people) identified by the review compared cadexomer iodine versus traditional dressings, but only three RCTs reported complete ulcer healing. Data pooling of these RCTs (181 ulcers) found that cadexomer iodine versus traditional dressings healed significantly more ulcers (31/60 v 15/75; RR 2.03, 95% CI 1.21 to 3.43), but the ulcers were smaller in people treated with cadexomer iodine, and results must be treated with caution as four RCTs could not be included in the data pooling. Two RCTs identified by the review compared enzymatic preparations versus traditional dressings (52 ulcers) and found no evidence of benefit.[23] Four RCTs identified by the review compared debriding agents versus each other, two compared cadexomer iodine versus dextranomer (69 people), one compared cadexomer iodine versus hydrogel (95 people), and one compared dextranomer versus hyaluronic acid (50 people). The RCTs found no significant difference in ulcer healing with different debriding agents, but may have been too small to detect a clinically important difference.[23]

Harms: It is unlikely that low adherent primary wound dressings cause harm, although dressings containing iodine may affect thyroid function if used over large surface areas for extended periods.[24] Many people (50–85%) with venous leg ulcers have contact sensitivity to preservatives, perfumes, or dyes.[25]

Comment: Simple primary dressings maintain a moist environment beneath compression bandages by preventing loss of moisture from the wound.[26]

OPTION THERAPEUTIC ULTRASOUND

One systematic review found insufficient evidence about the effects of therapeutic ultrasound in the treatment of venous leg ulcers.

Benefits: We found one systematic review (search date 1999, 7 RCTs, 470 people) comparing therapeutic ultrasound (see glossary, p 308) versus no ultrasound or sham ultrasound for venous leg ulcers.[27] Ultrasound improved ulcer healing in all studies, but a significant difference was found in only four of the seven RCTs, and heterogeneity precluded pooling the seven RCTs.

Harms: Mild erythema, local pain, and small areas of bleeding have been reported in some trials.

Comment: None.

OPTION SYSTEMIC DRUG TREATMENTS

One systematic review has found good evidence that oral pentoxifylline versus placebo significantly increases ulcer healing over 6 months in people receiving compression. Two RCTs have found that flavonoids versus placebo or standard care significantly increase the proportion of ulcers healed. One RCT found that injections of granulocyte macrophage–colony stimulating factor versus placebo significantly increased complete healing. One RCT found limited evidence that sulodexide plus compression versus compression alone significantly increased the proportion of ulcers healed after 60 days' treatment. One RCT found that systemic mesoglycan plus compression versus compression alone significantly increased the proportion of ulcers healed after 24 weeks treatment. RCTs found insufficient evidence on the effects of oral thromboxane α_2 antagonists, aspirin, or oral zinc supplements.

Benefits: **Pentoxifylline:** We found one systematic review (search date 2001, 9 RCTs, 572 people) comparing pentoxifylline (oxpentifylline) (1200 mg or 2400 mg daily) versus placebo or versus other treatments in the presence or absence of compression.[8] It found that, in the presence of compression, pentoxifylline versus placebo significantly increased the proportion of people with healed ulcers over 8–24 weeks (5 RCTs: 155/243 [64%] v 96/204 [47%]; RR 1.30, 95% CI 1.10 to 1.54; NNT for 6 months' treatment 6, 95% CI 4 to 14) (see table 1, p 310). One RCT identified by the review found no evidence of benefit for pentoxifylline compared with defibrotide in people receiving compression.[8] **Flavonoids:** We found two RCTs (245 people) comparing a flavonoid 1000 mg daily (900 mg diosmin and 100 mg hesperidin) versus placebo or standard care.[28,29] These RCTs had different lengths of follow up but were similar in other respects. When pooled in a random effects model (Nelson EA, Cullum N, Jones J, personal communication, 2001), flavonoids healed more ulcers than placebo (100/206 [48%] with flavonoids v 53/189 [28%] with placebo; RR 1.80, 95% CI 1.20 to 2.70). **Peri-ulcer injection of granulocyte macrophage–colony stimulating factor versus placebo:** One RCT (60 people) compared a 4 week course of injections around the ulcer of granulocyte–macrophage colony stimulating factor (400 µg) versus placebo and found a significantly increased proportion of people

Venous leg ulcers

whose ulcers had completely healed after 13 weeks' treatment (23/39 [59%] *v* 4/21 [19%]; RR 3.21, 95% CI 1.23 to 8.34; NNT for 13 weeks' treatment 2, 95% CI 1 to 7) (see table 1, p 310).[9] **Sulodexide:** We found one RCT (94 people). It found that significantly more ulcers healed after 60 days' treatment with sulodexide (daily im injection for 30 days and then orally for 30 days) in addition to compression treatment than with compression alone (35% *v* 58%; RR 1.61, 95% CI 1.03 to 2.63; NNT 4, 95% CI 2 to 64) (see table 1, p 310).[11] **Systemic mesoglycan:** We found one RCT (183 people) comparing systemic mesoglycan (daily im injection for 21 days and then orally for 21 wks) plus compression versus placebo plus compression.[30] It found that systemic mesoglycan versus placebo significantly increased the proportion of people with healed ulcers after 24 weeks' treatment (82/92 [89%] *v* 69/91 [76%]; RR 1.17, 95% CI 1.03 to 1.35). **Thromboxane α_2 antagonists:** We found one RCT (165 people) of an oral thromboxane α_2 antagonist versus placebo. It found no significant difference in the proportion of ulcers healed (54% *v* 55%).[31] **Oral zinc:** We found one systematic review (search date 1997, 5 RCTs, 151 people) comparing daily doses of 440–660 mg oral zinc sulphate versus placebo. The review found no evidence of benefit for oral zinc.[32] **Aspirin:** We found one small RCT of aspirin (300 mg daily, enteric coated) versus placebo. It found that more ulcers healed with aspirin versus placebo (38% *v* 0%), but the RCT had several methodological weaknesses so the result should be treated with caution.[33]

Harms: The systematic review of pentoxifylline found more adverse effects with pentoxifylline than with placebo, although the difference was not significant (RR 1.25, 95% CI 0.87 to 1.80).[8] Nearly half of the adverse effects were gastrointestinal (dyspepsia, vomiting, or diarrhoea). Adverse effects of flavonoids, such as gastrointestinal disturbance, were reported in 10% of people.

Comment: Sulodexide is not widely available, and daily injections may be unacceptable to some people.

OPTION   VEIN SURGERY

One RCT found insufficient evidence of the effects of vein surgery on ulcer healing.

Benefits: We found no systematic review. We found one RCT (47 people) comparing vein surgery (perforator ligation) versus no surgery or surgery plus skin grafting.[34] It found no difference in the proportion of ulcers healed after 1 year, or in the rate of ulcer healing. The RCT may have been too small to rule out a beneficial effect.

Harms: Vein surgery carries the usual risks of surgery and anaesthesia.

Comment: Several operative approaches are commonly used, including perforator ligation, saphenous vein stripping, and a combination of both procedures.

OPTION SKIN GRAFTING

One systematic review found insufficient evidence of the effects of skin grafting on ulcer healing.

Benefits: We found one systematic review (search date 1999, 6 RCTs, 197 people) of skin grafts (autografts or allografts) for venous leg ulcers.[35] In five RCTs people also received compression bandaging; two RCTs (98 people) evaluated split thickness autografts; three RCTs (92 people) evaluated cultured keratinocyte allografts; and one RCT (7 people, 13 ulcers) compared tissue engineered skin (artificial skin) with split thickness skin grafts. We found insufficient evidence to determine whether skin grafting increased the healing of venous ulcers.[35]

Harms: Taking a skin graft leaves a wound that itself requires management and may cause pain. We found no evidence of harm from tissue engineered skin.

Comment: None.

OPTION LOW LEVEL LASER TREATMENT

Systematic reviews found insufficient evidence of the effects of low level laser treatment on ulcer healing.

Benefits: We found two systematic reviews.[36,37] The first review (search date 1998) identified four RCTs (139 people).[36] Two RCTs compared low level laser treatment (see glossary, p 308) versus sham treatment and found no significant difference in healing rates over 12 weeks (17/44 [39%] v 14/44 [32%]; RR 1.21, 95% CI 0.73 to 2.03). One three-arm RCT (30 people) identified by the review compared laser treatment versus laser treatment plus infrared light or versus non-coherent, unpolarised red light. It found that significantly more ulcers healed completely after 9 months' treatment in the group receiving a combination of laser and infrared light compared with non-coherent, unpolarised red light (12/15 [80%] v 5/15 [33%]; RR 2.4, 95% CI 1.12 to 5.13) The fourth RCT identified by the review compared laser and ultraviolet light and found no significant difference in healing over 4 weeks.[36] The second review (search date 1999, 5 RCTs)[37] identified but did not fully describe the four RCTs identified by the first review. The review did not perform a meta-analysis. The additional RCT identified by the review (9 people, 12 venous leg ulcers) compared low level laser treatment versus sham treatment and found limited evidence that ulcer area reduction was greater with laser over 10 weeks (25% of ulcers remained unhealed in people receiving laser v 85% in people receiving sham treatment).[37] The RCT did not assess complete ulcer healing.

Harms: Eye protection is required when using some types of laser as the high energy beam may lead to damage of the retina.

Comment: The laser power, wavelength, frequency, duration, and follow up of treatment were different for all of the studies.

Cardiovascular disorders

Venous leg ulcers

QUESTION **What are the effects of interventions to prevent recurrence?**

OPTION **COMPRESSION**

We found limited evidence that compression reduced recurrence but non-compliance with compression is a risk factor for recurrence.

Benefits: **Versus no compression:** We found one systematic review of compression hosiery versus no compression (search date 2000, no identified RCTs),[38] and one subsequent RCT.[39] The RCT (153 people) found that compression stockings worn versus compression stockings not worn significantly reduced recurrence at 6 months (21% v 46%; RR 0.46, 95% CI 0.28 to 0.76; NNT for 6 months' treatment 2, 95% CI 2 to 5).[39] **Versus other forms of compression:** We found one systematic review (search date 2000, 2 RCTs).[38] One RCT (166 people) compared two brands of UK Class 2 stockings (see comment below) and found no difference in recurrence. The larger RCT (300 people) compared Class 2 and Class 3 stockings (see comment below). With intention to treat analysis, the RCT found no significant reduction in recurrence after 5 years with high compression hosiery (UK Class 3) compared with moderate compression hosiery (UK Class 2). This analysis may underestimate the effectiveness of the Class 3 hosiery because a significant proportion of people changed from Class 3 to Class 2. Both RCTs found that non-compliance with compression hosiery was associated with recurrence.

Harms: The application of high compression to limbs with reduced arterial supply may result in ischaemic tissue damage and, at worst, amputation.[8]

Comment: Compression hosiery is classified according to the magnitude of pressure exerted at the ankle; the UK classification states that Class 2 hosiery is capable of applying 18–24 mm Hg pressure and Class 3 is capable of applying 25–35 mm Hg pressure at the ankle. Other countries use different classification systems. Hosiery reduces venous reflux by locally increasing venous pressure in the legs relative to the rest of the body. This effect only takes place while hosiery is worn. The association between non-compliance with compression and recurrence of venous ulceration provides some indirect evidence of the benefit of compression in prevention. People are advised to wear compression hosiery for life and may be at risk of pressure necrosis from their compression hosiery if they subsequently develop arterial disease. Regular reassessment of the arterial supply is considered good practice, but we found no evidence about the optimal frequency of assessment. Other measures designed to reduce leg oedema, such as resting with the leg elevated, may be useful.

OPTION   SYSTEMIC DRUG TREATMENT

One systematic review found insufficient evidence on the effects of rutoside or stanozolol on ulcer recurrence.

Benefits: We found one systematic review (search date 1997, 2 RCTs, 198 people) comparing stanozolol or rutoside versus placebo in the prevention of leg ulcer recurrence.[40] **Rutoside:** The first RCT (139 people) identified by the review comparing rutoside versus placebo found no significant difference in recurrence at 18 months (32% v 34%; P = 0.93; no raw data available to calculate CI). **Stanozolol:** The second RCT (60 people) identified by the review comparing stanozolol versus placebo for 6 months found no significant difference in recurrence at the end of the study (length of follow up not specified; recurrence in 7/25 [28%] legs with stanozolol v 4/23 [17%]; RR 1.61, 95% CI 0.54 to 4.79).[40]

Harms: Stanozolol is an anabolic steroid; adverse effects included acne, hirsutism, amenorrhoea, oedema, headache, dyspepsia, rash, hair loss, depression, jaundice, and changes in liver enzymes. Tolerance of rutoside was reported to be good; adverse effects included headache, flushing, rashes, and mild gastrointestinal disturbances.[41]

Comment: None.

OPTION   VEIN SURGERY

One RCT identified by a systematic review found insufficient evidence on the effects of vein surgery on ulcer recurrence.

Benefits: We found one systematic review (search date 1997, 1 RCT, 30 people).[40] The identified RCT, which was poorly controlled, compared surgery plus compression hosiery versus compression hosiery alone for prevention of recurrence. It found a reduced rate of recurrence when surgery was carried out in addition to the use of compression hosiery (5% v 24%; RR 0.21, 95% CI 0.03 to 0.80).

Harms: Vein surgery has the usual risks of surgery and anaesthesia.

Comment: The results of the RCT should be interpreted with caution because it was small and poorly controlled.[40] The RCT randomised legs rather than people.

GLOSSARY

Cultured allogenic bilayer skin replacement Also called human skin equivalent. This is made of a lower (dermal) layer of bovine collagen containing living human dermal fibroblasts and an upper (epidermal) layer of living human keratinocytes.

Elastomeric multilayer high compression bandages Usually a layer of padding material followed by one to three additional layers of elastomeric bandages.

Intermittent pneumatic compression External compression applied by inflatable leggings or boots either over, or instead of, compression hosiery or bandages. A pump successively inflates and deflates the boots to promote the return of blood from the tissues. Newer systems have separate compartments in the boots so that the foot is inflated before the ankle, which is inflated before the calf.

Iontophoresis The delivery of an ionic substance by application of an electrical current.

Venous leg ulcers

Low level laser treatment Application of treatment energy ($< 10\,J/cm^2$) using lasers of 50 mW or less.

Short stretch bandages Minimally extensible bandages usually made of cotton with few or no elastomeric fibres. They are applied at near full extension to form a semi-rigid bandage.

Therapeutic ultrasound Application of ultrasound to a wound, using a transducer and a water based gel. Prolonged application can lead to heating of the tissues, but when used in wound healing the power used is low and the transducer is constantly moved by the therapist so that the tissue is not significantly heated.

Topical negative pressure Negative pressure (suction) applied to a wound through an open cell dressing (e.g. foam, felt).

Unna's boot An inner layer of zinc oxide impregnated bandage, which hardens as it dries to form a semi-rigid layer against which the calf muscle can contract. It is usually covered in an elastomeric bandage.

REFERENCES

1. Callam MJ, Ruckley CV, Harper DR, et al. Chronic ulceration of the leg: extent of the problem and provision of care. *BMJ* 1985;290:1855–1856.

2. Roe B, Cullum N, Hamer C. Patients' perceptions of chronic leg ulceration. In: Cullum N, Roe B, eds. *Leg ulcers: nursing management.* Harrow: Scutari, 1995:125–134.

3. Roe B, Cullum N. The management of leg ulcers: current nursing practice. In: Cullum N, Roe B, eds. *Leg ulcers: nursing management.* Harrow: Scutari, 1995:113–124.

4. Vowden KR, Barker A, Vowden P. Leg ulcer management in a nurse-led, hospital-based clinic. *J Wound Care* 1997;6:233–236.

5. Cullum N, Nelson EA, Fletcher AW, et al. Compression bandages and stockings in the treatment of venous leg ulcers. In: The Cochrane Library, Issue 1, 2002. Oxford: Update Software. Search date 2000; primary sources 19 electronic databases, hand searches, and personal contacts.

6. Meyer F, Burnand KG, McGuiness C, et al. Randomized clinical RCT comparing the efficacy of two bandaging regimens in the treatment of venous leg ulcer. *Br J Surg* 2002;89:40–44.

7. Partsch H, Damstra RJ, Tazelaar DJ, et al. Multicentre, randomised controlled RCT of four-layer bandaging versus short-stretch bandaging in the treatment of venous leg ulcers. *VASA* 2001;30:108–113.

8. Jull AB, Waters J, Arroll B. Oral pentoxifylline for treatment of venous leg ulcers. In: The Cochrane Library, Issue 1, 2002. Oxford: Update Software. Search date 2001; primary sources Cochrane Peripheral Vascular Diseases and Wounds Group, specialised registers, hand searches of reference lists, relevant journals and conference proceedings, personal contact with manufacturer of pentoxifylline, and experts in the field.

9. Da Costa RM, Ribeiro Jesus FM, Aniceto C, et al. Randomized, double-blind, placebo-controlled, dose-ranging study of granulocyte–macrophage colony stimulating factor in patients with chronic venous leg ulcers. *Wound Repair Regen* 1999;7:17–25.

10. Falanga V, Margolis D, Alvarez O, et al. Rapid healing of venous ulcers and lack of clinical rejection with an allogeneic cultured human skin equivalent. Human Skin Equivalent Investigators Group. *Arch Dermatol* 1998;134:293–300.

11. Scondotto G, Aloisi D, Ferrari P, et al. Treatment of venous leg ulcers with sulodexide. *Angiology* 99;50:883–889.

12. Callam MJ, Ruckley CV, Dale JJ, et al. Hazards of compression treatment of the leg: an estimate from Scottish surgeons. *BMJ* 1987;295:1382.

13. Chan CLH, Meyer FJ, Hay RJ, et al. Toe ulceration associated with compression bandaging: observational study. *BMJ* 2001;323;1099.

14. Nelson EA, Ruckley CV, Barbenel J. Improvements in bandaging technique following training. *J Wound Care* 1995;4:181–184.

15. Mani R, Vowden K, Nelson EA. Intermittent pneumatic compression for treating venous leg ulcers. In: The Cochrane Library, Issue 1, 2002. Oxford: Update Software. Search date 2001; primary sources The Cochrane Wound Group Trials Register and hand searches of journals, relevant conference proceedings and citations within obtained reviews and papers and personal contact with relevant companies

16. Bradley M, Cullum N, Nelson EA, et al. Dressings and topical agents for healing of chronic wounds: a systematic review. *Health Technol Assess* 1999;3 No17(Pt2). Search date 1997; primary sources Cochrane Library, Medline, Embase, and Cinahl.

17. Seeley J, Jensen JL, Hutcherson J. A randomised clinical study comparing a hydrocellular dressing to a hydrocolloid dressing in the management of pressure ulcers. *Ostomy Wound Manage* 1999;45:39–47.

18. Gherardini G, Gurlek A, Evans GRD, et al. Venous ulcers: improved healing by iontophoretic administration of calcitonin gene-related peptide and vasoactive intestinal polypeptide. *Plast Reconstr Surg* 1998;101:90–93.

19. La Marc G, Pumilia G, Martino A. Effectiveness of mesoglycan topical treatment of leg ulcers in subjects with chronic venous insufficiency. *Minerva Cardioangiol* 1999;47:315–319.

20. Stacey MC, Mata SD, Trengove NJ, et al. Randomised double-blind placebo controlled RCT of autologous platelet lysate in venous ulcer healing. *Eur J Vasc Endovasc Surg* 2000;20:296–301.

21. Evans D, Land L. Topical negative pressure for treating chronic wounds. In: The Cochrane Library, Issue 1, 2002. Oxford: Update Software. Search date 2000; primary sources Cochrane Wounds Group specialised register, experts, relevant companies, and a hand search.

22. O'Meara S, Cullum N, Majid M, et al. Systematic reviews of wound care management: (3) antimicrobial agents for chronic wounds. *Health*

Technol Assess 2000;4(No 21):1–237. Search date 1997; primary sources Cochrane Library, Medline, Embase, and Cinahl.

23. Bradley M, Cullum N, Sheldon T. The debridement of chronic wounds: a systematic review. Health Technol Assess, 1999; 3 (17 Pt 1). Search date 1997; primary sources 19 electronic databases (including the Cochrane Wounds Group Specialised Register) and hand searches of specialist wound care journals, conference proceedings and bibliographies of retrieved relevant publications and personal contact with appropriate companies and an advisory panel of experts.

24. Thomas S. Wound management and dressings. London: Pharmaceutical Press, 1990.

25. Cameron J, Wilson C, Powell S, et al. Contact dermatitis in leg ulcer patients. Ostomy Wound Manage 1992;38:10–11.

26. Wu P, Nelson EA, Reid WH, et al. Water vapour transmission rates in burns and chronic leg ulcers: influence of wound dressings and comparison with in vitro evaluation. Biomaterials 1996;17:1373–1377.

27. Flemming K, Cullum N. Therapeutic ultrasound for venous leg ulcers. In: The Cochrane Library, Issue 1, 2002. Oxford: Update Software. Search date 1999; primary sources Cochrane Wounds Group specialised register, and hand searches of citation lists.

28. Guilhou JJ, Dereure O, Morzin L, et al. Efficacy of Daflon 500 mg in venous leg ulcer healing: a double-blind, randomized, controlled versus placebo RCT in 107 patients. Angiology 1997;48:77–85.

29. Glinski W, Chodynicka B, Roszkiewicz J, et al. The beneficial augmentative effect of micronised purified flavonoid fraction (MPFF) on the healing of leg ulcers: an open, multicentre, controlled randomised study. Phlebology 1999,14:151 157.

30. Arosio E, Ferrari G, Santoro F, et al. A placebo-controlled, double blind study of mesoglycan in the treatment of chronic venous ulcers. Eur J Vasc Endovas Surg 2001;22:365–372.

31. Lyon RT, Veith FJ, Bolton L, et al. Clinical benchmark for healing of chronic venous ulcers. Venous Ulcer Study Collaborators. Am J Surgery 1998;176:172–175.

32. Wilkinson EAJ, Hawke CI. Does oral zinc aid the healing of chronic leg ulcers? A systematic literature review. Arch Dermatol 1998;134:1556–1560. Search date 1997; primary sources Medline, Embase, Cinahl, Science Citation Index, Biosis, British Diabetic Association Database, Ciscom, Cochrane Controlled Register of Clinical RCTs, Dissertation Abstracts, Royal College of Nursing Database, electronic databases

of ongoing research, hand searches of wound care journals and conference proceedings, and contact with manufacturer of zinc sulphate tablets.

33. Layton AM, Ibbotson SH, Davies JA, et al. Randomised RCT of oral aspirin for chronic venous leg ulcers. Lancet 1994;344:164–165.

34. Warburg FE, Danielsen L, Madsen SM, et al. Vein surgery with or without skin grafting versus conservative treatment for leg ulcers. Acta Dermatol Vereol 1994;74:307–309.

35. Jones JE, Nelson EA. Skin grafting for venous leg ulcers. In: The Cochrane Library, Issue 1, 2002. Oxford: Update Software. Search date 1999; primary sources Cochrane Wounds Group specialised register, hand searches of reference lists, relevant journals, conference proceedings, and personal contact with experts in the field.

36. Flemming K, Cullum N. Laser therapy for venous leg ulcers. In: The Cochrane Library, Issue 1, 2002. Oxford: Update Software. Search date 1998; primary sources 19 electronic databases, hand searches of journals, conference proceedings, and bibliographies.

37. Schneider WL, Hailey D. Low level laser therapy for wound healing. Alberta Heritage Foundation Report 1999. Search date 1999; primary sources Medline, HealthStar, Embase, Dissertation Abstracts, Current Contents, Cinahl, Cochrane library, the internet.

38. Cullum N, Nelson EA, Flemming K, et al. Systematic reviews of wound care management: (5) beds; (6) compression; (7) laser therapy, therapeutic ultrasound, electrotherapy and electromagnetic therapy. Health Technol Assess 2001;5(9). Search date 2000; primary sources Cochrane Wounds Group specialised register, 19 electronic databases (up to December 1999), and hand searches of relevant journals, conferences and bibliographies of retrieved publications, and personal contact with manufacturers and an advisory panel of experts.

39. Vandongen YK, Stacey MC. Graduated compression elastic stockings reduce lipodermatosclerosis and ulcer recurrence. Phlebology 2000;16:33 37

40. Cullum N, Fletcher A, Semlyen A, et al. Compression therapy for venous leg ulcers. Qual Health Care 1997;6:226–231. Search date 1997; primary sources 18 databases, including Medline, Embase, Cinahl with no restriction on date, hand searches of relevant journals, conference proceedings, and correspondence with experts to obtain unpublished papers.

41. Taylor HM, Rose KE, Twycross RG. A double-blind clinical RCT of hydroxyethylrutosides in obstructive arm lymphoedema. Phlebology 1993;8(suppl 1):22–28

E Andrea Nelson
Research Fellow

Nicky Cullum
Centre for Evidence Based Nursing
Department of Health Sciences
University of York
York
UK

June Jones
Clinical Nurse Specialist
North Sefton and West Lancashire
Community Services NHS Trust
Southport
UK

Competing interests: EAN has been reimbursed for attending symposia by Smith and Nephew, Johnson & Johnson, and Huntleigh Healthcare Ltd, and Convatec. EAN and NC are applicants on a RCT of compression bandages for which Beiersdorf UK Ltd is providing RCT related education. JJ has been reimbursed for attending symposia by 3M and Convatec.

TABLE 1	NNTs for healing of leg ulcers (see text, p 298).

Intervention	NNT (95% CI)
Elastomeric multilayer compression v non-elastomeric multilayer compression bandages	5 (3 to 12)[5]
Multilayer high compression v single layer compression bandages	6 (4 to 18)[5]
Pentoxifylline 400 mg three times a day v placebo (concurrent use of compression)	6 (4 to 14)[8]
Peri-ulcer injection of GM–CSF* (400 µg) v placebo	2 (1 to 17)[9]
Cultured allogenic bilayer skin equivalent v non-adherent dressing	7 (4 to 41)[10]
Sulodexide plus compression v compression alone	4 (2 to 64)[11]

*GM–CSF, granulocyte–macrophage colony stimulating factor.

Index

Subject index

Estimating cardiovascular risk and treatment benefit

Adapted from the New Zealand guidelines on management of dyslipidaemia[1] and raised blood pressure[2] by Rod Jackson

How to use these colour charts

The charts help the estimation of a person's absolute risk of a cardiovascular event and the likely benefit of drug treatment to lower cholesterol or blood pressure. For these charts cardiovascular events include: new angina, myocardial infarction, coronary death, stroke or transient ischaemic attack (TIA), onset of congestive cardiac failure or peripheral vascular syndrome.

There is a group of patients in whom risk can be assumed to be high (>20% in 5 years) without using the charts. They include those with symptomatic cardiovascular disease (angina, myocardial infarction, congestive heart failure, stroke, TIA, and peripheral vascular disease), or left ventricular hypertrophy on ECG.

To estimate a person's absolute five-year risk:
■ Find the table relating to their sex, diabetic status (on insulin, oral hypoglycaemics or fasting blood glucose over 8 mmol/L), smoking status and age. The age shown in the charts is the mean for that category, i.e. age 60 = 55 to 65 years.
■ Within the table find the cell nearest to the person's blood pressure and total cholesterol : HDL ratio. For risk assessment it is enough to use a mean blood pressure based on two readings on each of two occasions, and cholesterol measurements based on one laboratory or two non-fasting Reflotron measurements. More readings are needed to establish the pre-treatment baseline.
■ The colour of the box indicates the person's five-year cardiovascular disease risk (see below).

Notes: (1) People with a strong history of CVD (first degree male relatives with CVD before 55 years, female relatives before 65 years) or obesity (body mass index above 30 kg/m^2) are likely to be at greater risk than the tables indicate. The magnitude of the independent predictive value of these risk factors remains unclear—their presence should influence treatment decisions for patients at borderline treatment levels. (2) If total cholesterol or total cholesterol:HDL ratio is greater than 8 then the risk is at least 15%. (3) Nearly all people aged 75 years or over also have an absolute cardiovascular risk over 15%.

Charts reproduced with permission from The National Heart Foundation of New Zealand. Also available on http://www.nzgg.org.nz/library/gl_complete/bloodpressure/table1.cfm

REFERENCES

1. Dyslipidaemia Advisory Group. 1996 National Heart Foundation clinical guidelines for the assessment and management of dyslipidaemia. *NZ Med J* 1996;109:224–232.
2. National Health Committee. Guidelines for the management of mildly raised blood pressure in New Zealand: Ministry of Health National Health Committee Report, Wellington, 1995.

RISK LEVEL Five-year CVD risk (non-fatal and fatal)	BENEFIT (1) CVD events prevented per 100 treated for five years*	BENEFIT (2) Number needed to treat for five years to prevent one event*
Very High >30%	>10 per 100	<10
Very High 25–30%	9 per 100	11
Very High 20–25%	7.5 per 100	13
High 15–20%	6 per 100	16
Moderate 10–15%	4 per 100	25
Mild 5–10%	2.5 per 100	40
Mild 2.5–5%	1.25 per 100	80
Mild <2.5%	<0.8 per 100	>120

*Based on a 20% reduction in total cholesterol or a reduction in blood pressure of 10–15 mmHg systolic or 5–10 mm Hg diastolic, which is estimated to reduce CVD risk by about one third over 5 years.

RISK LEVEL: MEN

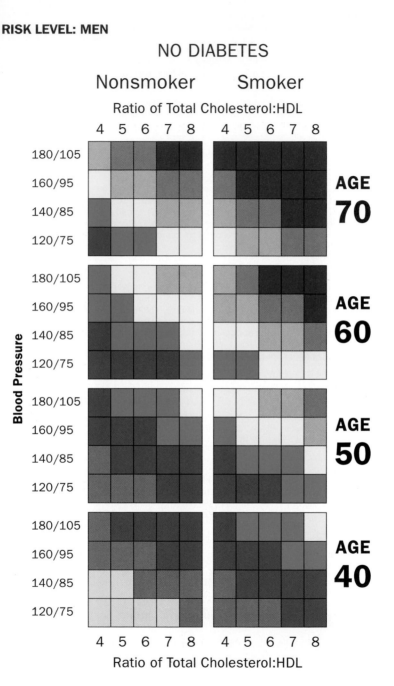

NO DIABETES

Nonsmoker   Smoker

Ratio of Total Cholesterol:HDL

Blood Pressure

AGE 70

AGE 60

AGE 50

AGE 40

Ratio of Total Cholesterol:HDL

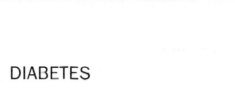

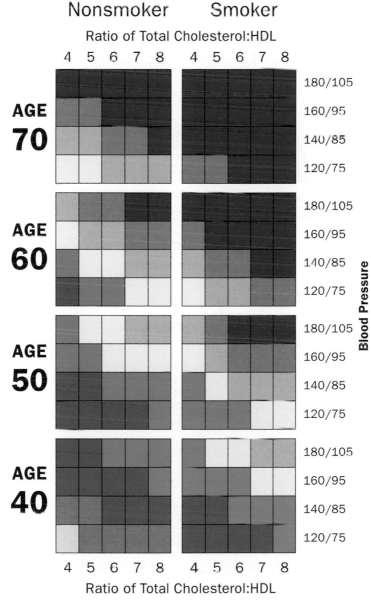

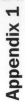

RISK LEVEL: WOMEN

NO DIABETES

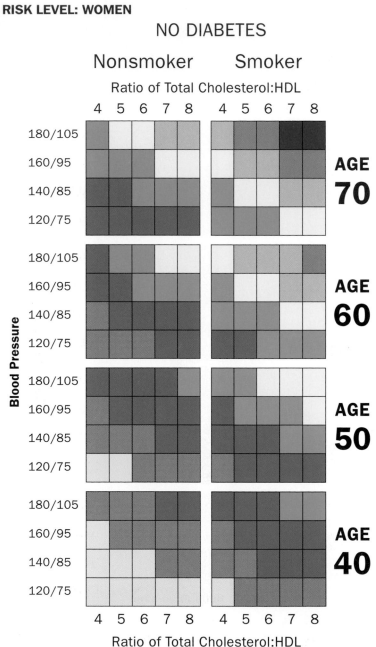

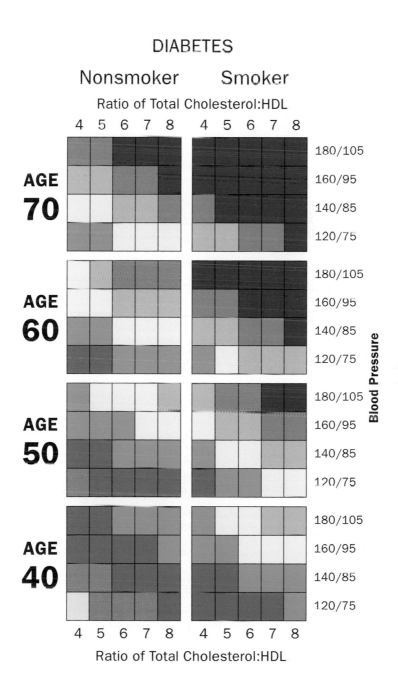

The number needed to treat: adjusting for baseline risk

Adapted with permission from Chatellier et al, 1996[1]

BACKGROUND

The number needed to treat (NNT) to avoid a single additional adverse outcome is a meaningful way of expressing the benefit of an active treatment over a control. It can be used both to summarise the results of a therapeutic trial or series of trials and to help medical decision making about an individual patient.

If the absolute risk of adverse outcomes in a therapeutic trial is ARC in the control group and ART in the treatment group, then the absolute risk reduction (ARR) is defined as (ARC − ART). The NNT is defined as the inverse of the ARR:

$$NNT = 1/(ARC - ART)$$

Since the Relative Risk Reduction (RRR) is defined as (ARC − ART)/ARC, it follows that NNT, RRR and ARC are related by their definitions in the following way:

$$NNT \times RRR \times ARC = 1$$

This relationship can be used to estimate the likely benefits of a treatment in populations with different levels of baseline risk (that is different levels of ARC). This allows extrapolation of the results of a trial or meta-analysis to people with different baseline risks. Ideally, there should be experimental evidence of the RRR in each population. However, in many trials, subgroup analyses show that the RRR is approximately constant in groups of patients with different characteristics. Cook and Sackett therefore proposed that decisions about individual patients could be made by using the NNT calculated from the RRR measured in trials and the baseline risk in the absence of treatment estimated for the individual patient.[2]

The method may not apply to periods of time different to that studied in the original trials.

USING THE NOMOGRAM

The nomogram shown on the next page allows the NNT to be found directly without any calculation: a straight line should be drawn from the point corresponding to the estimated absolute risk for the patient on the left hand scale to the point corresponding to the relative risk reduction stated in a trial or meta-analysis on the central scale. The intercept of this line with the right hand scale gives the NNT. By taking the upper and lower limits of the confidence interval of the RRR, the upper and lower limits of the NNT can be estimated.

REFERENCES

1. Chatellier G, Zapletal E, Lemaitre D, et al. The number needed to treat: a clinically useful nomogram in its proper context. *BMJ* 1996;321:426–429.
2. Cook RJ, Sackett DL. The number needed to treat: a clinically useful measure of treatment effect. *BMJ* 1995;310:452–454.

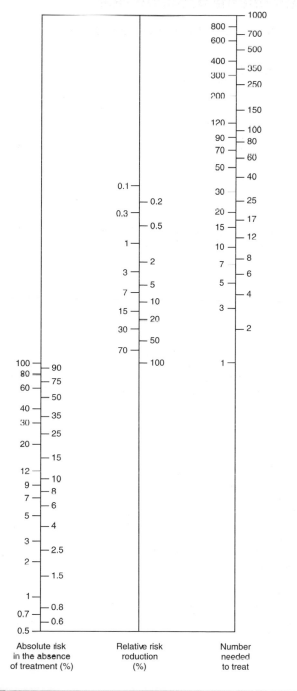

FIGURE Nomogram for calculating the number needed to treat. Published with permission[1]

Also from the BMJ Publishing Group

JOURNALS

Clinical Evidence Full edition
The original multidisciplinary version, covering a wide range of specialties.
ISSN: 1462-3846

Clinical Evidence Concise edition
New pocket-sized Concise edition allows for easy access to key messages and fast offline access to the full evidence detail on the companion CD-ROM.
ISSN: 1475-9225

Subscription price for full edition & online, or concise edition & online:
Personal - £85, €/$135
Student/Nurse - £40, €/$65
Institutional - £175, €/$280

Heart
A leading international clinical journal, which covers all aspects of cardiovascular disease and includes topical, authoritative editorials, comprehensive reviews, and case reports.
ISSN: 1355-6037 (print)
ISSN: 1468-201X (online)

Subscription price:
Personal print & online - £137, €/$218
Personal online only - £80, €/$125
Institutional print only - £334, €/$514

Institutional online only, and print with online rates are based on the number of full time equivalents at your institution. For further details please see: www.bmjjournals.com/subscriptions/institutional.shtml

BOOKS

The full range of cardiology titles published by BMJ Books is available at:
www.cardiology.bmjbooks.com

Cardiology Core Curriculum A Problem Based Approach
Covering all the main subspecialties in cardiology, including illustrative case studies.
ISBN: 0-7279-1690-4
£45.00

Evidence-based Cardiology
A ground-breaking text addressing the implementation of evidence-based medicine in the major cardiological subspecialties.
Second edition
ISBN: 0-7279-1699-8
£99.00

Evidence-based hypertension
Based on central questions the physician needs to ask when managing hypertensive patients.
ISBN: 0-7279-1438-3
£27.50

100 Questions in Cardiology
A compilation of the 100 most frequently asked questions answered by leading cardiologists from the UK and around the world.
ISBN: 0-7279-1489-8
£25.00